Writing and Publishing in Medicine

THIRD EDITION

Writing and Publishing in Medicine

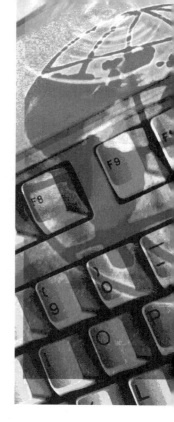

THIRD EDITION

PREVIOUSLY TITLED

How to Write and Publish Papers in the Medical Sciences

EDWARD J. HUTH, MD, MACP, FRCP

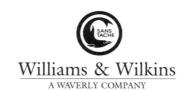

Williams & Wilkins
A WAVERLY COMPANY

BALTIMORE • PHILADELPHIA • LONDON • PARIS • BANGKOK
BUENOS AIRES • HONG KONG • MUNICH • SYDNEY • TOKYO • WROCLAW

Managing Editor: John Goucher
Project Editor: Ulita Lushnycky

Copyright © 1999 Edward J. Huth

351 West Camden Street
Baltimore, Maryland 21201-2436 USA

Rose Tree Corporate Center
1400 North Providence Road
Building II, Suite 5025
Media, Pennsylvania 19063-2043 USA

Printed in the United States of America

First Edition, 1982
Second Edition, 1990

Library of Congress Cataloging-in-Publication Data

Huth, Edward J.
    Writing and publishing in Medicine / Edward J. Huth.—3rd ed.
      p.   cm.
    Rev. ed. of: How to write and publish papers in the medical
sciences, 2nd ed. c1990.
    Includes bibliographical references and index.
    ISBN 0-683-40447-4
    1. Medical writing.   2. Medical publishing.   I. Huth, Edward J.
How to write and publish papers in the medical sciences. II. Title.
    [DNLM: 1. Writing.   2. Publishing. WZ 345H979w 1999]
R119.H87   1999
808' .06661—dc21
DNLM/DLC
for Library of Congress   98–35984
                                           CIP

To purchase additional copies of this book, call our customer service department at **(800)
638–0672** or fax orders to **(800) 447–8438.** For other book services, including chapter reprints
and large quantity sales, ask for the Special Sales department.

Canadian customers should call **(800) 665–1148,** or fax **(800) 665–0103.** For all other calls origi-
nating outside of the United States, please call **(410) 528–4223** or fax us at **(410) 528–8550.**

Visit Williams & Wilkins on the Internet: **http://www.wwilkins.com** or contact our customer service department at **custserv@wwilkins.com.** Williams & Wilkins customer service representatives are available from 8:30 am to 6:00 pm, EST, Monday through Friday, for telephone access.

99 00 01 02 03
1 2 3 4 5 6 7 8 9 10

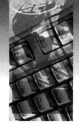

INTRODUCTION

···

with a Note on the Organization and Publication Style of This Book

Most of what we write goes onto a sheet of paper without our thinking much about how we are writing—shopping lists, routine letters, quickly scribbled clinical notes. We get to believe that writing is effortless. We forget that good scientific writing is hard work even for experienced authors. Read what an eminent gastroenterologist, Morton Grossman (1) had to say.

> I have not found . . . writing one bit easier today than it was 30 yrs. ago. I still have to work at it very hard and make many revisions, with a rare exception— once in a while something like an editorial or thought will come into my mind, and I'll write it out and be satisfied with the first draft. That's unusual, because the saying of Francis Bacon has always been deeply impressed in my mind . . . "Writing [maketh an] exact man." And we all have a head full of thoughts floating around that have not been formulated in a way that would withstand examination if they had been set forth in writing and allowed to be scrutinized by others. And I find this invariably so; with the general thought that I have at the start, I find that some of the premises were incomplete and incorrect and that things don't quite fit, so that the task of making things flow and putting things in their place, I still find very hard work, but work that I genuinely like . . . . I find it stimulating to write, but like any other person who does quite a bit of writing, there are times when I feel stuck, and I have to put something aside and let it mature before I get back to it.

These are words from a man who published 400 scientific papers, 134 editorials and other short papers, and 71 books or chapters in books. Writing will always be work if you wish to write well. But with the right approach it can become work you like or can at least tolerate.

In writing this book in its three editions I have tried to make it a broad but adequately detailed guide to decisions to be made by authors and to the processes of writing. I have offered as much practical advice as can be put into a not-too-long text, and I have tried to explain the basis for that advice.

This edition differs substantially from the preceding two editions. The sequence of steps in writing a medical paper for a journal has been moved from its previous position as an appendix in the second edition to its serving as Chapter 1. Because of the growing attention by journals to adequate reporting of research, this edition offers specific suggestions on content likely to be needed in papers reporting several types of research: in reports of clinical trials or of observational studies; in reports of laboratory research. The previous text on review articles has been heavily revised to also cover

v

metaanalyses. A chapter on difficulties for nonanglophone authors in writing English has been added. The formats for references used by over 500 medical journals throughout the world have been moved from one of the appendixes in the second edition into the chapter on scientific style. A chapter on writing or editing a book has been added. Chapters have been grouped into five parts to make more clear their relations to each other.

Inexperienced authors may wish to read this book from front to back. Experienced authors may wish only to dip into chapters that might expand what they already know, or they may use only some chapters or appendixes for reference.

With the suggestions in this book, the inexperienced author can develop skills in writing by mastering the main principles discussed, applying them in new work, and looking into books and papers recommended in Appendix E, "References and Reading: An Annotated Bibliography". Inexperienced authors can be helped to develop skills through workshops and seminars; defects in others' writing are usually seen more readily than those in one's own. The sequence of chapters suggests a sequence for teaching sessions. For example, Chapters 6 through 11 on the main kinds of formats can be used as a text for workshop sessions in which students analyze and criticize published papers for content and sequence. Teachers seeking explicit help in developing a syllabus for medical writing should consult *Scientific Writing for Graduate Students: A Manual on the Teaching of Scientific Writing* (2).

ORGANIZATION AND STYLE

The style conventions I have used—punctuation, abbreviation, citation, formats for references, and other details—come from *Scientific Style and Format* (3) and *Uniform Requirements for Manuscripts Submitted to Biomedical Journals* (4). Some of these are widely used in medical journals, but others are just being adopted; if authors wish to be sure of the publication styles specified by the journals for which they are writing, they must consult their information-for-authors pages.

In accordance with the requirements for bibliographic references specified by the International Committee of Medical Journal Editors (4), references are cited by reference numbers within parenthesis marks on the line in the citation-sequence style; the references for each chapter follow its text. Note that the citation numbers in the text, which are the numbers of the cited references, begin anew with "1" in each chapter carrying references.

The placement of quotation marks in relation to commas and periods (full stops) follows the British style.

The term *metaanalysis* is not hyphenated ("meta-analysis"), a recommendation in the CBE style manual (3).

Footnotes for tables are indicated with superscripts a, b, c, and so on rather than the older sequence * † ‡ § and so on.

Note that when Internet Web site addresses ("URLs") are at the end of a sentence, the sentence closes as usual with a period (full stop). This closing period is not part of the Web site address and should be omitted in using the address.

REFERENCES

1. Boyle JD. Morton I Grossman, MD, PhD: an oral history. Gastroenterology 1982;83:285–324.
2. CBE Committee on Graduate Training in Scientific Writing. Scientific writing for graduate students: a manual on the teaching of scientific writing. Bethesda, Maryland: Council of Biology Editors; 1968. Reprinted 1983. As of 1998 a new edition was in preparation.
3. Style Manual Committee, Council of Biology Editors. Scientific style and format: the CBE manual for authors, editors, and publishers. 6th ed. New York: Cambridge University Press; 1994.
4. International Committee of Medical Journal Editors. Uniform requirements for manuscripts submitted to biomedical journals and supplemental statements from the International Committee of Medical Journal Editors. 1997. Available at various Web sites such as the Web site of *The Lancet:*(http://www. thelancet.com/lancet/writing/uniform.html) and the American College of Physicians Web site (http://www.acponline.org/journal/resource/resortoc. htm); note that the ACP Web site also gives access to the list of journals that subscribe to the uniform requirements specified in this document. The uniform-requirements document has also been published in the *Annals of Internal Medicine* 1997 Jan 1;126:36–57. An abridged version is in Appendix 2.

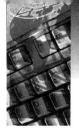

ACKNOWLEDGMENTS

I continue to be grateful to those many persons who reviewed parts of the first and second editions of this book; their help undoubtedly contributed to whatever values this third edition may have. They were named in the Acknowledgments section of the second edition.

For this edition I am grateful to the anonymous peer reviewers who provided, via Williams & Wilkins, detailed and truly useful criticisms of various parts of the first draft and offered many excellent recommendations for deletions, changes, and additions. I am equally grateful to Mohan Alladi, Kim Burton, Margaret Corbett, Dong Geng, Sarah Edmunds, Sue Edwards, Gregory W Froehlich, Stuart Handysides, Roderick Hunt, Barbara J Kuyper, Derek G Land, Thomas A Lang, Kathleen Lyle, Ana Marusic, Arjan Polderman, Anne Parry, Peush Sahni, Angela K Turner, David Roberts, and Gilbert Welch for specific and useful suggestions and information. The criticisms and recommendations of Sheldon Kotzin, National Library of Medicine, were especially valuable for my revising Chapter 3. Hiroaki Itoh provided some materials useful for Chapter 18. Please note, however, that none of these persons should be charged with any responsibility for any errors in this edition.

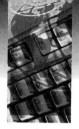

CONTENTS

PART 1

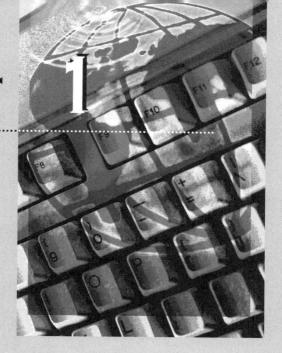

Before Writing

CHAPTER 1

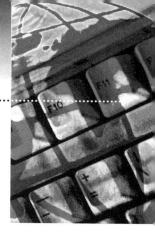

A Systematic Method for Writing and Publishing Papers

Writing scientific papers is hard work. Inexperienced authors trying to get started can be so intimidated by it that they feel paralyzed. Days or weeks may pass before they can bring themselves to get down to the task. If, however, they can see that the task can be broken down into steps, many of which will not be too difficult to get through, the task ahead may seem less intimidating.

Most of this book has a sequence that corresponds to the steps any author should go through in planning and preparing a paper for journal publication. These steps are laid out below and the chapters dealing with them are indicated. Many of these steps are also relevant to writing chapters for a book.

NINETEEN STEPS IN PLANNING, WRITING, AND PUBLISHING A PAPER

1. Decide on the message of the paper. What is the main point you hope to make? Can you state it in a single sentence? With case reports and reviews, you may not be sure of the exact message until you have searched the literature. (Chapters 2 and 3)

2. Decide whether the paper is worth writing. Have similar findings been reported? Is there a need for another report? Will your research findings be more convincing? Even if it is a report of a "negative-results clinical trial", it may merit being published. If you are planning to write a review, has your literature search turned up similar reviews? Will your review be more thorough and more rigorous? (Chapters 2, 3, and 9)

3. Decide on the importance of your paper. Apply the "so-what" test; how would the paper change concept or practice? (Chapter 2)

4. Decide on the audience for the paper; apply the "who-cares" test. (Chapter 2)

5. Select the journal for which you will prepare the paper. (Chapter 2)

6. Search the literature or update a previous search: for a firm decision on writing the paper and on its message; for documentary materials. (Chapter 3)

7. Decide on authorship or review previous decisions on authorship. (Chapter 4 and Appendix A)

8. Assemble the materials needed to write and eventually publish the paper: protocols, data, graphs, illustrations, references, permissions. If you are writing an invited review paper or editorial, make sure you know the conditions accompanying the invitation and request any you believe should be met before you accept it. Decide on technical tools needed to help you with the mechanics of writing: software for word processing, bibliographic references, graphs. (Chapter 4)

9. Look up the manuscript requirements for the journal. (Chapter 4)

10. Consider the proper structure for the paper before you begin to outline it and write the first draft. (Chapters 5–11)

11. Develop an outline or informal sketch of the paper for the first draft. (Chapter 12)

12. Write the first draft (Chapter 12) and prepare tentative versions of the title and abstract (Chapter 13) and of tables and illustrations (Chapters 14 and 15).

13. Revise the first draft and subsequent drafts (with any coauthors) until you are fully satisfied with the content of the paper. (Chapter 16)

14. Revise the prose style of your text for fluency, clarity, accuracy, economy, and grace (Chapter 17). If English is not your native language, look for mistakes you have made in trying to write good English or get the paper read by someone for whom English is the native language. (Chapter 18)

15. Make sure that the details of scientific style and the formats of citations and references are correct for the journal to which the paper will be submitted. (Chapter 19)

16. Review, and revise if necessary, the last complete draft; prepare the final choices and right presentations for tables and illustrations. Prepare the final complete manuscript. (Chapter 20)

17. Assemble the manuscript copies and accompanying materials to send to the journal's editor with a submission letter. (Chapter 21)

18. Respond to the editor's decision: Revise a provisionally accepted paper as requested by the editor and peer reviewers; if necessary, defend not making any requested changes. Send a rejected paper to another journal only after making needed revisions; or give up trying to get the paper published. (Chapter 22)

19. If the paper is accepted, correct proof carefully as soon as it arrives, return it promptly or telephone in corrections, and await publication of the paper. (Chapters 23 and 24)

In writing multiauthor papers, responsibility for these steps can be divided among two or more authors, but all authors should be informed of how these steps have been allotted and of who is going to do what. All authors should not only have the right to see the paper at any stage, but should be expected to review each draft, at least after the first, and to approve it or make specific recommendations for further revision.

WRITING BOOKS OR BOOK CHAPTERS

Many of the steps outlined above are also those to be taken by authors preparing individual chapters for a multiauthor book. There are, however, additional steps to be taken by an author of a single- or multi-author book or someone organizing a contributor text and planning to be its editor. These steps are considered in Chapter 25.

PREPARING YOURSELF FOR YOUR FUTURE WRITING

As you go through this book you might come to feel that you may not have all the intellectual and practical skills needed to become a truly effective scientific author. Keep in mind, however, that the more you write and the more you get real criticism from colleagues and peer reviewers, the more you will become aware of what skills are indispensable. Let me suggest a list of those needs.

- Knowing what makes up scientific evidence
- Knowing how scientific evidence is gathered
- Knowing how scientific evidence should be judged: statistical methods; reference standards
- Knowing the elements of critical argument and how they should be applied in decisions on the content of a scientific paper and its arrangement
- Knowing how to get honest and thorough critical judgments of your writing
- Knowing how to read your own writing closely and revise it thoroughly

- Knowing how journals are run and how this knowledge should be applied in your seeking publication

Keep firmly in mind that the more you write the better a writer you will become.

CONCLUSION

Writing a journal paper or a book chapter is likely to seem less intimidating to the inexperienced author if he or she will work through the task systematically. The task can be divided into 19 steps. How to proceed in each step is considered in the following chapters.

CHAPTER 2

The Paper, the Audience, and the Right Journal

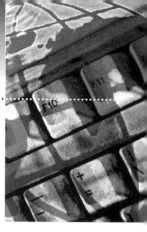

Before sitting down to write a paper or even to just plan a paper, answer six questions.

> Question 1: What do I have to say? What will be the message?
> Question 2: Is the paper worth writing?
> Question 3: Have I already published such a paper or any part of its probable content?
> Question 4: What will be the right format?
> Question 5: Who are the audience for the message?
> Question 6: What is the right journal for that audience?

You or coauthors may be able to answer some of these questions, but consider also putting at least some of them to a more experienced colleague. Authors can easily overestimate the importance of what they have to say and the size of the audience for the message. These overestimates may lead to writing a paper that should not be written or sending a paper to a journal unlikely to publish it. As one sage put it: mothers love their own babies.

In working out a complete answer to question 1, you may be tempted to move toward writing the first draft of the paper you have in mind, but a first-step, short answer to the question is a powerful test of whether you have a message and are really ready to write. There may be lesser questions you will be able to answer, but you must be sure that your paper will have a leading, most important message.

WHAT DO I HAVE TO SAY?

What will be the message of the paper? Papers likely to be read are those that are useful to readers because they answer their questions or likely future questions. An effective paper deals with a question important for an audience clearly answered with adequate evidence for the answer. Can you state the main question your paper will aim to answer? Do you have an answer, an answer that can be stated in one sentence? Your being able to state the answer in a single short sentence is a powerful test of whether your paper will have a clear and strong message. That answer should be the clear focus of your paper.

The Research Paper

You have carried out a study designed to answer a specific question: Is antibiotic A more effective than antibiotic B in treating disease X? The study has yielded a clear answer amply supported by statistically sound data: "Treatment with antibiotic A is more effective in reducing mortality from disease X than treatment with antibiotic B". The paper with that message will make that main point; you know what you have to say.

The chief of your surgical service has been reviewing his last 50 cases of total colectomy for treatment of severe ulcerative colitis. He asks you to join him in writing a paper on his findings. You ask him what point the paper is going to make. He gets irritated. He is not "trying to make a point", he is just going to "report his experience" because his "colleagues elsewhere will be interested". Your surgical chief does not have a clear message in mind for his paper; he does not know what he has to say.

Data-gathering not organized to answer a specific question may or may not lead to papers worth writing. The probability that a paper with a clear message will emerge from research is determined more by how the research was conceived, planned, and executed than by how well the paper is written. A clear question must be posed before the research is planned, the design of the research plan must be adequate, and the data must be properly collected and appropriately analyzed.

Well-conceived and well-executed research does not necessarily lead, however, to an answer important to a large audience; that assessment is covered by question 5.

The Case Report

Exactly what message a case report will carry is usually not clear until the literature has been searched for reports of similar or closely related cases. A clinician's feeling that a case is unique or so uncommon as to merit description may impel him or her to describe it in a case report. But the uniqueness of a case is rarely the message of an important case report; the importance lies more in the extent to which the report will enlarge our concepts of disease and our skills in practice. These judgments should determine the exact message of the case report, and they cannot be reached without a search of the literature for reports of similar cases.

The Review Article or Metaanalysis

An author of a research paper is ready to consider questions 2 through 6 posed above after having concluded that it will have a clear message: He or she examined data from the study and came up with an answer to the question for which the research was designed. But a decision to write a review article, like the decision to write a case report, usually follows a search of the literature that has turned up no review of the kind intended. That literature search will not necessarily lead to an exact message for the review until the literature relevant to the review's topic has been thoroughly digested. The initial search of the literature will have to be guided, however, by a tentative decision on what question or questions the review might answer.

A review may not be worth writing if you cannot frame one or more important questions it will aim to answer. What if the chief of your medical service suggests that you join him in writing a review on the neurologic manifestations of lupus erythematosus? The two of you must discuss exactly what questions such a review might answer. What are the various neurologic manifestations that may develop in patients with this disease? How can these be identified as due to the disease rather than to treatment? What is the effect of treatment on these manifestations? With these questions you can consult some up-to-date textbooks and search the literature for reviews of lupus erythematosus to see what answers they already give.

The same considerations apply to writing a contemplated metaanalysis. Has the question you propose to answer with a metaanalysis already been answered with an adequate metaanalysis? If it has, do you have in hand data from clinical trials not covered by preceding metaanalyses that may change the conclusion previously reached?

The Opinion Paper

You may have views on some question of current importance that you cannot answer with research data. You might consider writing a review article dealing with the question, but there are not enough reliable data for a formal analysis of the kind readers would expect in a review article or metaanalysis. Your paper would have to rely heavily on speculation or a personal hypothesis. Perhaps you could prepare a paper that would give your opinion, your judgment, your personal analysis of the question tackled. Some journals are willing to consider publishing informal papers of this kind in a section of the journal designated with a heading such as "Opinion Piece", "Sounding Board", "Perspective", "How I See It", or some similar title. As suggested below under "What Is the Right Journal", you should check the information-for-authors page(s) of journals you think might publish a paper of this kind to see if in fact the journal will consider it for possible publication.

IS THE PAPER WORTH WRITING?

Writing is hard work. Why write a paper if it is unlikely to get published?

What Is in the Literature?

Whether a journal accepts a paper often hinges on whether its message is new to the medical literature, or at least new to the journal's audience. Even if the message is not new, the paper may get published because it expands on, or firms up, a previously published message. So deciding to write a paper may depend in part on what you find in a new search of the literature. Research you started 3 years ago that was preceded, of course, by a literature search may have reached conclusions already reported in five papers published in the past year. The unusual, perhaps unique, case you think of describing in a case report has already been described in 10 papers published in three countries. The kind of review article you think is needed has already been published as two only slightly different reviews in two major journals.

If your search of the literature turns up no paper of the kind you are planning, you have a green light. Or the search may tell you that the findings in an apparently unique case you wish to report have been described in a French journal but not in an English-language journal. You may find a review on the topic you have in mind, but it is insufficiently critical. So a search or re-search of the literature can also tell you much about the factors determining the odds that your paper, if you write it, will be accepted for publication: the newness and importance of its message in the entire medical literature, or for particular audiences.

The "So-What" Test

How important will the paper's message be? One editor of a major journal frequently applies the "so-what" test. What if the paper's message is correct? What may happen if the paper is published? May the paper change concepts of a disease? May the paper change treatment? May the paper at least stimulate further research on an important problem? The "so-what" look at your message is a powerful, if crude-sounding, measure of its importance. What effect is the message likely to have? If the paper stands little or no chance of changing anyone's thinking, it is probably not worth writing. Be sure not to confuse what you think the paper should change with what will probably happen. You may benefit from getting opinions from colleagues on the "so-what" question.

There is a kind of paper that can be called an "everybody knows it" paper. Current opinions widely held about the best treatment for a particular clinical problem agree on one treatment; "everybody knows" that this is the best treatment! You and some colleagues were not able to find any adequate research evidence supporting this current opinion. So you conducted a clinical trial that does rigorously support it. When you search the relevant literature again you still cannot find any research reports that have come up with evidence as strong as yours. Is this a paper some journal will publish? A leading journal that prides itself on publishing new information will probably turn it down. But a journal of lower rank, especially a journal in the relevant subspecialty, may be quite happy to consider the paper for possible publication; it could become widely cited in textbooks.

HAVE I ALREADY PUBLISHED A PAPER OF THE KIND I HAVE IN MIND?

Scientific publishing is costly. Many editors do not wish to give space to papers representing content already published, whether only in essence or in exactly the same form. And authors are ethically obliged not to waste space in the journal literature. For many years the difficulties in becoming aware of new developments in fields other than one's own may have justified repetitive publication in journals with different audiences. No longer; electronic bibliographic databases now make rapid searches for new information easy. New data added to already published data may yield new conclusions and justify a new paper, but resist temptations to try repetitive publication of the same data. The odds are going up that the attempted repetition will be detected by peer reviewers and that at best you have wasted your time. If the paper is accepted and published, the repetition will probably be discovered and your reputation sullied.

Some circumstances may justify repetitive publication. Editors do expect, however, that any kind of repetitive publication will be agreed to by them and that the repetitive paper carry clear indications of what in its content has been published before and where. This topic is also discussed below in the section "Fractionated Publication" and in Chapter 21, "Submitting the Paper to the Journal".

WHAT WILL BE THE RIGHT FORMAT?

Your message and the materials your paper will carry for its support may point to the right format (the structure of a paper). The clinical trial comparing antibiotic A with antibiotic B for treatment of disease X has yielded a new message (the conclusion reached from the trial) that is new or, if not entirely new, important to a large audience. Critical readers will want to know many details about the trial so they can judge whether the conclusions are sound. They will want to know the criteria for case selection, how patients were assigned to treatment, and other details of study design and data assessment. They will expect a formal report of the trial (see Chapter 7, "The Research Paper: Reporting Clinical Trials").

The best choice of format may not be immediately apparent. The surgeon who reviewed his 50 cases of total colectomy for severe ulcerative colitis without first asking himself what question he expected his case review to answer wound up with no clear message. Without a message that is new or valuable in some other way, he is unlikely to get his paper published in a high-ranking journal. But the surgeon may be able to use a format other than the case-series analysis (see Chapter 10). Analysis of the large body of data from his 50 cases does not yield any new important findings, but the data do firm up previously published views. Further, while analyzing his cases, the surgeon reviewed the relevant journal literature. He probably has as much information on this subject as any other surgeon and perhaps more. If the subject has not been comprehensively surveyed in a review article in the past 5 years, many younger surgeons and surgical residents may find a new review useful. With this line of thinking, the surgeon may be able to develop a plan for a comprehensive review article incorporating his case data that he could not get published standing alone in a "me-too" paper.

Choose the shortest format for what you have to report. A case report of a new, but probably uncommon, adverse effect of a drug may be accepted by a large-circulation journal despite intense competition among authors to get their papers into it if the report is very concise, prepared as a letter-to-the-editor or in one of some other short but formal formats known variously as "brief reports", "clinical notes", or "short communications".

WHO ARE THE AUDIENCE: THE "WHO-CARES" TEST

A powerful test of the potential audience for a paper is "who cares", a close relative of the "so what" test. You should look at the message of your paper and ask, "Who will care?" when they see it in print. Who will want the answer the paper offers for the question it tackled? Will it be most practitioners, or specialists in a small field, or a handful of technicians?

Any author is likely to think that his or her paper will merit the attention of far more readers than in fact it will get. This human trait can lead to tactically poor decisions in writing a paper and selecting a journal to which to send it. If you are satisfied that the paper will have a definite, valuable message, ask yourself who are really likely to read it, not who in your opinion should read it. Remember that papers are read mainly by persons who need answers to questions. Your decision can be crucial for prompt publication. If you overestimate the probable audience, you may prepare the paper for, and send it to, a prestigious large-circulation journal likely to reject it; you will have lost valuable time.

Do not confuse the probable audience with the audience you feel "needs" the paper. Practitioners and investigators are busy persons with heads already full of facts. Just because your paper will carry facts unknown to them does not mean that they will make room in their brains for its message, if they do read it.

WHAT IS THE RIGHT JOURNAL?

Choosing the right journal is an early step in planning the paper. Journals differ widely, even within the same scientific discipline or clinical specialty. They differ in scope, in balance of topics, in their variety of formats, and in the balance of research reports and synoptic papers like reviews and editorials.

If you work in a narrow specialty or a subspecialty of your field, only a few journals may be appropriate choices. But most of the fields of medicine are represented by large numbers of journals. You should draw up a list of journals that seem to be suitable choices. The list should be short enough to allow for considering each journal carefully. Apply these questions to each journal.

1. Is the topic of the proposed paper within its scope?
2. Is the topic represented in it frequently or only rarely?
3. Would it offer the best match of audience with that topic?
4. What formats does it accept?
5. Does it publish an information-for-authors page or issue a similar sheet or booklet?

How do you get answers?

The most direct way to sizing up which journals on your list might be interested in your paper is to look closely through recent issues, perhaps at least a year back. But the answers you come up with are going to be only your judgments. A more direct source may be the journal's information-for-authors page or pages (which may be differently named, for example, "Instructions for Contributors", "Advice for Authors"). The information-for-authors page(s) in many journals describes the topics the journal is interested in covering and the kinds of articles (research reports, reviews, and so on) it publishes. This page may also give information on the journal's acceptance rate, the time to decisions, and other factors that may be important to you in selecting a journal for eventual submission of your paper. For information on how to find a journal's information-for-authors page(s) in the journal or at a Web site reached via the Internet, see the section "Manuscript Requirements" in Chapter 4, "Preparing to Write". Many of these pages are carried in *The Author's Guide to Biomedical Journals* (1) and the collection by Atlas (2).

MATCH OF TOPIC, JOURNAL, AND AUDIENCE

You may know all the journals appropriate to your topic. But if you are in a young and quickly growing field, you may profit from getting more information on possible choices before you try to answer the questions posed above.

Colleagues may be able to suggest new journals not known to you. You may be able to get suggestions from a librarian in your medical sciences library.

Some compilations of biomedical-journal titles list them by fields; some also describe their scope and other characteristics.

Journal Citation Reports (3), an annual compilation in *Science Citation Index,* lists in its "Subject Category Listing" the indexed journals grouped by subject field and gives their "Impact Factors". For further detail on this source, see the note at the end of reference 3.

List of Journals Indexed in Index Medicus (4) includes a list of over 2600 journals grouped by subject field in the section "List of Journals Indexed: Subject Listing". This list does not, however, give impact factors; its main value is indicating which journals in a subject field are indexed for *Index Medicus* and MEDLINE. The journals listed in *Journal Citation Reports* are not necessarily indexed for *Index Medicus.*

Another route to identifying suitable journals is searching MEDLINE for references to papers on a topic identical with, or closely similar to, the topic of your proposed paper. You will have to be careful in formulating your search for this purpose because a single relatively common term such as *diabetes mellitus* or *pneumococcal pneumonia* could lead to hundreds or thousands of references

How can you judge a journal's quality and influence? *Journal Citation Reports* (3) provides several kinds of data useful for assessing the intellectual importance of journals and the range of their influence. The "Impact Factor" indicates how many times, on average, a journal's papers are cited in other journals covered by *Science Citation Index.* The impact factors for two or more journals in a particular field give a quantitative clue to their relative intellectual influence and hence their probable audiences. What if, for example, you are preparing to write a paper about a study on an aspect of lung function? If you consult *Journal Citation Reports*'listing of "Respiratory System" journals (in the 1995 issue, as an example), you will find a list of 21 journals arranged by descending impact factors. At the top is *American Review of Respiratory Disease* (subsequently renamed *American Journal of Respiratory and Critical Care Medicine*) with an impact factor of 6.421, a quite high factor. At the bottom of the list is *Revue des Maladies Respiratoires* (the French journal, "Review of Respiratory Diseases") with a relatively low impact factor of 0.135. In between are 19 other journals, many of which may be as suitable choices as the top-ranking journal. Your choice among these 21 journals might be determined mainly by their apparent preferences for papers on basic research or clinical problems, which you can identify by searching recent issues. Keep in mind that the ranking of journals by impact factor is not necessarily the same as a ranking by circulation. Some journals with high impact factors have relatively small circulations; they are usually journals that publish highly important papers, each of which is of interest mainly to a small group of investigators. Other journals have high impact factors because their papers are frequently cited by academic authors, but they are not widely read by nonacademic clinicians.

Do not feel compelled to choose the most prestigious journal in your field. A normal and leading motive for publishing is to build one's reputation among peers. Getting a paper published in a journal with a high ranking raises your reputation. But submitting a paper to the most prestigious journal in your field also raises the risk that the paper will not be accepted and that you will have lost the weeks, and sometimes the months, the journal needed to process the paper, sometimes with peer review, before rejecting it. High-prestige journals also have high rejection rates. Because they receive 1000 to 4000 manuscripts per year and can publish only a fraction of these papers, their rejection rates run as high as 90%. Should you aim lower in the ranks of relevant journals and swap possible prestige for faster publication?

Are some journals apparently out of your field worth considering as possible outlets for your paper? How can you identify them? *Journal Citation Reports* (3) offers a compilation, "Cited Journal Listing", that gives the number of citations of a journal's papers in a calendar year. This total is broken down by journals carrying the citations and the number of citations in each journal. Impact factors are given before each journal. The listing for *American Journal of Respiratory and Critical Care Medicine* will show, for example, that many of its papers are cited in wide-scope journals like *Annals of Internal Medicine* and *The New England Journal of Medicine*. This means that these two journals also publish papers on respiratory system topics. You must be aware, however, that their relatively high impact factors means that competition for publishing in them is also high.

For all of these reasons, your best choice of journal for your paper on an aspect of lung function may be one in the *Journal Citation Reports'* listing for "Respiratory System" but not the top journal. Probably most of the journals in the list are known by your intended audience, even if not regularly scanned by them, and the journals below the top two or three represent a lower risk for rejection of your paper.

Match of Format and Journal

The journals of your choice may be right for the topic, but do they publish papers with the format you have chosen? You are planning to write a detailed, critical review of diagnosis and treatment of gonococcal urethritis. Gonorrhea is a widespread clinical problem; surely a good choice would be a journal with a large audience of practicing physicians. Why not *Journal of the American Medical Association?* This choice might be wrong; this journal occasionally carries short summaries of diagnosis and treatment but not long, detailed, heavily referenced reviews.

As recommended above, scan many issues of the journals you are considering. Also check the journals' information-for-authors page(s) again to see if your format is mentioned. Without thus assuring yourself about this question of format, you could spend 6 weeks writing a paper in a format not used by the journal to which you send the paper. You would then have to put in more time in revising it to another format for that journal or in sending it to a second-choice journal that may require revision of it to yet another format.

Even if the journal publishes papers on the topic and in the format you have chosen, the journal may carry other clues that the odds are high against acceptance of your paper. A PhD candidate in clinical psychology wrote a long term paper on the usefulness of psychological tests in assessing emotional problems in women with breast cancer. Her faculty adviser praised the paper and urged her to try to publish it as a review article. The student picked out six journals in her field. Two of them publish only original research papers, two publish some reviews, but mostly research papers, and all the reviews they had published in the preceding 3 years were by authors preeminent in their field, not academic nobodies. She concluded that her review probably would not be accepted because she was then an academic nobody. This left two journals. Of the two, one publishes short, relatively informal reviews of currently important topics. She chose this journal, revised her turgid and academically flavored term paper to a short, informal discussion of her topic, and got the paper accepted immediately.

A Query to the Editor

If you have gone through all of these steps and still feel unsure of whether you have picked the right journal and the right format, write or call the journal's editor and raise the question. Be sure you frame your query the right way. The question "Will you publish a review of the diagnosis and treatment of gonococcal urethritis?" does not tell the editor whether you are talking about a two-page concise summary of the topic or a 50-page detailed review. And when you ask, "Will you publish . . .", no editor is going to commit the journal in advance to publishing the paper; ask instead, "Are you willing to consider for publication a 50-page detailed review of the diagnosis and treatment of gonococcal urethritis?". The replies may be various. You may learn that the editor has just accepted such a review or that the journal never publishes such long reviews. Replies like that may disappoint you for the moment, but they can save you time and work later. The reply you are more likely to get is, "Send it in and we'll look at it."

FRACTIONATED PUBLICATION ("SALAMI SCIENCE")

You may be tempted to try to publish more than one paper from the data collected in one study. This impulse is understandable, given the pressure to publish for academic appointments and promotions. Some studies do justify more than one paper. A study of an epidemic of a serious infection caused by a newly identified bacterium could legitimately yield a paper on characteristics of the bacterium appropriate for a journal in bacterial taxonomy. A separate paper on newly developed culture methods for the bacterium might go into a journal on laboratory methods in microbiology. A clinical journal would be a suitable outlet for a third paper detailing the clinical manifestations of the infection. Each of these papers would have a clear message and a particular audience. A single paper describing all of the findings might be much too long. Keep in mind, however, that papers which represent arbitrary carving up of clearly related aspects of a single study have been called "salami science" (5). An example is a study of the cardiovascular effects of a new drug. Is it legitimate to divide presentation of the data into three papers: one on cardiac effects, one on effects in the pulmonary circulation, and one on the peripheral circulation? The answer is probably "no" if all of the findings together yield a message that can be presented in a paper of normal length. The answer may be "yes" if the three aspects of the study yield different messages and if combined would yield a paper too long for any journal to accept. If you do proceed to prepare the contemplated three papers, each of the papers should carry reference to the other two. Further, you should inform the editors to whom you submit the papers on how information from the study is divided among the three. Some of these points are also discussed in Chapter 21, "Submitting the Paper to the Journal".

A related question is whether to try to publish in an informal symposium paper the findings from a study and then to seek subsequently to publish the same material in a formal journal paper. If you tell the editor about the symposium paper, he or she may be willing to publish the second paper. But if the editor does not have this information and a consultant reviewing the manuscript is aware of the symposium paper and points it out to the editor, the chances of rejection go up sharply.

CONCLUSION

If you think you have a paper to write, ask yourself some questions. What will be its message? Can I put the message into one sentence? What is likely to be the value of the message? Test its importance with the "so-what" test; what may the paper's message change? If it passes the "so-what" test, try the "who-cares" test and ask "important to whom?".

If you still think you have a paper to write, decide on the right format: a formal research paper, a detailed review, a concise letter-to-the-editor. Inspect closely recent issues of the journals you have in mind for the paper; consult their information-for-authors pages; query the editors if necessary. Is your topic within their scope? Do they accept the format you believe will be right?

continued

Conclusion continued.

If you are thinking of writing a paper as only one of several representing the same study or presenting the same data, can you justify this step as necessary for effective presentation? Or will you be multiplying publication not for the sake of readers but for selfish motives?

REFERENCES

1. The author's guide to biomedical journals: complete manuscript submission instructions for 185 leading biomedical periodicals. 2nd ed. New York (NY): Mary Ann Liebert; 1997.
2. Atlas MC. Author's handbook of styles for life science journals. Boca Raton (FL): CRC Press; 1996.
3. Institute for Scientific Information. Journal citation reports. Philadelphia: Institute for Scientific Information. Published annually as a part of *Science Citation Index*. Note that *Journal Citation Reports* is no longer issued as a printed volume in the *Science Citation Index* set. It is issued in a separate binder that carries the detailed pages of data in a microfiche format, but the microfiches are accompanied by a printed manual that explains the *Reports* in detail and carries lists of journals covered by *Science Citation Index*, including the list referred to here of journals grouped by their subject fields.
4. National Library of Medicine. List of journals indexed in *Index Medicus*. Bethesda, Maryland: National Library of Medicine. Published annually.
5. Huth EJ. Irresponsible authorship and wasteful publication. Ann Intern Med 1986;104:257–8.

CHAPTER 3

Searching the Literature

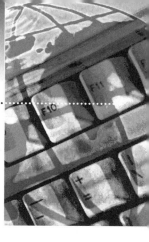

If the paper you are about to write is a research report, you reviewed the relevant literature before you started the research. You probably searched the literature from time to time as the research proceeded, to keep aware of newly published relevant papers. Reports of similar findings might influence whether you will report your research in a paper and, if so, how. You will, of course, periodically look for new reports until you prepare the final version of your paper. This chapter may not be useful to you; you probably have had a search strategy and have applied it in relevant databases. You may not, however, have searched all of the possibly relevant sources.

Potential authors of other kinds of papers usually have to carry out a new search of the literature before they commit themselves to starting to write.

If you are thinking of reporting an unusual, or possibly unique, case, you must find out whether any similar cases have been described. If some have been, how similar are they? Is the report really worth writing?

If you are thinking of writing a review article, you must find out whether any similar reviews have been published recently. If any have been, do they give adequate answers? Are they out-of-date? Are they in foreign languages? If you do see a need for the review, you will have to search carefully for all papers not previously seen by you that might be relevant for your review.

Detailed instruction on searching the literature through computerized databases is well beyond the scope of this chapter. Such instruction is best sought in your nearest medical library and in manuals describing online access to databases (including Internet access), the use of databases in the CD-ROM format, or both. Appendix D, Searching *Index Medicus*, describes some tactics that can be used by persons for whom that index is the only available resource for searching the medical literature.

DECISIONS TO BE MADE FOR A SEARCH

Unless you are thoroughly familiar with search methods and tactics, do not first rush to sit down at your computer or in the nearest medical sciences library to access any of the now widely available online databases. Regardless of what databases you plan to use, you should first take five steps to organize your search tactics.

1. Decide on the subject of your search: the topics and how they relate to each other, what terms will adequately represent these topics.

2. Decide on the extent of your search: how broad and how far back your search should go.

3. Decide on whether you will do your own search or will seek help from a professional searcher.

4. Decide on the bibliographic databases through which you will search for relevant papers. A professional librarian or information specialist can offer valuable advice on where to search. Keep in mind that the Internet can give access to nonbibliographic specialized databases that may be much faster routes to information you need; an example from clinical genetics is the database Online Mendelian Inheritance in Man.

5. Decide on how you will record the references from your search.

THE SUBJECT OF THE SEARCH

Terms Representing the Subject

What terms you select to represent your subject and how they relate to each other are critically important for an effective search. The problem is akin to selecting a diagnostic test. One set of search tactics can be highly sensitive but low in specificity; it picks up all papers relevant to your subject but also many irrelevant papers. Another set can be insensitive and miss many relevant papers while being highly specific, picking up only highly relevant papers. Different strategies may each be best for a particular need. Note that some professional searchers would refer to *sensitivity* by the term *recall ratio* and to *specificity* by *precision ratio*.

High-sensitivity, low-specificity searches may be best when you do not want to risk missing possibly relevant papers, as in preparing to write a review article, a metaanalysis, or a report of a possibly unique case. You must be willing to put in the time to weed out many irrelevant papers for the sake of "complete" coverage.

Low-sensitivity, high-specificity searches may be adequate for papers such as scientific editorials, "teaching" articles, and textbook chapters in which you need to draw only on important papers from major journals.

Start by writing down the terms that could represent aspects of the subject of your paper. Suppose you wish to review the clinical problems of cytomegalovirus infection of the gastrointestinal tract in persons with the acquired immunodeficiency syndrome. Your first list may look like this.

cytomegalovirus infection
gastrointestinal tract
acquired immunodeficiency syndrome (AIDS)

Then you should start to think of other possible terms. Are there other related terms? Are there specific techniques that might be relevant?

treatment?   diagnosis?   duodenoscopy?   gastric aspiration?

What about synonyms? *Paget disease of bone* is equivalent to *osteitis deformans.* Is your subject to cover only human aspects? Might some animal research be relevant? Continue this process until you think you have exhausted the possibilities. You can help to ensure that you have developed a complete list by drafting a tentative outline of your paper (see Chapter 12). At this stage you need as full a list as you can compile; you will refine it later.

If you have in hand some papers that cover the same subject as your proposed paper, by searching MEDLINE (the National Library of Medicine's index of biomedical literature) for its citations of those papers you can get the terms by which those papers were indexed; these may be especially efficient terms to use in your search.

Adequate Forms of Terms

Medical vocabulary is by no means standardized in the medical literature. Variant forms of terms turn up in journals of different countries and in journals of any one country. If your list of search terms does not include variant forms, you might miss some truly relevant papers. For example, *acquired immunodeficiency syndrome* was represented for several years by variant forms.

acquired immuno-deficiency syndrome
acquired immune deficiency syndrome
acquired immune-deficiency syndrome

Such synonyms are usually eventually discarded in favor of a single form—in this case it was *acquired immunodeficiency syndrome*—but the earlier forms may still appear in older paper-published indexes. Remember that eponymic terms can appear in nonpossessive, as well as possessive, forms.

the Cushing syndrome   Cushing's syndrome

Some search systems make it easy to deal with variants like this, but some do not and you should be prepared to use all possible variants of terms.

Do not forget that many complex terms are represented by abbreviations. *Acquired immunodeficiency syndrome* is widely represented by AIDS as pointed out above, *human immunodeficiency virus* by HIV. Journals in general do not allow the use of such abbreviations by themselves without the terms they represent, but you cannot be sure that you will not miss papers relevant to these topics if you do not include such abbreviations among your search terms in some systems.

At this point keep your terms in the form in which they occur to you. You should remember, however, that in search vocabularies (thesauri) your terms could appear in an inverted form.

depression, chemical	depression, involutional	injections, epidural	injections, intralesional

The inverted form keeps together in an index those terms that share a word representing the more general concept they represent.

Relations of Terms

After you have compiled the terms that seem to represent adequately all possibly useful topics within your subject, assemble these terms and modify them to indicate the relations you want them to have to each other. These relations will determine how a search is specifically formulated for an online bibliographic database or its equivalent on a CD-ROM disk. Even if you are going to search a "paper-format" bibliographic index such as *Index Medicus* (see Appendix D), you should take this step of putting together your search terms in a precise formulation. The formulation for your review on gastrointestinal cytomegalovirus infection in AIDS might look like this.

clinical aspects of gastrointestinal cytomegalovirus infection in men and women with the acquired immunodeficiency syndrome, including symptoms and signs, findings on examination, diagnostic methods, treatment, and autopsy findings

Such a formulation will be asked for by a professional searcher you engage.

Logical (Boolean) and Proximity Operators: The Combining of Search Terms

If you are going to carry out the search yourself in an online or CD-ROM database, you must be sure that you know how to combine your search terms with the possible connecting "operators".

The logical (or "Boolean") operators *and, or,* and *not* indicate to the computer how you want your terms treated in relation to each other during the search. (*Boolean* refers to Charles Boole, 1815–1864, the British logician and mathematician.) *And* usually indicates that both of the terms it connects must be found in each reference or document (such as an abstract) searched. *Or* indicates that terms it connects are synonymous for the search; either one must be found. *Not* excludes references and documents (such as abstracts) containing the term it precedes. How carefully you use these operators can determine the efficiency of your search. In a cytomegalovirus-AIDS search, "cytomegalovirus *and* acquired immunodeficiency syndrome" would retrieve only references to papers on both subjects, probably a good specific yield. Keep in mind, however, that some retrieval systems automatically link different terms together with "and"; if too many terms are thus linked, no citations might be retrieved. A linkage of terms with "or", as in "cytomegalovirus *or* acquired immunodeficiency syndrome", would also yield references to papers on either subject by itself, a much greater total number of papers, most of which would not have to do with these subjects considered together.

The proximity operators *same* and *with* used in some online systems indicate how closely the terms they connect must be linked in a document. In general, the closer that two terms appear together in a document, for example, an introductory paragraph, the more likely the document will have major content in which both subjects are closely related. The value of proximity operators is mainly in searching full-text databases.

Professional searchers are familiar with these operators. If you are going to do your own online or CD-ROM searches, be sure you consult the manuals for the systems so that you understand their operators thoroughly; if you do not, you can make costly errors in searching.

THE EXTENT OF THE SEARCH

The medical literature is enormously large. No one can, or should have to, search all of it. You have not fully formulated your search until you have defined what kind or kinds of literature you are looking for, what languages you can deal with, and how far back in time you need to go.

Kinds of Literature

Most searches are for journal papers and review articles. Searches for other kinds of sources may need special strategies and specific databases. Books can be sought through card and online catalogs, but searches into what librarians call "ephemeral literature" can be difficult. Ephemeral literature is that usually judged to have a short period of usefulness and only for a small audience and hence to be not worth indexing or cataloging: examples are public-health statistical reports by small governmental entities like counties, surveys of regional health problems, annual reports of organizations, proceedings of conferences, and so on. Other kinds of literature difficult or impossible to find through the most frequently used indexes include technical reports and grant summaries. If you need to search these kinds of literature, you will probably need the help of a professional librarian.

Keep in mind that the efficiency of online searches of some versions of MEDLINE can be raised for some kinds of searches by designating the kind of article sought (designated in the MEDLINE vocabulary as "publication type" [pt]). For example, someone wishing to find all review articles on a particular topic can specify "review". Reports of clinical trials are identified as "clinical trial" or, even more specifically, "clinical trial, phase III" or "randomized control trial". The terms for publication types used in MEDLINE can be found in the introduction to the annual edition of the Medical Subject Headings (MESH) compilation of the National Library of Medicine (1).

Language

Are you going to look for papers in languages other than English? A truly thorough search, as for a definitive review article, calls for a review of the non-English as well as the English literature. Bibliographic indexes usually indicate the language in which papers have been published, even when the index uses English translations of titles. If you read only English, are you going to search for papers in other languages and be willing to pay someone for translations of non-English papers? Many non-English journals do publish English abstracts that give enough of the content of papers for a judgment on whether translations are worth getting.

If English is your native language but you can read other modern languages, for example, French and Spanish, you can specify in some databases the languages you wish to include in the search.

Period of Time

How far back are you going to search? If the paper you are planning is a report of research, you reviewed the literature before you wrote the protocol for your research. The search now needed is a check to be sure that in your routine scanning of literature in your field you have not overlooked relevant papers published since that first search. If you are planning a review on a recent development in practice—for example, a drug introduced 3 years ago—the search may not have to run more than 6 years from the present. Searches going back farther than 5 years can sometimes be avoided by finding review articles and published bibliographies that have already sifted through the older literature.

CONSULTATION WITH A PROFESSIONAL SEARCHER

Twenty years ago a search was much simpler to plan. The number of indexes was small. Online computer searches were unheard of or uncommon. Today we have many indexes. Although technical improvements have made the use of online systems much simpler, many online searches are still best conducted by persons trained in search strategies. Librarians, who are most likely to be the professional searchers whose help you can get, are now not yesterday's custodians of book and journal collections; they are now experts in information sources and accesses to systems for literature searches. No matter how well you think you are equipped for a search, you are likely to benefit from consulting a librarian for suggestions on the most efficient way to find the literature you need. He or she will also be able to recommend the right person to carry out the search if you want it done for you. For most authors such a consultation is indispensable for searches into literature other than journals and books.

The searcher will need your help. One experienced searcher (2) suggests that the person requesting a search follow a checklist to be sure that the searcher gets all the help needed. The checklist below includes her recommendations with some updating detail added.

- Work directly with the searcher, not through your secretary or laboratory assistant.
- Complete the search request form with information it calls for. Be sure you include billing information.
- Write your terms out as a statement or question. Do not give the searcher just a list of keywords. Be prepared to explain in detail exactly what you are looking for.

> How terms relate to each other
> Synonyms, variant forms of terms, abbreviations
> Subject limits on the search: human, animal, or both; age periods; any other kinds of limits
> Extent-of-search limits: kinds of literature; languages, years

- Suggest, if you can, a recent journal article that is the best example of the kind of paper you wish to find.
- Indicate the degrees of sensitivity ("recall ratio") and specificity ("precision ratio") you need in the search. A librarian can help in selecting strategies for your preference.
- Provide any relevant information not requested on the search-request form.
- Be sure the searcher knows how to reach you by telephone, fax, or e-mail.
- Review the results (printout) of a search before you leave the library; raise questions and discuss any dissatisfactions immediately. You may also wish to have the search findings loaded onto a diskette for transfer into your bibliographic file maintained by a bibliographic software program (see "Managing References" later in this chapter).

WHAT INDEXES TO SEARCH

Most authors in the medical sciences and clinical medicine will be able to carry out searches adequate for their needs in one, or a combination, of three major database resources: The National Library of Medicine's MEDLINE, the Institute for Scientific Information's SCISEARCH, or Excerpta Medica's EMBASE. Searchers in some regions of the world have to use the paper equivalents of these databases (for example, *Index Medicus* instead of MEDLINE); search tactics for *Index Medicus* are described in Appendix D. Even these major resources differ in scope, and some subjects may call for searches into other biomedical indexes and the indexes for other disciplines. (See further comment on this point in the section "Searches in Overlapping Services" near the end of this chapter.) Some bibliographic databases can, or must, be entered through "gateway" systems, the computer online systems that serve as intermediate connections between searchers and particular databases.

The remaining sections of this chapter describe briefly the major indexing and abstract services and indexes in related fields.

THE NATIONAL LIBRARY OF MEDICINE'S BIBLIOGRAPHIC SERVICES

The National Library of Medicine (NLM; Bethesda, Maryland, United States of America) offers two main groups of bibliographic services.

* The MEDLARS online databases (MEDLINE and related databases)
* Print resources, including *Index Medicus* and other documents helpful for searchers

The National Library of Medicine's MEDLINE

The National Library of Medicine database and computer system was originally named MEDLARS (**MED**ical **L**iterature **A**nalysis and **R**etrieval **Sys**tem). The MEDLARS system includes a number of separate databases, of which the best known is MEDLINE.

MEDLINE (**MED**LARS on**LINE**) is the most broadly useful database of the Library. Its coverage includes roughly 3900 journals in clinical medicine, medical sciences, dental medicine, nursing, and veterinary medicine (as it relates to human health). It should be noted, however, that for some fields, for example, dental medicine and veterinary medicine, the indexing may not cover aspects of their literature that deal mainly with practical matters, such as technical procedures and equipment. Its files cover mostly articles published from 1966 to the present. Current references to English-language journals are about 80% of the total. MEDLINE is updated weekly. The citations include abstracts when they are published with an article (about 75%). MEDLINE can be searched via terms in article titles and abstracts, not only via Medical Subject Headings (MeSH) terms. MEDLINE is searchable by novices and many other nonprofessional searchers in two versions accessible free at the Library's World Wide Web site (http://www.nlm.gov): PubMed and Internet Grateful Med.

PubMed, a free service, includes sets of related articles precomputed for each article cited in MEDLINE. It offers a choice of search interfaces from simple keywords to advanced Boolean expressions. Field restrictions and MeSH (Medical Subject Headings) index terms, both main topics and sub-headings, are supported. Linkage to some journal sites for full-text retrieval is available. It offers a clinical inquiry form with search filters for diagnosis, therapy, and prognosis. Linkages are available to some molecular biology databases. PubMed will soon include citations from files that had long been separate databases, for example, AIDSLINE, BIOETHICSLINE, CANCERLIT, TOXLINE. These specialized databases are described briefly in Appendix C. PubMed will also provide the Loansome Doc feature that allows requests for delivery of documents identified in a MEDLINE search. For an up-to-date picture of all services offered in PubMed, consult the Library's Web site.

Internet Grateful Med offers free access (without a user identification code [ID]) to MEDLINE, including its citations from the previously separate databases. Its Loansome Doc document delivery service is available for domestic US and Canadian health-professional users, but a user ID code is required and local charges may apply. The search engine uses the full range of Medical Subject Headings (MeSH terms) and the Unified Medical Language System Metathesaurus (UMLS). Searches can be limited by language, publication type, age groups, and other limiters by using pull-down menus.

Searchers without access to the Library's Web site via the Internet but having available a personal computer with a modem can access MEDLINE with Grateful Med, the easily run software program that can be run with computers running the Windows operating system or with Macintosh computers. Grateful Med can also be used to access CATLINE for book references. It has many advantages over the paper index *Index Medicus:* speed of retrieval, access to 550 more journals, availability of abstracts for many references, searching by non-MeSH terms in titles and abstracts, linkage of terms to raise the specificity of references retrieved. Experienced searchers can use Grateful Med to access NLM databases with the standard MEDLINE command language. Purchase of Grateful Med brings a detailed manual as well as the software diskettes. Further information on Grateful Med versions, hardware and software requirements, and how to obtain Grateful Med and the needed User ID and Password can be obtained from the fact sheet "Grateful Med" at the Web site address, http://www.nlm.nih. gov/pubs /factsheets/grateful_med.html. This Grateful Med service may be discontinued at some future time in favor of the Internet access version. Telephone inquiries can be made through the NLM's customer service at 1-888-346-3656.

Keep in mind that despite the ease of use of PubMed and Internet Grateful Med, searches with them by inexperienced searchers can result in inadequate retrievals (missing probably relevant references) or excessive retrievals (many irrelevant references). These failures usually occur because of the use of only single-concept searches and failures to use the MeSH vocabulary adequately, including failure to use the MeSH subheadings such as "Complications", "Therapy", and failure to use synonyms for search concepts. An especially helpful search device is what the Library calls "exploding". If one selects a fairly broad term such as "goiter" and has requested in the search interface that "More Specific Terms" be used, the more specific terms below the more general term will also be applied in the search. For "goiter", these would include, for example, "goiter, endemic" and "Graves disease". The MeSH display can give you these more specific terms for your own selection. A thorough knowledge of how to use MeSH terms in online searches of MEDLINE can substantially improve your results. The manuals for Grateful Med versions are helpful but an especially detailed guide is a paper by Lowe and Barnett (3). Searchers inexperienced with PubMed and Internet Grateful Med should seek some initial training in their use by professional librarians or guidance in launching a particular search.

Two special files are useful for finding very recent citations or citations before 1966:

PREMEDLINE carries bibliographic information on new citations before index terms have been added to them. The file is updated each weekday.

OLDMEDLINE carries citations in electronic form from *Cumulative Index Medicus,* the print index. This file is gradually being extended back in time and should be useful in finding older citations not available in MEDLINE. Currently the file has citations from the period 1962–65.

Files from MEDLINE are available in many libraries on disks of the CD-ROM format ("compact disk-read only memory") for local, offline searching in the library or through a local-area computer network ("LAN"). These CD-ROM files of MEDLINE reduce the cost of searching. Their search engines can make searches easier for novices. MEDLINE is also accessible. through dial-up systems of some online vendors.

The full potential of MEDLINE is usually realized, however, only through the services of professional searchers in the National Network of Libraries of Medicine, in libraries in health science centers and independent hospitals, and in companies in the health science industries.

Detailed information on MEDLINE and access to it can be obtained through several routes. At the National Library of Medicine's Internet Web site (http://www.nlm.gov) one can obtain numerous detailed fact sheets covering such topics as PubMed, Internet Grateful Med, the other NLM databases and databanks, and Medical Subject Headings (MeSH), the Library's indexing vocabulary. Inquiries on MEDLINE and other NLM online databases can also be directed by mail to the MEDLARS Management Section, Building 38A, National Library of Medicine, Bethesda, MD 20894, USA and to the

NLM's customer service at telephone number 1-888-346-3656 (1-888-FIND-NLM). Information about services available through the National Network of Libraries of Medicine can also be obtained by calling 1-800-338-7657.

SEARCHES IN OLDER LITERATURE

The MEDLINE files currently extend back only to 1966 (but will be extended back in the future). *Index Medicus* runs back only to 1960. Searches farther back may have to go into the predecessor print-indexes.

> *Current List of Medical Literature* 1952–1959
> *Quarterly Cumulative Index Medicus* 1927–1956
> *Quarterly Cumulative Index to Current Medical Literature* 1916–1926
> *Index Medicus:* the first three series 1879–1899, 1903–1920, 1921–1927

Other resources available in large medical-science libraries include the *Index Catalogue of the Library of the Surgeon General's Office,* particularly valuable for the 19th century and early 20th century.

SCIENCE CITATION INDEX AND SCISEARCH

Another major and valuable bibliographic resource for authors in medicine is *Science Citation Index*, published by the Institute for Scientific Information (ISI), and its online equivalent, SCISEARCH. *Science Citation Index* differs markedly from *Index Medicus* in its approach to subject searches. It can be searched as *Index Medicus* is searched, that is, backward year by year by subject for papers published shortly before each yearly compilation. It differs from *Index Medicus* in that you can start with an important paper published in the past and find more recently published papers that cite it. Thus you can readily trace and consider the evolution of concepts and findings from their origin and early development.

Science Citation Index has four parts: the *Citation Index,* the *Source Index,* the *Permuterm Subject Index,* and the *Corporate Index.* The *Citation Index* lists articles and other documents referred to (cited) in the bibliographies of just-published articles, with sublisting of the current citing articles. Thus it links current subjects of articles to their conceptual predecessors. The *Source Index* lists the just-published articles analyzed for citations indexed in the *Citation Index* and gives full bibliographic identification for these articles. The *Permuterm Subject Index* uses pairs of terms from the titles of articles indexed in the *Source Index* to index the articles by subject. The *Corporate Index* lists publications by institutions of origin.

Science Citation Index can be searched by subject through two primary routes. If you are aware of an author whose past work is important for the subject of your search, you can start the search by looking for that author's name in the *Citation Index.* If you find the name, it will be followed by brief identifications of the author's articles cited in recently published articles and the names of the citing authors. These recently published articles that cite the earlier articles relate in subject to the earlier articles and can be identified with more detail in the *Source Index.*

The second primary route by subject to articles recently published is through the *Permuterm Subject Index.* You will probably find in it almost any of the terms jotted down in your list of subjects for your search. Beneath the terms given as primary terms are coterms that appeared with the primary terms in the titles of index articles. Beside the coterms are listed the authors of indexed articles. These author names can then be found in the *Source Index* with their articles fully identified.

Any term that occurred to you when you jotted down topics for your search is likely to be found in the *Permuterm Subject Index* because the index is built up from words in the titles of articles indexed, not from a standard vocabulary. You should be sure, however, to search with all the synonyms you can think of; articles on the same subject may use different synonyms or near-synonyms. Failure to search under all terms (and their variants) likely to be used in the modern medical vocabulary can cause you to miss relevant articles.

The pages on the inside of the covers of *Science Citation Index* illustrate tactics for searching by subject and by author and explain the structure and content of entries on the indexes. These explanatory pages are especially helpful if you think you know how to use *Science Citation Index* but forget some details of its structure.

The Compact Disc Edition of *Science Citation Index* makes it available in a CD-ROM format for local searching. This format enables both experienced and novice searchers to take advantage of unique accession methods. A new version of *Science Citation Index,* Web of Science, is available via the Internet.

ISI also publishes four specialized citation indexes relevant to the medical sciences: *Biochemistry & Biophysics Citation Index*, *Biotechnology Citation Index*, *Chemistry Citation Index*, *Neuroscience Citation Index*.

ISI publishes other broad indexes akin to *Science Citation Index: Social Sciences Citation Index* and *Arts & Humanities Citation Index*. These can be highly useful in some fields of medicine, for example, psychiatry, social medicine, humanities studies in medicine.

SCISEARCH, the online computer-based service that is the counterpart of *Science Citation Index,* covers 5000 journals indexed in *Science Citation Index* (plus additional journals covered in the *Current Contents* series) in the natural and physical sciences; more than 50% of indexed articles are related to biomedicine. This online index offers access to research-front specialties via a unique indexing method that groups papers into active areas of research identified through their citation and cocitation patterns. SCISEARCH is available through the Knight-Ridder DIALOG, Knight-Ridder DATASTAR, DIMDI, and STN systems.

Current Contents Search, the online version of the 5 *Current Contents* editions (including *CC/Clinical Medicine*) provides online access to tables of contents of more than 4500 biomedical and other scientific journals. This database consists of a 3-month rolling file that is updated weekly.

The Institute for Scientific Information offers other computer-based services useful to authors.

Research Alert services are search services that provide weekly reports on new articles in your field of interest that have just been processed by the Institute for Scientific Information. The standard profiles of interests include such topics as allergies, asthma, clinical immunology; cancer chemotherapy, emphysema; monoclonal antibodies, hybridomas; recombinant DNA, gene cloning and sequencing; systemic lupus erythematosus. Individual profiles of interests can also be specified and thus tailored to specific needs for tracking new literature. This service could be especially useful to authors who have completed major literature searches in *Index Medicus* or *Science Citation Index* before starting research and want to keep up-to-date on relevant papers as they proceed with their own research interests. This service was formerly titled *ASCA-Automatic Subject Citation Alert*. A list of journals covered by this system can be obtained from ISI: "Source Publications for Research ALERT".

Further information on these and other services can be obtained from the Institute for Scientific Information, 3501 Market Street, University City Science Center, Philadelphia, PA 19104, USA or via ISI's Web site (http://www.isinet.com); telephone inquiries can be made to (215) 386-0100.

EXCERPTA MEDICA SERVICES

The Excerpta Medica system will be searched by most authors for article references in its online database EMBASE or one or more of its many separate print-format abstract journals and literature indexes. EMBASE draws on over 3600 journals and is notably strong for searches for drug and pharmacoeconomic information. EMBASE-related products include EMBASE Alert, a current awareness service, and EMBASE CD-ROMs available from Ovid Technologies and SilverPlatter. EMBASE records date from 1974. The printed abstract journals total in number 41, most covering a clinical or basic science field of the medical sciences—for example, *Adverse Reactions Titles, Arthritis and Rheumatism, Cancer, Endocrinology, Psychiatry, Surgery*. Some cover areas more peripheral to clinical and basic medical science—for example, *Health Policy, Economics and Management*. Each volume of a section includes abstracts arranged by relatively general subject groupings indicated by a table of contents and an alphabetical subject index. The subject-index entries are opened by a boldface entry term, followed by other entry terms that, with the first entry term, give an indication of the scope of the indexed article; the reference number for the abstract of the indexed article completes the entry. Each of the abstracts referred to by the index is headed by the abstracted article's title, its authors, the institutional origin, the journal title, year of publication, volume and issue number, and inclusive page numbers.

Excerpta Medica publishes a number of aids that provide guidance in how to use both its print and online products: *EMTREE Thesaurus* (the controlled subject vocabulary to be used in online searches), *EMBASE User Manual* (guide to searching EMBASE online in the various systems through which it is available), and various free user aids and guides.

Further information on Excerpta Medica products can be obtained from Elsevier Science, Secondary Publishing Division, 245 West 17th Street, New York, NY 10011, USA; telephones 800-457-3633 and (212) 633-3980; fax (212) 633-3975; e-mail usembase-f@elsevier.com. Inquiries in Europe can be addressed to Elsevier Science, Secondary Publishing Division, Molenwerf 1, 1014 AG Amsterdam, The Netherlands; telephones 31 6022 6525 and 31 20 4853 507; fax 31 20 485 3222; e-mail embase-europe@elsevier.nl. Inquiries in Japan can be addressed to Elsevier Science Japan, 9-15 Higashi-Azubu 1-chome, Minato-ku, Tokyo 106, Japan; telephone 81 3 5561 5036; fax 81 3 5561 5047.

ADDITIONAL INDEXES AND ABSTRACT SERVICES IN HEALTH SCIENCE FIELDS

The services described above are all useful in many of the health science fields, but additional services may be valuable for some needs.

Bioengineering

Many aspects of bioengineering are covered by MEDLINE and the services of BIOSIS and Chemical Abstracts (see descriptions below). Specialists in bioengineering may find additionally useful *Engineering Index* (published monthly as *Engineering Index Monthly* and annually as *Engineering Index Annual*). The related online system is Ei Compendex which is available through a number of gateway systems, among which are Knight-Ridder DataStar, Knight-Ridder Dialog, and STN International. CD-ROM versions of Ei Compendex and of more specialized derivatives of this main database are also available. Aids in the use of these services include *Ei Thesaurus; Ei Thesaurus, English-Deutsche Ausgabe; Ei Thesaurus, Edición Español-Inglés;* and *PIE* (*Publications in Engineering*). For detailed information, write Engineering Information, Inc, 345 East 47th Street, New York, NY 10017, USA, or consult the Ei Web site (http://www.ei.org).

Dental Medicine

The main index to dental journals and relevant nondental journals is *Index to Dental Literature,* produced from the National Library of Medicine MEDLARS system and published quarterly by the American Dental Association, 211 East Chicago Avenue, Chicago IL 60611, USA, with citations also available through MEDLINE. Issues are cumulated annually. The format is like that of *Index Medicus* and includes subject and author sections. The preface explains construction and use of the index. Further information can be obtained from the Internet Web site http://www.ada.org/p&s/catalog or from the ADA Publishing Company by telephone (312) 440-2867 or fax (312) 440-3538.

Hospital Administration and Services

Hospital and Health Administration Index covers journal literature on the administration and economics of hospitals and other health care institutions. It is issued quarterly, with a format like that of *Index Medicus* and subject headings based on the MeSH system. The Index is produced in cooperation with the National Library of Medicine but is published by the American Hospital Association, 840 North Lake Shore Drive, Chicago, IL 60611, USA.

Nursing

Cumulative Index to Nursing and Allied Health Literature (CINAHL) covers a large number of journals (including many not covered by other indexes) and many popular-type magazines. CINAHL is available for online searching through gateway systems and a search guide is available from the publisher. For information on journal coverage by alphabetic listing and by main categories (such as "Core Nursing", "Peer Reviewed"), by country of publication, by discipline or field, and by subject, consult the specific CINAHL Internet Web site http://www.cinahl.com/data/journals.htm. CINAHL is published by Cumulative Index to Nursing and Allied Health Literature, 1509 Wilson Terrace, Glendale, CA 91206, USA which can be reached by telephone (in the US) 800-959-7167; its Internet Web site is http://www.cinahl.com.

Pharmacy

Both MEDLINE (and *Index Medicus*) and *Science Citation Index* cover literature relevant to clinical pharmacy. Only generic and drug-class names can be used to search *Index Medicus* because its MeSH vocabulary does not include trade names; MEDLINE can be searched for trade names used in article titles and abstracts. As mentioned above, EMBASE is strong in representation of pharmaceutical literature.

Coverage of many topics relevant to pharmacy but not covered thoroughly in the indexes described above can be found in *International Pharmaceutical Abstracts* (IPA), issued semimonthly by the American Society of Health-System Pharmacists (ASHP), 7272 Wisconsin Avenue, Bethesda MD 20814,

USA ([301] 657-3000; customer service [301] 657-4383, fax [301] 664-8888). Such topics include drug analysis, pharmaceutical manufacturing and chemistry, the practice of pharmacy, and the economics of the pharmaceutical industry. IPA covers over 600 journals, including many, such as state pharmacy journals, not covered in MEDLINE. IPA is also available for online searching through several gateway systems, including DIALOG (File 74), STN (File IPA), DATA-STAR (File IPAB), DIMDI (File IPA), and EBSCO (File IPA).

International Pharmaceutical Abstracts is also available in the CD-ROM format in versions sold by SilverPlatter, OVID, and DIALOG OnDisc.

The ASHP publishes two guides helpful in searching both the paper and online versions of IPA, *IPA Users Guide* and *IPA Thesaurus and Frequency List.*

Information on these products is available from the ASHP Web site at http://www.ashp.org.

Veterinary Medicine and Science

Much of the journal literature pertinent to the basic-science aspects of veterinary medicine is covered by the MEDLARS system, including *Index Medicus.* But this coverage is biased toward journals oriented mainly to human medicine and does not extend into much of the journal literature on veterinary practice.

Full coverage of veterinary science and practice can be obtained only by searching online databases in addition to those of the National Library of Medicine. The two main additional relevant databases in the United States are AGRICOLA (**AGRIC**ultural **O**n-**L**ine **A**ccess), a database produced by the National Agricultural Library, US Department of Agriculture, and *BIOSIS Previews* (see description below). AGRICOLA covers 1400 journals and other serials, monographs, conference papers, reports, and US government publications. Online access to AGRICOLA can be obtained through commercial vendors, including DIALOG Information Services and DIMDI (Germany). Information on AGRICOLA can be obtained through the Internet Web site http://www.nalusda.gov/general_info/agricola/agricola.htm or from the National Agricultural Library, Education and Information, Beltsville, MD 20705, USA. CD-ROM versions of AGRICOLA are produced by several commercial vendors.

The widest veterinary coverage in a single database is probably that of CAB ABSTRACTS, by CAB International (formerly the Commonwealth Agricultural Bureaux), the online counterpart of 26 abstract journals published by CAB International. The coverage extends to over 8500 journals in 37 different languages and to books, conference proceedings, technical reports, theses, government reports, and patents. Americans searching CAB ABSTRACTS must remember that some of its terms may have British spellings and that failure to use these alternative spellings in searches could lead to missing many relevant references; the same point applies to British preferences for some chemical and drug names. CAB ABSTRACTS is available in the United States through the Knight-Ridder ScienceBase source. CAB publishes the important paper-version index, *Index Veterinarius,* a monthly and annually cumulated index with author and subject entries.

INDEXING AND ABSTRACTING SERVICES IN RELATED SCIENCES

Indexes of the literature in other scientific fields may be especially useful to searchers in the basic medical sciences and psychological medicine.

Biology

BioSciences Information Services (BIOSIS) prepares abstracts and indexes of literature relevant to biology and closely related sciences (including, to a degree, medical sciences). *Biological Abstracts*, issued semimonthly and cumulated semiannually, provides abstracts to journal research papers, book reviews, editorials, and other types of documents. *Biological Abstracts/RRM,* also published semimonthly and cumulated semiannually, provides summaries of research reports, reviews, and meetings. These two publications can be searched through four indexes.

- Author index, for searches by name of author or corporate body
- Subject index, for searches by more specific subjects such as chemicals, diseases, drugs, organisms (identified by common name)
- Generic index, for searches on an organism identified by genus-species name
- Biosystematic index, for searches by biological classifications (phyla down through families)

The print products *Biological Abstracts* and *Biological Abstracts/RRM* are also available in the CD-ROM format as *Biological Abstracts on CD* for searching with Ovid or SilverPlatter software. The online computer services (*BasicBIOSIS* and *BIOSIS Previews*) are available through a number of gateway services.

BIOSIS provides free courses on how to use its computer services, including a full-day Med/BIOSIS course of particular value for the medical sciences. BIOSIS provides free-of-charge several unusually detailed and helpful booklets about its publications and services and how to use them: "How to Use Biological Abstracts and Biological Abstracts/RRM", "How to Search BIOSIS Previews and BIOSIS Previews/RN", and "How to Search Biological Abstracts and Biological Abstracts/RRM". An extensive and detailed search manual of all of these BIOSIS services is available for purchase: "BIOSIS Search Guide".

Searches in *Biological Abstracts* for older literature have to be conducted with the Cumulative Indexes, which began publication in 1927.

Detailed information is available from BIOSIS, User Communications Group, 2100 Arch Street, Philadelphia, PA 19103-1399, USA; telephone 800-523-4806 (USA and Canada) or (215) 587-4847 (worldwide); fax (215) 587-2016; e-mail info@mail.biosis.org; Web site http://www.biosis.org. In Western Europe and the Middle East, requests for information can be directed to BIOSIS, U.K., 54 Micklegate, York, North Yorkshire, YO1 1LF, United Kingdom; telephone 44 (0) 1904 644269; fax 44 (0) 1904 612793; e-mail helpdesk@york.biosis.org.

Chemistry

Very wide coverage of all fields of chemistry, including those in the medical sciences such as biochemistry and pharmaceutical chemistry, is provided by *Chemical Abstracts* and its thorough and numerous indexes; 80 sections cover 8000 titles per year. In addition to journals, monitoring also covers patents, symposia, conference proceedings, dissertations, technical reports, and new books in chemistry. Subject searches can be carried out through the weekly and semiannual (volume) indexes. The weekly subject index is built of keywords from article titles, abstracts, and texts. Search of the volume indexes by subject should begin with a check into the *CA Index Guide* and its supplements (issued annually) to find out whether the subject terms you have selected are in the subject indexes or whether you must use synonyms. The General Subject Index for each volume is built of main entry terms beneath which are arranged multiterm entries for the abstracts that serve in effect as miniabstracts.

The online equivalent of *Chemical Abstracts* is CAS ONLINE, available through STN International Search Service (accessible through Macintosh and IBM PC-type personal computers).

Various user guides for *Chemical Abstracts* and CAS ONLINE are available, some free, some for purchase. Copies of *How to Search Print CA* in Windows and Macintosh versions can be downloaded through the CA Web site. The *CAS Catalog* is available as a PDF file ($\sim$ 2.3 MB). Information on *Chemical Abstracts* and related services can be obtained from Chemical Abstracts Service, Post Office Box 3012, Columbus, OH 43210, USA; telephones 800-753-4227 (only in North America) and (614) 447-3731; fax (614) 447-3751; e-mail help@cas.org. The CA Web site is http://www.cas.org.

Psychology and Related Disciplines

Many subjects relevant to the medical sciences are covered in *Psychological Abstracts* (PA), its related publications, and its indexes: psychometrics; consciousness states, including sleep, hypnosis, and meditation; physiological states and interventions; communication; development and growth; medically relevant social processes including drug and alcohol abuse, abortion, and birth control; and physical and psychological disorders, including disease states. Most searches of PA will begin in the volume indexes for the years up to the current year. For the current year, the monthly issues must be consulted individually through the brief monthly subject index. The subject terms are drawn from the *Thesaurus of Psychological Index Terms,* a psychology counterpart to the *Index Medicus* thesaurus, *Medical Subject Headings.* Terms you have selected for your subject search should be checked against the terms in the *Thesaurus,* which offers additional guidance, with synonymous terms and terms for related but broader or narrower concepts. The *Cumulative Subject and Author Indexes to Psychological Abstracts* cover successive 3-year periods through 1983 and are more efficient for longer searches than the volume indexes. PA for 1974 to the present is available in CD-ROM formats. A specialized CD-ROM, *ClinPSYC,* covers mental disorders and treatments, psychological aspects of physical disorders and treatments, professional issues in the mental and physical health fields, experimental and clinical neuropsychology, psychopharmacology, and health and illness assessment methods.

The online counterpart to *Psychological Abstracts* is PsycINFO, which is available through gateway services, including DIALOG, DataStar, and Ovid Online, and through the Internet.

User aids include, among others, *Searching PsycINFO on CompuServe Knowledge Index, PsycINFO News,* and the *Thesaurus* mentioned above. Additional information on PsycINFO, *The Pocket Guide to PsycINFO,* is available at the American Psychological Association's Web site, http://www.apa.org. For more detailed information on *Psychological Abstracts* and its related publications and services contact User Services, American Psychological Association, 750 First Street NE, Washington DC 20002-4242, USA; telephones 800-374-2722 and (202) 336-5650; fax (202) 336-5633; e-mail psycinfo@apa.org.

Sociology and Other Social Sciences

Akin to *Psychological Abstracts* is *Sociological Abstracts* (SA), published six times annually. Among the subjects covered are the sociology of medicine, social psychiatry, and substance use–abuse and compulsive behaviors. Subject searches are most efficiently carried out through the *Cumulative Subject Index* for each volume. The subject index is similar in structure to that for *Psychological Abstracts:* main entry terms have listed below them grouped descriptors that serve as mini-abstracts. SA's counterpart to MeSH compilation of *Index Medicus* indexing terms is the *Thesaurus of Sociological Indexing Terms.*

SA is available for online searching through the gateway systems of Knight-Ridder Information, Ovid Technologies, OCLC, CompuServe, and DIMDI (Germany).

CD-ROM versions are available from EBSCO Publishing, National Information Services Corporation (NISC), Ovid Technologies, SAI CD-ROM Products, and SilverPlatter Information. Further details on SA products can be obtained from the Sociological Abstracts Web site http://www.socabs.org.

Also available for searches in sociology and related fields is *Social Sciences Citation Index,* already mentioned above under *Science Citation Index.* This index, structured like its sister, *Science Citation Index,* covers journals and multiauthored books in a wide range of fields that includes not only sociology but also such fields as economics, education, geography, law, psychology, and urban studies. Its coverage overlaps with that of *Science Citation Index* through indexing for drugs and addiction, geriatrics and gerontology, health policy services, nursing, and rehabilitation. *Social Sciences Citation Index* provides four indexes structured like their four equivalents in *Science Citation Index.*

SEARCHES IN OVERLAPPING SERVICES

All of the major indexing services overlap in coverage to some degree, so searches in two services will usually turn up some of the same articles. Data published in 1984 (4) indicated that about 90% of articles indexed in *Index Medicus* were also indexed in *Science Citation Index* and about 50% in *Chemical Abstracts.* Although the percentages have probably changed since then, this degree of overlap is probably still characteristic of the index products of this kind. Authors who want to carry out an exhaustive search should use both MEDLINE and one or more of the other services, preferably one covering journals not indexed by the National Library of Medicine. A search on a subject in medical sociology might, for example, include either *Psychological Abstracts* or *Social Sciences Citation Index* or *Sociological Abstracts.* A comprehensive search on a subject in clinical pharmacy might properly use, in addition to MEDLINE, *Excerpta Medica,* and *International Pharmaceutical Abstracts.* These combinations could also be searched, of course, in their online equivalents.

A major advantage in searching databases in addition to MEDLINE is that some of the other databases index not only journals but also conference proceedings, symposia, dissertations, technical reports, and other print sources.

RECORDS TO KEEP IN CONDUCTING A SEARCH

Your search will proceed most efficiently if you have kept records, in any preceding searches on the same subject, of what services you have used and how.

Before you start a search, record on cards or in a computer file all the subject terms you think you will need (including synonyms, variants, and abbreviations) and the date of the record; if you add terms or delete terms later, record the dates of the changes. Terms drawn from index-term compilations (like the Medical Subject Headings of MEDLINE and *Index Medicus*) should be so identified.

In using each service, record any synonymous terms you found were needed for its index as substitutes for your original terms. Record the services searched, the years searched; also record limitations you placed on your search, such as only English-language journals or "human only". If in using online services you record the date you searched, you will easily be able subsequently to get an updated search covering later citations.

In examining original articles or abstracts to which you have been directed, keep a record of those you have decided not to use so that in conducting a search with a second service you do not go back to articles you have already seen.

When you find articles you expect to use later in writing your paper, make xerographic or scanned copies of them. This precaution will enable you later to verify both the content of each article and its bibliographical details that will be needed in your references. Be sure, however, that the pages you copy have all the data you will need for the references (such as journal title, volume number, and year).

MANAGING REFERENCES

References can be managed with greater efficiency and versatility if they are kept in a computer file organized with specifically bibliographic software rather than on file cards ("3 by 5s"). Many flat-file (nonrelational) database programs are readily adapted for this use. You can develop a bibliographic file yourself with one of these programs, but you would find it more advantageous using one of the numerous specifically bibliographic, more versatile management programs available for Macintosh and IBM PC-type computers; two examples are EndNote and Reference Manager. In selecting a software program of this type, you should try to make sure that the one you select has the features that the most versatile of them offer. Some of the programs of this type can be used to automatically assign citation numbers to references in the final version of a paper and arrange them in the order of their initial citation. They generally provide a range of formats for the citations and references themselves (for example, citations and reference formats in the citation-sequence system ("Vancouver ") widely used in clinical journals and citation and reference formats in the name-year system ("Harvard style") used in many basic-science journals. A further advantage of some bibliographic software programs is their being able to take references retrieved from a database like MEDLINE and input them accurately into a personal bibliographic file. The availability of a "keywords" field that you fill in for each inputted reference means that you could later search your own bibliographic file for references relevant to topics other than those of your current interests. Demonstration versions ("demos") of some of these programs are available and will give you a chance to try them out for their ease of use as well as their versatility. "Demos" for ProCite and Reference Manager are available at ISI's Web site http://www.isinet.com/prodserv/refman.html. "Demos" for EndNote (Macintosh, Windows, and DOS versions) are available at Web site http://www.niles.com.

CONCLUSION

Before you start a search of the literature, prepare a list of all the subject terms that may be relevant, including variant forms, synonyms, and abbreviations. Decide on how exhaustive a search you need, taking into account such limits as English-language journals only, years, kinds of subjects (human only, animal only), and disciplines (medical sciences only or other fields such as sociology, law, economics). Consider using the services of a professional searcher. If you have to use a conventional on-paper index (such as *Index Medicus*) rather than one or more of the online database systems, be sure at the start of the search that you are familiar with the indexes' structure and terminology. The main indexes differ greatly in their structure and, hence, in how they are searched. In addition to searching the main indexes for the medical sciences, you might profitably search indexes to literature in related disciplines, including biology, chemistry, psychology, and sociology. As you proceed with your search, keep adequate records of the terms used, the services searched, and the limits of subject. Use of a bibliographic program in your computer can simplify your capture of references found in searches, preparation of your manuscript, and future needs for bibliographic information.

REFERENCES

1. National Library of Medicine. Medical subject headings—annotated alphabetic list. Bethesda (MD): National Library of Medicine; [annual publication]. Available from Government Printing Office (GPO): Superintendent of Documents, PO Box 371954, Pittsburgh, PA 15250-7954; phone (202) 512-1800; fax (202) 512-2250. This valuable comprehensive version of the MeSH vocabulary can be usefully supplemented with 2 other publications: *Medical Subject Headings—Tree Structures* (also published annually) and *Permuted Medical Subject Headings* (also published annually). These 3 publications can be found in medical libraries.
2. Calabretta N. Educating the online search requester: a checklist. Med Services Ref Quart 1983;2:31–9.
3. Lowe HJ, Barnett GO. Understanding and using the Medical Subject Headings (MeSH) vocabulary to perform literature searches. JAMA 1994;271:1103–8.
4. Poyer RK. Journal article overlap among Index Medicus, Science Citation Index, Biological Abstracts, and Chemical Abstracts. Bull Med Libr Assoc 1984;72:353–7.

Chapter 4

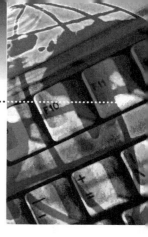

Preparing to Write: Materials and Tools

Before you start to write the first draft of your paper (see Chapter 12, "The First Draft: Text"), take four steps to prepare for that task.

1. Decide on authorship: If you will not be the sole author, come to an agreement with other potential authors on who will be authors. Then come to an agreement with the coauthors on the order for authors' names on the published paper. Coauthors should also agree on who will be the author responsible for settling any later disputes on authorship, for managing any revision of the paper, and for dealing with the journal editor. If you think disputes on authorship may arise later, you might consider getting agreement on a potential referee outside the author group for such a dispute.

2. Make sure you know the manuscript requirements of the journal to which you will submit the paper.

3. Assemble research data (tables, analyses), case records, photographs, references, and any other documentary evidence you will need to have before you while writing the first draft. Assemble documents you may need in submitting the paper to the journal, such as permissions to reproduce figures or to cite personal communications.

4. Select a word-processing program with which to write and revise the paper in its several drafts or arrange for typing of drafts and the final manuscript.

This chapter discusses these steps in detail.

AUTHORSHIP

In research studies, authorship is preferably decided on at their outset. Even if that was done, the decisions should now be reexamined and revised, if necessary, or affirmed. Some investigators may have dropped out, others added, or responsibilities within the research may have changed.

Why decide so early on who will be the authors? Why not wait until the title page is about to be typed for the final version? Do not wait, do not wait, do not wait! No failure in scholarly procedure is more likely to breed ill will and wreck friendships than putting off decisions about authorship to a time when failure to agree may bring unpleasant consequences and even damage careers. If you are to be the sole author, you are probably ready to move on to Step 2. Be as sure as you can, however, that no one else will have a claim to authorship before you send your paper to the journal and that designated authors can legitimately accept authorship.

Criteria for Authorship

What is a fair claim to authorship? Editors wish to see authorship conferred only on legitimate authors but rarely have any way of knowing which authors have had legitimate claims. Decisions on authorship must be made by authors themselves. The decisions should be guided by a central ethical principle: The reader takes the authorship statement on the paper's title page as honestly representing the person or persons who can take public responsibility (1) for its content.

Two points follow from this premise; its two key words are responsibility and content. First, persons who cannot take responsibility for defending the content of the paper if it were challenged by a reader should not be authors. Content does not refer only to data but also to intellectual content: development of concept and interpretation of data.

Second, no one is likely to be able to take responsibility for a paper's content without having taken part in writing the paper or revising it for content (2). These considerations are the basis of three criteria by which to judge claims to authorship.

1. An author should have generated at least a part of the intellectual content of a paper.
   a. This work could have been conceiving of or designing the study reported, if the paper is a research report, or identifying the particular features of a case that justifies a case report. If the paper is a review article or editorial, the equivalent work would have been identifying the question or questions to be answered and developing a plan for the paper.
   b. This work could have been collecting reported data (including clini-

cal observations) and interpreting them for the paper's conclusions. Note that interpreting data is required; the collecting of data does not by itself justify authorship.

2. An author should have taken part in writing the paper, or reviewing it for possible revision, or revising its intellectual content (not just its technical content), in two or three of these steps. The author among coauthors who is taking overall responsibility for preparing the paper should have records indicating that either a coauthor has made specific recommendations for changes in any of the drafts or has recorded a judgment that no change is needed.

3. An author should be able to defend publicly in the scientific community all of the intellectual content of the paper. In kinds of research that have used highly specialized methods, only one author may be able to defend aspects of the paper that depend on that specialized work. If this is the case, the paper should indicate, perhaps in an "Acknowledgments" section at the end of the paper, that "Dr. Xmmm has responsibility only for the use of the xxxxxxxx procedure and interpretation of the data collected with it." or some similar statement. Also note that all technical and interpretive aspects of a paper must be represented by at least one author; in other words, a paper should not contain any content for which none of the authors can take responsibility.

Only persons who qualify by all three criteria—participation; writing, reviewing, or revising; and responsibility—should be authors on a paper. Table 4.1 illustrates how these criteria can be applied for decisions on the legitimacy of what might justify authorship. For additional comment on criteria for authorship see Appendix A.

Authorship for Reports of Multicenter Studies

Difficult questions on authorship can arise with research reports by large, multicenter, cooperative teams. Multicenter studies have become more frequent in the past two decades, in part because of increasingly frequent arrangements between pharmaceutical firms and academic departments. Many multicenter studies will probably continue to have Federal support, especially those organized for getting interpretable data on uncommon diseases and treatments of uncertain value. Some editors would like to see authorship for such reports credited by group titles, such as "The National Cooperative Gallstone Study", rather than by listings of 15, 25, 50, or more "authors". The "authors" prefer, understandably, having their individual names listed for visibility in tables of contents and in the reference lists of subsequent papers. The truly important claim to authorship for the sake of career is the one on the personal bibliography attached to a curriculum vitae.

TABLE 4.1. Justifications for authorship

Basis for authorship	Legitimate	Not legitimate
Rationale for the paper		
Research report	Development of a testable hypothesis or specific question	Suggestion that legitimate author(s) work on the problem
Case report, clinical observation	First notice of previously unobserved phenomenon	Physician's, nurse's, pharmacist's routine referral, care, or service
Review article	Critical interpretations of reviewed papers and assembled data	Suggestion that the review be written
Research tasks	Development of study design	Suggestion of use of standard study design
	Development of new method (laboratory, field, statistical) or critical modification of previous method	Observations and measurements by routine methods
	Personal collection *and* interpretation of data	Collection of data without interpretation
Clinical studies	New diagnostic and therapeutic efforts	"Routine" diagnostic and therapeutic efforts that would have occurred even if the paper had not been written
Interpretation of findings	Explanatory insight into unexpected phenomena	Routine explanations such as electrocardiographic and radiologic reports
Writing a paper	Writing the first draft or critically important revision of concept or interpretation in a later draft	Solely criticizing drafts and suggesting revision of presentation, not ideas. Revision limited to technical changes, as in details of prose style or table structure.
Responsibility for content	Ability to justify intellectually the conclusions of the paper, including defense of the evidence and counterevidence weighed in reaching them	Solely attesting to accuracy of individual facts reported

Unfortunately, claims to authorship in such studies may represent a continuous range of contributions from minor to major. The difficulties in discussions about authorship among participants in multicenter studies can be settled not by agreeing on which 15, 25, 50 persons, or some other fraction out of everyone in the enterprise, should be authors but by coining a group title for "author", listing the members of the group in a title-page footnote, and agreeing that persons so identified could legitimately list the paper in personal bibliographies. If a group, or collective, title is agreed on, decisions should also be made about who might be identified in an Acknowledgments section (or in a footnote on the title page) as writers of the paper, collectors and interpreters of the data, and other kinds of participants.

Division of Authors' Work

Aside from avoiding last-minute squabbles, discussing authorship early on—either before starting a research study or, at the latest, before the paper is written—has another practical value. When authorship has been agreed on, the authors-to-be can then decide on how to divide the work of writing the paper. With relatively short papers the first draft is probably best written by only one author, but with long and complex papers the work may be shared to advantage. For example, the sections on study design and statistical analysis in a paper reporting a large cooperative study are probably best written by its statistician. With such division of work on early drafts, agreement should also be reached on their deadlines and who will pull them together for a single, integrated manuscript.

MANUSCRIPT REQUIREMENTS

If you have taken the advice in Chapter 2, you have already consulted the information-for-authors page(s) of the journal for which you have decided to write the paper, to get information on topics and formats. The journal may set limits on the acceptable numbers of tables, illustrations, and references. There may be other restrictions. If you ignore any of these until you prepare the final version of the paper, you will face the painful job of revising at the last minute to meet the journal's specifications for manuscripts, with the risks of errors introduced by hasty revision and more keyboarding. If you do not prepare the paper to meet the specifications, it may be published only after delay due to your having to revise the provisionally accepted version on request of the editor.

The journal's information-for-authors page(s) may not state a limit on numbers of tables and illustrations. You can estimate what the limits might be by looking at articles in some recent issues and calculating the ratio of the numbers of their tables and illustrations to the number of words in their texts. In one major journal, for example, the limit is 1 table or illustration to each 750 words of text (about three pages of manuscript text typed double-spaced). Knowing the probable limit early can spare you the distasteful work of revising tables or discarding figures late in the preparation of the paper or at the request of the editor.

Where can you find the journal's information-for-authors page(s)? Most journals publish this page or group of pages at least in the first issue of each volume; a few publish it in every issue. Some journals not publishing the page(s) in every issue do indicate in the table of contents of each issue in which issue the page(s) can be found. These pages may have slightly different titles, for example, "Information for Contributors" or "Advice to Authors" rather than "Information for Authors". Increasingly, journals' information for authors can be found at a journal's Web site, the address ("URL", Uniform Resource Locator) for which is likely to be given on the journal's table-of-contents page or its "officers' page" (the listing of the editors, the editorial board, the journal's managers). An especially useful Web site is "Instructions to Authors in the Health Sciences" of the Raymon H. Mulford Library, Medical College of Ohio; this document (found at http://www.mco.edu/lib/in-str/libinsta.html) lists alphabetically the titles of several hundred journals in clinical medicine and biomedical sciences; clicking on a journal title takes you to that journal's Web site and its information for authors. Another convenient source for journal Web sites is the so-called "Wilma" Web site, http://www. edoc. com/jrl-bin/wilma/spr. See Table 4.2 for examples of Web site URLs for a few journals.

What is found in a typical information-for-authors page?

A good example is the content of "Information for Contributors" at the Web site (http://www.sciencemag.org/misc/con-info.shtml) of *Science,* the weekly journal of the American Association for the Advancement of Science.

- Categories of signed papers: General articles, research articles, reports, policy forums, perspectives, letters, technical comments. For each category, advice is given on suitable length, the character of papers in the category, and other details.
- Manuscript preparation: Details on titles, abstracts, text, figures and tables, informed consent, animal welfare, permission to reprint, copyright transfer.
- The section "Manuscript Selection" briefly discusses manuscript assignments for editorial processing, reviewing, and other decisions.
- Additional useful information appears in "Conditions of Acceptance" and "Printing and Publication".
- The central section is the "Science Style Sheet", which specifies many technical details on manuscript components, photographs, table structure, and other matters in publication style.
- The closing section, "Checklist for Submission" defines what should be in a submission letter and what to include with the manuscript.

Similar information is found in the information-for-authors pages of other journals.

Note that the information-for-authors pages of many journals draw heavily on the *Uniform Requirements for Manuscripts Submitted to Biomedical Journals*

TABLE 4.2. Information-for-authors pages

Journal issues

    Weekly journals   Usually found in the first issue of each volume, which typically is the first issue in January and the first issue in July.

    Monthly journals   Usually found in the first issue of each volume, which is typically the January issue and the July issue. The first issue of the volumes of bimonthly and quarterly journals may be in other months.

    [Note that some journals list the location of its information-for-authors page(s) in the table of contents of each issue.]

Web sites of journals carrying their information-for-authors documents

    Constantly available. Getting to the information-for-authors document may call for going through several steps after accessing the opening Web home page for a journal. Examples of Web URLs[a] for information-for-authors documents for some well-known journals

        American Journal of Clinical Nutrition http://www.faseb.org/ajcn/inform.htm

        Annals of Internal Medicine http://www.acponline.org/journals/resource/info4aut.htm

        Journal of Immunology http://www.at-hom.com/JI/submission_of_manuscripts.html

        The Lancet http://www.thelancet.com/lancet/writing/index.html

The Web site of the Mulford Library of the Medical College of Ohio

    This Web site carries "Instructions to Authors in the Health Sciences", a comprehensive alphabetic listing of several hundred journal titles that serve as links to Web sites providing their information-for-authors documents. The URL for the journal listing is http://www.mco.edu/lib/instr/libinsta.html

The Web site "Wilma" Directory of Scientific and Technical Journals

    A Web site listing hundreds of scientific and technical journals with Web sites. Some of the sites are little more than advertisements for the journal but many provide links to their information-for-authors document. The URL for the "Wilma" listing is http://www.edoc.com/jrl-bin/wilma/spr

[a]A "URL" is a "Uniform Resource Locator", the Internet address for a Web site.

issued by the International Committee of Medical Journal Editors (3). But also note that some journals subscribing to the requirements set forth in this document only indicate thereby that they will not require revision of the manuscript for technical matters by the author, if the paper is accepted, if the manuscript has been prepared in accordance with the document's requirements. The journal is free to modify technical aspects of the paper (such as references formats) so that they conform to its own publication style.

A comprehensive print source of journals' information-for-authors content is the collection assembled by Atlas (4).

ASSEMBLING EVIDENCE

Virtually all papers published in professional journals—research reports, case reports, reviews, editorials—support their conclusions with evidence: observational data, case descriptions, photographs, citations of published papers, and other kinds of evidence. When you sit down to write, you should have the evidence before you and not rely on memory. Not all of the evidence need be in final form at this point. You may need a series of chest radiographs to illustrate how a malignant tumor of the lung regressed under treatment. Photographs of these radiographs have not been taken; you may wish to have the photographer crop the original images to emphasize the area and features of interest, or the prints may have to be trimmed so they can be assembled in a multipart, single illustration. You should at least have the original radiographs, or full copies of them, so that as you write you will be describing what you see before you, not what you think you saw a few months ago.

Citing published papers from memory is risky. If you try to recall from your computer-maintained bibliographic file, or your "3 by 5" file cards, or other notes the contents of papers you read a year ago in preparing your research protocol, you may not see points that have new relevance in view of your experience in the interval. It is safer to assemble copies or reprints of the papers you expect to cite. If you do not have copies, get them made now. Be sure you have thoroughly digested the papers you plan to cite; do not cite them from abstracts or secondary sources.

The Research Paper

Papers reporting research that get published might be said to have been written long before the first draft goes onto paper. This apparent paradox means that research with findings important enough to report in a published paper very likely has been properly conceived to answer an important question that can be framed as a testable hypothesis. The research has been carried out with appropriate design and methods, including statistical analysis. You have valid data and a conclusive answer.

The tabulated data should be complete and clearly organized before you start the first draft. Tables should include evidence of statistical analysis used to show the strength of the data as evidence for the conclusion. If statistical analysis is deferred until after you have written the first draft, you may have to revise its content heavily to accommodate changes in conclusions. At worst, you may write the first draft and then find out you do not really have an answer to the research question.

If the research was supported by a grant or at least was described in a written protocol for review by a research committee, the grant application or protocol probably contains sections describing proposed study design and methods that may be readily adapted for parts of the first draft. The list below includes these and additional kinds of evidence and documentation likely to be needed for most research papers.

- Papers to be cited (copies or reprints rather than notes): papers read before and while drawing up the research proposal; papers that came to your attention during the research; papers found in a final search of the literature immediately before you decide to report the research in a paper
- Descriptions of study design and methods: papers to be cited for methods; grant application or protocol approved by an institutional review committee
- Copies of signed informed-consent forms
- Tables of data: analyzed data, with statistical assessments
- Preliminary graphs, with statistical assessments if needed
- Case summaries
- Other kinds of illustrations: radiographs, electrocardiographs, and similar records; preliminary sketches for art work

Do not overlook the ethical need (2) to cite in your paper those pertinent reports that appeared after you started your research.

Preliminary illustrations will be adequate for the first draft. Properly drawn graphs can be prepared by you or an artist when you are sure, after the first or second draft, that you will use the graphs in the final version. The same point applies to radiographs, electrocardiographs, drawings of surgical procedures, and similar records.

Chapters 6–8 describe suitable structures for research papers and the principles on which they are built. You may wish to read these chapters before you start to write your first draft.

The Case Report

The documentary needs for a case report are fewer and simpler than for research papers.

- Hospital, clinic, and office records: case summaries from these records; letters
- Tables of data: data illustrating clinical course; data from special studies
- Preliminary graphs: illustrating clinical course; illustrating special studies
- Papers to be cited: copies and reprints
- Photographs and permission to use them; radiographs, electrocardiographs, and similar records

If you plan to use photographs that show a patient's identity and do not have written permission from the patient (or a responsible agent) for publication, now is the time to get that permission (see below, "Permissions"). The journal accepting the case report will need to have the permission in hand before publishing the paper. If the patient has moved to another region or country, you may need a good bit of time to get that permission. Clinical records may have to be requested of other physicians or institutions; do not delay in asking for them.

Chapter 10, "The Case Report and the Case-Series Study", has a section that describes the structure you should have in mind before you start to write the first draft of a case report.

The Review Article and the Editorial

Review articles and most scientific editorials are similar in that they look analytically and critically at important questions with the aim of providing justified answers. Thus the kinds of materials to be gathered before writing their first drafts are likely to be much the same. Many reviews and most editorials are invited by editors; for such papers the author has special needs.

- A firm understanding with the editor on whether you are free to take your own position or must develop a specified position.
- Agreement on whether you may have one or more coauthors if you wish to have any. If the paper is to be an editorial, will it be published over your name as author?
- Agreement with the editor on a deadline.
- A firm understanding of the conditions for publication: possible peer review; guaranteed acceptance or not; an honorarium?
- If the paper is an editorial to be linked to another paper in the same issue, an agreement that you will be given an advance copy of that paper.

For all reviews and editorials, some additional steps are needed.

- Sharpening as much as possible your concept of the central message of the editorial or review; state it in a single sentence before you outline and write.
- Finding out any limit on length and on number of references, and whether tables or figures will be acceptable (and if so, what number).
- Assembling references likely to be cited and any tabulated data.

The structure of reviews and metaanalyses is discussed in Chapter 9; that of editorials, in Chapter 11.

PERMISSIONS

You may have to use various kinds of documentary evidence in support of conclusions in your paper other than your own tables and illustrations. If a journal is going to publish your paper, it will probably expect you to submit written permissions for use of such materials.

- Previously published items: extensive quotations from text; illustrations; tables of data
- Photographs of patients; photomicrographs
- Letters and other "personal communications", such as unpublished papers

Some materials may be protected by copyright and cannot be used without permission of the copyright holder. You can avoid possible delay in completing your paper if you take steps to get such permission as you prepare to write. Most journal papers are copyrighted by the publisher of the journal, from whom permission should be sought even for use of single tables or figures. Note that the journal may specify in its instructions to authors or its "officers page" (listing editorial staff, giving business information, and so on) to whom requests for permissions should be addressed. An example of a letter requesting permission is illustrated in Figure 4.1. If a journal article has been copyrighted by the author, his or her copyright will be indicated on the title page of the article. The copyright holder for a book is given on the page that follows the title page. Even though the copyright holder gives permission for use of copyrighted materials, it is ethically desirable also to get agreement for their use from the authors who assigned copyright to the publisher.

Previously unpublished photographs of patients, whether of their faces or other parts of the body by which they might be identified, are unlikely to be covered by copyright, but use of them without documented express permission could leave you open to legal action. A patient may have signed a blanket permission for reproduction of the photograph when it was taken, but this permission may not be adequate. It is safer to request permission for use of the photograph specifically in the article you are planning (Figure 4.2).

Letters or other "personal communications" (including informal verbal communications, talks, lectures) are sometimes cited in scientific papers, although this kind of usually unverifiable evidence is rejected by some editors. If you hold a letter or unpublished paper you plan to cite, you should ask its author for permission to cite it, whether or not you quote from it. Such a citation without permission would be unlikely to lead to a legal action against you, but unauthorized citations of a letter may embarrass or irritate its writer; seeking permission is, at least, a courtesy.

Use of text taken from other publications may or may not need permission of the copyright holder. In general, the factor determining the need for permission is the effect of quoting on the economic interests of the copyright holder. Some quotations are generally regarded as "fair use" under copyright law and permission to use them is not needed. If the quotation is a small fraction of the original text, permission is usually not needed. If the quotation is of the entire original text—an entire poem, for example—per-

The Editor
Annals of Internal Medicine
6th Street at Race
Philadelphia PA 19106-1572

Sir:

I wish to quote a paragraph of an editorial published in your journal in 1976. The quotation is to be used in a paper, "The Next 100 Years of American Medicine", I am preparing for the Journal of American Medical Economics and Sociology or a similar scholarly journal devoted to medical economics. The reference for the editorial from which I wish to quote is as follows:

> Smith A. Medical things to come. Ann Intern Med 1976;
> 99:921-3.

The paragraph to be quoted begins "If H. G. Wells were alive today ...". This is paragraph 3 on page 922.

I am also separately requesting Dr Smith's permission to use this quotation from his editorial. Acknowledgment of permission to quote the editorial will be given in the review. You may wish to specify the form of acknowledgment.

Thank you for considering this request.

Carolyn Janavel, PhD

4321 Sequestra Street
Birch Woods ME 01234

FIGURE 4.1.   Typical letter requesting permission to use copyrighted material.

mission clearly is needed. Uses between these limits are harder to sort out as to possible copyright infringement. A safe procedure is to request permission if you expect to quote more than 4 or 5 consecutive sentences. Most scholarly journals will give permission for generously long quotations, but some commercial publishers will charge royalty fees for even relatively short quotations from novels, biographies, and similar literary works written by professional authors and published for profit. A helpful discussion of fair use can be found in the section 3.6.6, "Copying, Reproducing, and Adapting", in Chapter 3 of the American Medical Association style manual (5).

Persons whose names are to be mentioned in the Acknowledgments section of a paper should be asked to give permission for use of their names.

Mr John Doe
141 Wolfe Road
Montcalm MO 00001

Dear Mr Doe,

I am writing an article on the treatment of burns for possible publication in the <u>North American Review of Surgical Nursing</u> or a similar journal. I would like to reproduce in the article the pictures of your face taken by the hospital photographers immediately after the burns and six months later. Copies of the photographs are enclosed. These photographs would help readers greatly in appreciating the problems of patients with severe burns.

If you are willing to let me use those photographs in my article, please date and sign at the indicated points below and return this letter to me in the enclosed stamped envelope. A copy of this letter is enclosed for your records.

Thank you for considering this request.

Sincerely,

I L Hauser, MD

ILH:dw

DATE:_____   _____
                              Signature of patient John Doe

FIGURE 4.2.   Typical letter requesting permission to use photographs.

You should provide them with a copy of the text of the Acknowledgments section so that they can see the context in which their name would appear. The presence of such names in a paper may be taken by some readers as endorsement of its content, and the potentially named persons should be free to avoid such implications if they wish.

SELECTING A WORD-PROCESSING PROGRAM

If someone else will type your paper (on a typewriter or through a word-processing program) you need not be concerned with exactly how the typescript and tables will be produced. But if you are dexterous at a computer keyboard, you may decide to type your own paper, both the drafts and the final version. If this is your choice, you should try to select a word-processing program that will make easier some of the more complex operations in preparing the manuscript of a scientific paper.

Manuscripts of short and simple papers like editorials and book reviews can usually be prepared easily enough with the cheaper and most simple programs. These programs can be used for longer and more complex manuscripts, but the larger word-processing programs with more features simplify some of the tasks in constructing tables, writing equations and scientific notation like subscripts and superscripts, and repeatedly revising text.

Some features of a word-processing program can be highly useful in preparing the manuscript of a scientific paper. If you are about to acquire a new word-processing program, check on whether it has some or all of these capacities.

- Producing headers and footers so that each page can carry identification of the manuscript, including a short "running title" and page numbers.
- Inserting automatically into a header or footer the date you are working on the manuscript—the so-called "auto date/time" feature. This date will indicate unambiguously where a draft version of the paper sits in a sequence of drafts.
- Numbering the lines of a manuscript; this can facilitate reference to specific points in a manuscript by coauthors or other readers wishing to make critical comments.
- Writing mathematical equations.
- Preparing tables.
- Checking spelling with a "spell checker", preferably one to which you can add scientific and technical terms you will be using frequently.

It is also desirable to have a font in your computer with characters frequently used in scientific writing, such as Greek letters and characters that serve as footnote signs (for example, * † ‡ §).

CONCLUSION

Four steps will prepare you to write: deciding on authorship, getting the manuscript requirements of the journal, pulling together the data and documentary materials needed to write the paper, and either selecting a suitable word-processing program or arranging for adequate typing services. The documentary materials may include not only papers turned up in literature searches you are going to cite, but also radiographs, pictures of patients, and similar clinical evidence. Permissions to use several kinds of materials, such as photographs of patients, text from other publications, and letters, should be sought well in advance. The authors of invited reviews and editorials must be sure of the conditions accompanying the invitation before beginning to write.

REFERENCES

1. Huth EJ. Guidelines on authorship of medical papers. Ann Intern Med 1986; 104:269–74. Also see Appendix A.

2. [Huth EJ]. Ethical conduct in authorship and publication. In: CBE Style Manual Committee. CBE style manual. 5th ed. Bethesda (MD): Council of Biology Editors; 1983: 1–6.

3. International Committee of Medical Journal Editors. Uniform requirements for manuscripts submitted to biomedical journals. Ann Intern Med 1997;126:36–47. Note that this document is also available at various Web sites, for example, the American College of Physicians' Web site (http://www.acponline.org/journals/resource/resortoc.htm); the Web site of *The Lancet,* the Web site of the Mulford Library, Medical College of Ohio (see Table 4.2).

4. Atlas MC. Author's handbook of styles for life science journals. Boca Raton (FL): CRC Press; 1996.

5. Iverson C, Flanagin A, Fontanarosa PB, Glass RM, Glitman P, Lantz JC, Meyer HS, Smith JM, Winker MA, Young RK. American Medical Association manual of style. 9th ed. Baltimore (MD): Williams & Wilkins; 1998.

PART 2

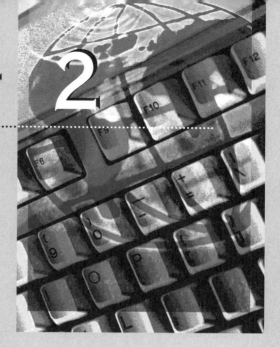

The Content and Format of Papers

CHAPTER 5

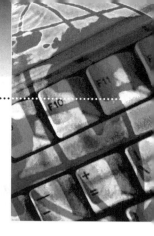

Critical Argument and the Structure of Scientific Papers

The questions most often asked in workshops on medical writing are on the right content for sections of scientific papers and its sequence. What should be in the Introduction? What should open the Discussion section? Should validation of a method be in the Methods section or in Results? Such questions are usually asked about research reports but sometimes about other kinds of papers: the sequence of sections in a review article; the arrangement of comments in a book review. This manual might simply give you cookbook answers, setting out exact recipes for each kind of paper. But you will be a more resourceful author, one more able to work out your own answers, if you understand some principles that should control the content and structure of virtually all scientific papers, be they research reports, case reports, review articles, editorials, book reviews, or some other type of paper.

WHAT THE READER NEEDS

Why do we read scientific journals? Few of us read journals cover to cover when they arrive. We scan them as we scan newspapers, to keep aware of what is going on in our fields, to get a sense of new developments that may become important to us. But sometimes we really read selected papers closely. Then we are looking for more. We are looking for answers to questions; we are looking for solutions to problems, problems we face now or expect to face in the future. A clinician needs to know the best antibiotic for treatment of an unusual bacterial pneumonia. A nursing instructor needs to know the best way to teach the surveillance of obstetric labor. The microbiologist wants to know what characteristics of *Legionella pneumophila* have justified creating a new genus and species in bacterial taxonomy. The physiologist wants to know how substance X mediates renal vasoconstriction. The clinical pharmacist wants to know the pharmacokinetic variables that should determine how the dose of a new psychotropic drug should be adjusted.

But close readers are looking for more than just answers to questions and solutions to problems. If this is all they want, they probably need not read entire papers; the answers and solutions are usually stated clearly in an abstract at the head of the paper or at the end in a Conclusion section. What we need as close readers is to be convinced that the message of the paper— its answer to our question, its solution for our problem—is correct, is valid. We are not going to apply the message in how we think and work unless we are persuaded that we can rely on it. Scientific papers are not just baskets carrying unconnected facts like the telephone directory; they are instruments of persuasion (1). Scientific papers, even if they are based on sound research, must argue you into believing what they conclude; they must be built on the principles of critical argument.

WHAT IS CRITICAL ARGUMENT?

The "argument" in critical argument is not "argument" in its popular sense. It is not a Republican and a Democrat shouting at each other on the Senate floor about the welfare state. It is not a married couple having a row about whether to squeeze the toothpaste tube in the middle or at the end. Argument here is "a coherent series of reasons, statements, or facts intended to support or establish a point of view" (2). And critical means assessing evidence for its validity, what evidence to accept and what evidence to reject. In their classic book on clear statement and the graces of prose, *The Reader Over Your Shoulder: A Handbook for Writers of English Prose*, Graves and Hodge (3) set forth "the natural arrangement of ideas in critical argument".

- Statement of problem
- Marshaling of evidence, first on main points, then on subsidiary ones— the same sequence kept throughout the argument
- Credibility of evidence examined
- Statement of possible implications of all evidence not wholly rejected
- The weighing of conflicting evidence in the scale of probability
- Verdict

At first reading, Graves and Hodge's outline of the structure of critical argument, their "natural arrangement of ideas", sounds more like an agenda for a judge conducting a murder trial than an outline of a research paper.

This "arrangement" makes more sense for authors of scientific papers if it is restated thus.

- Statement of problem: posing of a question or stating a hypothesis
- Presentation of the evidence
- Validity of the evidence
- Implications of the evidence: initial answer or judgment on the validity of the hypothesis
- Assessment of the answer's validity in the face of conflicting evidence
- Conclusion

Note that the location of these elements in a scientific paper may differ from the sequence just outlined above; this point is expanded in the paragraph immediately below and in Chapter 6.

Consider how these elements of "critical argument" can be found in a paper reporting a study of an antibiotic treatment.

Antimycin is often effective against the infectious disease called K fever, but it has a high rate of adverse effects. A new antibiotic, megamycin, has been found to inhibit the growth of the causative bacterium in vitro. But for clinicians a vital question remains to be answered: Is megamycin more effective than antimycin A in treatment of K fever? The investigators draw up a protocol for a clinical trial to answer the question. The trial gets under way. Antimycin and megamycin appear for a while to have the same efficacy, but then megamycin begins to look better. The investigators carefully monitor the results of treatment statistically so that the comparative trial can be stopped when a significant answer is reached. Finally megamycin is found to be definitely better, a conclusion reached with statistically supported evidence. The trial is completed. Then the investigators write and get published a paper reporting the trial. The paper makes clear in the Introduction why the study was carried out: the question that had to be answered. The paper describes the findings in a Results section: the evidence. The validity of the findings is established through description of study design and methods, through statistical statements, and through assessment of possible alternative conclusions. A conclusion is reached; the answer is clear: "Megamycin is more effective for treatment of K fever than antimycin". The reader who needs the answer and wants to know whether the answer is reliable gets in the paper all that he or she needs. The reader is persuaded; the reader has been argued into accepting the answer.

The concept of critical argument includes more than just the content of argument. Graves and Hodge's outline also specifies a sequence for the argument. The evidence is not stated first, with the question to which it is applied posed later. The question is made clear at the beginning. This principle should apply to all scientific papers, be they research reports or reviews. The reader needs to know at the beginning exactly what the paper is about, what question or questions it is setting out to answer. The sequence of its content thereafter may not follow exactly that in Graves and Hodge's outline. The sequence in a research report is likely to be that of a mainly forward narrative and in a review article, a "flashback" akin to a historical review. But authors must keep in mind that the sequence must be made clear to readers. As discussed in the following several chapters, the sequence of content in a paper is usually indicated by dividing it into sections with text headings, such as "Methods", "Results", and other kinds of headings. Conventional headings of this kind do help orient readers to a paper's structure but they do not necessarily correspond directly to the elements of critical argument. Chapters 6–11 try to show how the elements of critical argument should be presented in various kinds of papers and where in the usual format used for the presentation. Note, however, that not all possible types of papers are covered in these chapters, but only the most common types.

CONCLUSION

The reader of a scientific paper is looking for the answer to a question, the solution to a problem. The author of the paper must first make clear the question the paper proposes to answer or the hypothesis the research has tested. The author must convince the reader, through critically sifted evidence arranged in a clear sequence, that the conclusion of the paper is correct. This content, that of critical argument, is appropriate for other kinds of papers as well as for the research report. The sequence of the content may, however, properly differ in some kinds of papers discussed in the following chapters.

REFERENCES

1. Weiss EH. The writing system for engineers and scientists. Englewood Cliffs (NJ): Prentice-Hall; 1982:116.
2. Gove PB, ed. Webster's third new international dictionary of the English language, unabridged. Springfield (MA): G & C Merriam; 1961:117.
3. Graves R, Hodge A. The reader over your shoulder: a handbook for writers of English prose. 2nd ed. New York (NY): Random House; 1979:125.

CHAPTER 6

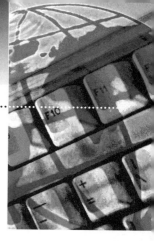

The Research Paper: General Principles for Structure and Content

Papers reporting research are the most frequently published kind of scientific paper. The huge number of research papers being written has forced authors into competing intensely for space in journals. You can compete most effectively when your paper reports your research clearly and completely, but efficiently, when you select the right content, when you select the right format.

A conventional format for research papers has come to be widely used: the "IMRAD" format (**I**ntroduction, **M**aterials and Methods, **R**esults, **a**nd **D**iscussion). This format is not arbitrary; it is based on principles derived from the content and sequence of critical argument discussed in the preceding chapter. If you master these principles, you will often be able to decide for yourself on how to structure your papers and when you might properly modify this conventional format. Indeed, some journals do not require that authors use this conventional format; the alternatives will be discussed later in this chapter. Note that the "IMRAD" format is recommended by the International Committee of Medical Journal Editors (1) as the usually desirable format for papers reporting experimental and observational studies.

The "IMRAD" format is essentially a format only for research reports such as reports of clinical trials, of observational studies, or of laboratory research. Other kinds of formats are needed for other kinds of articles, such as reviews, metaanalyses, case reports, editorials, opinion papers. These are discussed in Chapters 9–11.

THE CONVENTIONAL FORMAT: "IMRAD"

What do readers want to find in a paper reporting research? The eminent biostatistician, A. Bradford Hill, said (2) the answers to four questions: "Why did you start?" "What did you do?" "What answer did you get?" "What does it mean anyway?" His questions ask for more than their simple form implies, but these points and their sequence do clearly indicate what readers expect.

> *Why did you start?*
> The question to be answered must be stated or clearly implied; the alternative is the hypothesis to be tested. But preceding this statement should be the answer to Hill's first question: Why did you start? Where did the question come from? These points make up the paper's Introduction.
> *What did you do?*
> How the answer was sought, or the hypothesis tested, must be specified in convincing detail. This content makes up what is conventionally labeled "Materials and Methods", or "Subjects and Methods", or some other similar heading.
> *What answer did you get?*
> The evidence bearing on the final answer is described: your findings and other supporting evidence, counterevidence. This content is usually distributed between the "Results" section and the "Discussion", as noted below. The answer to the question (or judgment on whether the hypothesis was supported) is given after assessment of all evidence.
> *What does it mean anyway?*
> The meaning of the research's answer for further research or use in practice is considered in the "Discussion."

You can see that this sequence is, in essence, a narrative sequence, the "story" of the research: where you started; what you did; what you ended up with. The elements of critical argument in research papers do not follow exactly the usual sequence in "critical argument" (see Chapter 5) but are usually divided to fit into the "story" format; this point is summarized in Table 6.1. As noted above, you may need to vary the sequence in response to the preference of a particular journal; it may not, for example, allow use of a closing Conclusions.

The Introduction

When you go to an interview for a job, your clothes and behavior may determine right away whether you get hired. Likewise, the Introduction to your paper may immediately influence how the paper is sized up by an editor, a manuscript consultant, or, if the paper gets published, by a reader. If the Introduction is too long, it can irritate or bore; if it is too short, it may not make clear why the research was needed. The Introduction quickly gives an impression of your skill as an investigator and writer. Four rules may help you in deciding what to put into the Introduction.

TABLE 6.1.   Structure of the research paper as critical argument

Sequence of the research	Format	Elements of critical argument[a]
Where the question to be answered came from; the question (or hypothesis) itself	Introduction	The "problem" (question)
How the answer was sought	Material and Methods	Credibility of evidence
Findings	Results	Evidence (the data); initial answer
Your findings considered for their validity; considered in relation to the findings of other investigators; the final answer	Discussion and Conclusion	Your valid evidence; supporting evidence from others; contradictory evidence; final assessment of all evidence. Answer

[a]See Chapter 5, "Critical Argument and the Structure of Scientific Papers".

Tell the Reader Why the Research Was Started

What was the gap in knowledge to be filled by the research? What question has not been settled by previous research? Answers to these questions justify the research; the Introduction thus puts a probable value on what the paper provides. Gaps in knowledge may be of several kinds. There may have been a need to account for a new phenomenon: A study of the pharmacokinetics of a new antibiotic in patients with inadequate renal function may have been launched because a serious side effect of the drug had been found to occur only in patients with renal disease. There may have been a need to reconcile conflicting previous observations: A drug for treatment of congestive heart failure has been described in one paper as highly effective and in another paper as effective in only about half of the patients. To what is the difference due—to different doses, to differences in the severity of the heart failure?

Do Not Explain What Can Be Found in Any Textbook in the Field

In justifying your research go back no farther in citing the relevant literature or explaining the problem than is needed by the intended audience. Do not use the Introduction to try to show off wide knowledge; the audience for the paper should be expected to know almost as much as you. If the paper reports a comparative trial of two drugs for treatment of metastatic breast cancer, you need not explain to an intended audience of physicians that metastatic breast cancer is a frequent and serious clinical problem; you need not describe its characteristics. Physicians know all of this; you start the Introduction simply by reviewing why a new treatment is needed and why the drugs studied were selected.

Do Not Elaborate on Terms in the Title of the Paper

If the title is "The Prevalence of Hypercalcemia in Patients with Sarcoidosis", do not start with explaining hypercalcemia and sarcoidosis. Readers of the title who do not know what you mean by these terms are not likely to be interested in going on to read the paper.

Make Clear What Question the Research Was Designed to Answer

You need not state the question as a question, but what you state as the purpose of the research should be translatable as a question. For a trial of a new multidrug chemotherapeutic regimen for metastatic breast cancer, you state, "This study was designed to compare the efficacy for treatment of metastatic breast cancer of the new multidrug therapeutic regimen, cobracin-IL2 with the present standard therapy, CLOPP, in women under the age of 50". The reader readily translates this statement into a question: "Is cobracin-IL2 a better treatment for metastatic breast cancer in women under age 50 than CLOPP?". The statement "was designed to compare" is not, however, specific enough; the reader needs to know what yardstick was used to define "better". A more specific statement would be "The new multidrug therapeutic regimen, cobracin-IL2 was compared with CLOPP, the present standard therapy, for its effect on survival at 1 year after treatment".

The purpose of a research study can also be stated as testing a hypothesis: "This clinical trial tested the hypothesis that the cumulative mortality from metastatic breast cancer at 1 year after treatment will be lower in women under age 50 with cobracin-IL2 than with CLOPP".

A clear statement of the question to be answered or the hypothesis to be tested is indispensable in planning research; without it, the research may not yield useful conclusions (a symptom of this failure can turn up as a vague statement of purpose at the close of an Introduction). But even if you did pose a specific hypothesis at the beginning of your research and have found a clear and useful answer, some readers may regard a "tested-the-hypothesis" statement as pedantic, artificial, and not in clinical idiom. Even if a hypothesis was formally proposed, most clinical readers will be more comfortable with your posing the research purpose as a question.

The Introduction should also make clear what population (represented almost invariably by a sample of that population) the study aimed to have as the subjects of the intervention studied or the observations to be made and the measure of outcome chosen.

In closing the Introduction with a statement of research purpose, some authors include a brief summary of the study design: "The two regimens were compared in a double-blind trial with randomized assignment of patients." This kind of summary lengthens the Introduction very little; if the journal for which you are preparing your paper uses smaller type for the Materials and Methods section than for the rest of the text, a concise summary of study design at the end of the Introduction emphasizes to readers how the research was carried out.

Some authors close the Introduction with a short statement of the research findings, the paper's answer. This practice has been justified as a device to hold the reader's attention; it has been criticized as moving the conclusion from its logical place—at the end of the paper—in the sequence of argument. A better reason for not stating the conclusion at the end of the Introduction is that many journals now publish papers' full summaries or abstracts—with the papers' conclusions—on their title pages. Why give the answer twice at the beginning of the paper?

Avoid a temptation to load up the end of the Introduction with more than the central question to be answered. Many research efforts are aimed at answering more than one question, but the focus of the paper should be sharply on the main question. The subsidiary questions considered can be presented in the Results section. For example, a clinical trial of a new drug comparing it with the present standard drug may properly look at the relative kinds and degrees of adverse effects found and at the relative costs of the two treatments with a cost–benefit analysis. But the main question was probably the efficacy of the new drug in reducing mortality or morbidity compared to that of the present standard drug. This is the question most readers will wish to have answered first. The subsidiary questions and their answers can be developed in the Results and Discussion sections. The focus of the report is kept sharply on the efficacy question.

Note that the kind of question asked for the research can depend on whether it was an interventional study, such as a clinical trial, or an observational study, such as a longitudinal study that sought to identify risk factors for a disease. But the central need for readers in an Introduction is a clear statement of the question.

The Materials and Methods Section

How did you carry out your research? The critical reader will want to know exactly what you did, in enough detail to be able to judge whether the findings reported in the Results section support your conclusions reliably.

Properly designed research has a logical sequence.

- The study design is selected (after the central question and any subsidiary questions have been formulated or the hypothesis to be tested has been posed).

- The state, condition, or intervention to be studied (disease, physiologic state, drug treatment) is defined.
- The subjects (patients, normal persons, animals, plants) to be studied are defined.
- The methods for selecting subjects are designed.
- The interventions, if any (such as treatment), are decided on in detail.
- All observations to be made are specified, including the methods for making them.
- The statistical procedures to be used to assess the implications of recorded data are selected.

The Materials and Methods section should follow such a sequence. Each part of the section must expand with relevant detail each of these aspects of the study as it was actually executed.

Content

The paragraphs immediately below do not specify all possible details relevant to a complete description of research design, methods, and procedures. Many of these details are considered in the next two chapters, Chapter 7, "The Research Paper: Reporting Clinical Trials and Observational Studies", and Chapter 8, "The Research Paper: Reporting Laboratory Research".

Study Design and Protocol. Some study designs are so well known that they need be specified only by a descriptive phrase. Unusual designs that have been described in the literature may be specified by a phrase but with a citation of the reference to the source. New designs should be described in detail. The study groups should be described briefly but adequately and identified, as appropriate, by kinds of intervention. Additional details are likely to be needed; see the next two chapters.

Subjects. Well-designed studies use subjects carefully specified and selected to represent properly the population under study and to minimize variations caused by subject characteristics. Results can be interpreted accurately for effects due to treatment or another kind of intervention only when other effects on results (such as physiologic effects, ethnic, or sex differences) can be excluded. Hence, subjects must be characterized as fully as possible so there will be no questions about uncontrolled variables. For animals, the sex, age, species, breed, and physiologic state should be given. For microorganisms, identify species, strain, serotype, and any other characteristics. If the effect of a drug on a disease has been studied, the criteria used in diagnosis of the disease should be specified. Ethical controls used should be mentioned: informed consent, review of the research protocol by an institutional committee, conformity of procedures to requirements of a granting agency.

Interventions (Treatment). Drugs, hormones, other chemicals, and any other agents used for experimental intervention or treatment should be described fully: the specific preparation (including details such as commercial source, trade name, drug vehicle, placebo composition) and administration (dosage, route, method). Some therapeutic trials include statistical controls to prevent unjustifiable morbidity or mortality; such a control may be described with the details of treatment rather than in the description of statistical assessment.

Measurements and Other Observations.   Standard methods for chemical and other laboratory procedures need to be identified only by name and citation; variations from these should be described in enough detail to enable another investigator to duplicate your results. Previously unpublished methods must be described in detail, with evidence that they have been validated. If the description of a new, previously unpublished method is long, the journal may be interested in having it shifted to the end of the paper as an appendix. Functional tests need to be identified or described similarly. Other relevant description may include blindness of outcome assessment and of assessment of treatment complications.

Statistical Analysis.   Specify the statistical methods. For methods (including computer programs) well known in your field, simply name the methods and give citations to standard sources. Unfamiliar methods should be described in detail. Information relevant to judging the power of the statistical assessment should be included. But note that data in the Results section with critical importance to the paper's main conclusions should be accompanied there by short specific statements of the methods for their statistical assessment.

Title, Placement, and Format of the Methods Section

The phrase "Materials and Methods" is widely used for the section of the research paper that describes how a study was carried out. Some more specific titles for this section may better fit what you have done: "Study Design, Subjects, and Methods" or "Study Plan, Patients, and Procedures". Do not be surprised, however, if a rigid editor forces you back to the tried-and-true "Materials and Methods"; sometimes old habits are not easily broken.

Most Materials and Methods sections indicate the author's sequence (study design, subjects, and so on) only by paragraphing each unit. If the section is long, you may wish to insert text headings for each unit. This device will also help to ensure that all of the content is appropriately placed within each headed section.

Where do you place the Materials and Methods section if your paper reports an unusual case—perhaps a new syndrome—and special investigations carried out to identify mechanisms responsible for the disorder or some of its manifestations? The case is of great interest, but so are the special studies. The paper is a hybrid: part case report, part research report. The solution? Tell the story. After the introduction, describe the case under the heading, Case Report. Then describe what you did under the heading Special Studies to distinguish them from the routine hospital studies.

In this sequence, "Case Report" corresponds to "Subject"; "Special Studies" corresponds to "Interventions, Measurements, and Other Observations". "Special Studies" will then be followed logically by the next major section, "Results".

Length

What do you do if the study was long and complex? Your paper appears to need a very long and detailed Materials and Methods section. Many of your readers may not want to read through all of the detail. One solution is to write a synoptic Materials and Methods section in which you give only the main points of design and procedure, with a more detailed description placed at the end of your paper as an appendix. You should try, however, to get the editor of the journal for which you are writing the paper to agree to this structure before you begin to write; relocating the detailed description in revising the paper might call for a complicated shift of references.

The Results Section

The evidence you need to answer the question that prompted your research may come partly from previously published work, but if your research has been concerned with a new question or has used a new approach to an old question, most of your evidence will be your own observations, data, and statistical assessment. This new evidence is what should be reported in the Results section.

New evidence should be described as efficiently as possible. Numeric data can usually be presented more effectively in tables or graphs than in text; the text should present no more than a summary or otherwise critically important data (for example, mean values with appropriate statistical assessments). For therapeutic trials in a very small number of cases of a rare disease, brief case descriptions may be convincing if the natural course of the disease is well known, but tables of case characteristics may be adequate.

The content of the Results section should follow the sequence the reader will expect. If the report is of a clinical trial, most readers will want to know, first, whether the trial was properly designed; second, whether the design was effective; and, third, the effects of the new drug compared to those of the standard of comparison, namely, the drug that has usually been used.

Readers are assured of the proper study design by the Materials and Methods section, but did the design accomplish what was expected of it? For example, in a clinical trial comparing two drugs, the two groups of patients in which they were used must be shown, if possible, to have been closely similar in all characteristics so that any differences in treatment results can be attributed to the drugs and not to patient–group differences. Therefore the first section of Results presents data bearing on the similarity or dissimilarity of the two groups. The possible consequences of apparent dissimilarities are analyzed later in considering actual confounding in the data.

What comes next in a Results section? The general rule to follow here is that the "known" findings come before the "unknown" findings. In a laboratory study the "known" might be the findings in control animals; in a clinical trial, the "known" would be the results of treatment with the drug that represents current standard treatment. In a laboratory study the "unknown" would be the findings in the animals treated with an intervention whose value is being assessed; in a clinical trial, the "unknown" would be the results with the new drug that is being compared with the standard drug. With such sequences you are proceeding from the old to the new, from the "known" to the "unknown". Such sequences do not necessarily call for separate paragraphs for each study group.

The Results section should give as clear an answer to the question posed for the research as the data from the study will permit. Thus, statements in the text summarizing data gathered in the research should include unequivocal statements of findings in statistical analyses applied to the data, be they confidence intervals for estimates of measures, correlation coefficients, or other kinds of statistical variables. You will not enhance your reputation by hiding the meanings of your results behind weaseling phrases like "tended to be greater" and "showed promising trends". Be sure to include with statements of statistical findings a brief mention of the methods by which they were derived (for example, "Fisher exact test", "Student's t test"). A good source for guidance in reporting statistical information is Lang and Secic's detailed guidelines (3).

The Discussion and Conclusions Sections

The opening pages of this chapter emphasize that the research paper is, in essence, a special kind of argument. The evidence gathered in your research is the evidence that should give the answer to the question posed for the research. This section should include thorough self-criticism of your own reported work. There may be evidence from other sources that appears to support your answer or that appears to be at odds with your answer. This other evidence, your assessment of its validity, and your judgment as to whether it supports your answer or contradicts it may have to be a major part of the Discussion section.

The opening of the Discussion should give the answer to your research question that comes from the research you are reporting. In the first paragraph of the section, state concisely the central conclusion, or answer, to be drawn from the data presented in Results. Remember, however, that the answer may not be fully supported until you have cited additional evidence, such as research findings previously reported by you or by others. Give full credit for this evidence by citing published reports; do not omit supporting evidence from others in an effort to make your present research appear unique or more important. If a previously published paper on the same question arrived at the same answer, do not try to pump up the importance of your findings by burying the citation of it in the Discussion, the "Reference 13" treatment (4). Avoid this devious practice; such citations should be in the Introduction.

Evidence from other papers supporting your own data may not be the only evidence you must present in the Discussion. Any counterevidence must be presented and assessed. What if another therapeutic trial led to an answer differing from that found in your trial? If you are an ethical scientist (5), you will assess this counterevidence—you will not ignore it. Perhaps it can be dismissed because the other trial tested the compared drugs in patients at a different stage of disease, but perhaps the counterevidence cannot be thus dismissed. What if the previous investigator found a different result, apparently because a different experimental animal was used? The honest Discussion considers all evidence bearing on the argument even if it is evidence that appears to lead to a conclusion different from yours. You should, if you can, logically resolve the apparent difference in findings, but even if you cannot, the difference should not be left in obscurity.

There are several ways to close the Discussion. You may need to discuss to what extent findings in a therapeutic trial can be generalized to all patients with the disease. If you cannot resolve conflicting evidence from your trial and trials by others, you may wish to suggest how the discrepancy could be resolved in a new trial. Do not extend implications and speculations too far; readers of scientific papers are looking for firm conclusions supported by fact. If you are reporting laboratory research that has tested a hypothesis and supported it, you may wish to end the Discussion section with what you see as implications for further research in the field of your topic.

If you accept the view that a research paper is a special kind of argument, you will close it with "the verdict", the answer to your research question. For many years virtually all research papers did close with a Conclusions statement in addition to the Discussion. Today many journals do not keep readers in suspense, forcing them to go through papers to the end to learn the answer; instead they put the conclusions up front in an abstract or summary on the title page. A few journals do carry papers with a title-page abstract and a terminal Conclusions. This detail is one of the many that you should check in the manuscript-requirements statement of the journal for which you are preparing the paper.

TITLE AND ABSTRACT

Whether your paper is read can depend on the accuracy and adequacy of its title and its abstract. A paper with a vague title and an unclear abstract may be quickly passed over by the reader of a journal who only scans its contents page for items of possible interest. A title with inadequate detail can lead to the paper's not being detected in a bibliographic search. For a detailed discussion of the needs, see Chapter 13, "The First Draft: Titles and Abstracts".

CONCLUSION

The research paper is based on the principles of critical argument. In the research you are reporting, you have raised a question, gathered evidence bearing on the question, and produced an answer. Therefore, the content of your paper should include all the elements needed for clear and fair argument, and its structure should be built on the natural sequence of question, evidence, and answer fitted into a narrative format that reproduces the sequence of steps in the research.

REFERENCES

1. International Committee of Medical Journal Editors. Uniform requirements for manuscripts submitted to biomedical journals. Ann Intern Med 1997;126:36–47. Note that this document is also available at various Web sites, for example, the American College of Physicians' Web site (http://www.acponline.org/journals/resource/resortoc.htm); the Web site of *The Lancet*, the Web site of the Mulford Library, Medical College of Ohio (see Table 4.2).
2. Hill AB. The reasons for writing. Br Med J 1965;2:870.
3. Lang TA, Secic M. How to report statistics in medicine: annotated guidelines for authors, editors, and reviewers. Philadelphia (PA): American College of Physicians; 1997.
4. [Anonymous]. Reference 13. Br Med J 1985;291:1746.
5. [Huth EJ]. Ethical conduct in authorship and publication. In: CBE Style Manual Committee. CBE style manual: a guide for authors, editors, and publishers in the biological sciences. 5th ed. Bethesda (MD): Council of Biology Editors; 1983:1–6.

CHAPTER 7

The Research Paper:
Reporting Clinical Trials
and Observational Studies

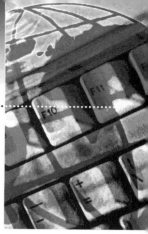

The preceding chapter shows how the content of a research report represents a specific "type" of "critical argument" and how its elements are usually arranged within the "IMRAD" structure of Introduction, Methods, Results, and Discussion. It did not indicate, however, many of the details a reader of a paper reporting a clinical trial or other types of clinical or epidemiologic studies expects to find. These details will be needed by any reader who wants to be sure that the reported research was so designed, carried out, and analyzed that he or she can feel confident that what is presented in the paper can be relied on.

CLINICAL TRIALS AND OTHER TYPES OF INTERVENTIONAL STUDIES

Probably no other kind of research in clinical medicine has more influence than clinical trials on how physicians treat patients and what patients get as outcomes of disease or injury. That influence can come from physicians' reading of trials reports themselves. But more and more, it comes from critical reviews or metaanalyses of all the available trials reports pertinent to judgments on drugs or other methods of treatment for particular diseases or syndromes. Authors preparing reviews or metaanalyses need to know a large number of details on how a trial was designed, executed, and analyzed if they are going to be able to conclude the trial's findings are worth incorporating into their analysis and the review's conclusion. It is your task to report your trial with the detail they will need.

The term "clinical trials" most often applies to research aimed at finding how a drug or some other kind of treatment changes or does not change a patient's disease, syndrome, or some other kind of undesired physical or mental state. It is, however, also conveniently applied to other kinds of studies that have in common with research on drugs or other treatments investigating how some intervention or "agent" changes or does not change some measurable variable not relevant to patient care. An example is an experimental, controlled study of how a change in the medical school curriculum might change student performance in standardized examinations. The rest of this section will discuss clinical-trial reporting in terms of drug or other treatment studies, but the principles that apply to reporting such trials are useful in reporting trials of nonclinical-type interventions.

The Title

If your title does not represent all the main elements of your trial, it may be overlooked by searchers of MEDLINE or other bibliographic databases. These minimally needed elements are the name of the disease, syndrome, other clinical state, or other target which the intervention was intended to cure or improve, the population sampled (for example, age, sex, ethnic group), a term indicating the intervention (for example, drug, drug form, supportive treatment, training, and so on), and the trial design. These designations should, if possible, use standard nomenclature. As discussed in Chapter 13, the most important elements in the title should be placed first. Some journals may allow subtitles; these can help to ensure that all needed elements are visible at the head of the paper.

> "A New Treatment for Mild Hypertension in Elderly Persons" [What treatment? A drug? What drug? What was the study design?]
> "A Randomized Controlled Trial of Hypotensol in Elderly Patients" [Will all readers know that hypotensol is a drug for treatment of hypertension? Won't most physicians' eyes be more likely to be caught by placing the condition being treated up front rather than the study design? What is the control treatment?]
> "Mild Hypertension in Elderly Patients Treated with a New Drug, Hypotensol, Compared with Oligotensin: A Randomized Controlled Trial" [Isn't this a more detailed and specific title with the more important elements in a stronger sequence?]

If the journal allows titles cast as declarative statements, you might consider building into the title a concise statement of the trial's findings.

> "Hypotensol, a New Drug, Controls Mild Hypertension in Elderly Patients as Effectively as Oligotensin: A Randomized Controlled Trial"

Some journals may put a limit on the length of titles; such limits will usually be stated in the information-for-author page(s).

The Abstract

Representing all of the important content of a clinical-trial report in its abstract can be difficult or even impossible. Most journals put limits on the length of abstracts they will accept. Even if they do not, you should keep in mind that bibliographic databases carrying abstracts along with the rest of a paper's bibliographic data may cut off abstracts at an arbitrary limit, and the closing part of your abstract may be lost if its length exceeds what they will carry. MEDLINE, for example, truncates abstracts at 250 words if they exceed that limit as published in the journal. To hold the abstract to an allowed length may force you to leave out some details. What should certainly be kept and what can be dropped is up to you, but you can help yourself to come to a decision by drawing up an outline of what elements you think should be present and in a descending order of importance. Here is a possible outline.

Background justifying the trial
The main objective of the trial: the outcome desired
The interventions, trial and control: drug, procedure, or other agent
The study design
Main methods: outcome measurement, laboratory tests, statistical procedures
Specific details on the intervention, such as specific drug by trade name
Specific outcome measures: most important first
Results in the outcome measures: most important first
Other useful findings, for example, adverse effects
Conclusion on the main objective of the trial
Important implications and limitations

You can see that this list is similar to the sequence you will have used in the report itself. If you cannot present all of this information within the allowed length of abstract, you will have to drop some elements. If your trial had more than one outcome measure, present only the most important, that named as the main objective of the trial. If you found numerous kinds of adverse effects, present only the most frequent or serious.

Keep in mind that you should check on the kind of abstract desired by the journal for which you are writing the report and the length allowed. As discussed in Chapter 13, some journals require structured abstracts with a specific format in preference to the older conventional single-paragraph abstract.

The Introduction

The content needed in the introduction in a clinical-trial report has already been suggested in Chapter 6. It is the answer to Bradford Hill's first question, "Why did you start?" and at least a condensed answer to his second, "What did you do?".

A clinical trial may be launched for one or more of many possible reasons. Currently used drugs are frightfully expensive; a much cheaper drug of the same kind is now available. Is it just as effective, or more effective? Present surgical procedures have a substantial morbidity and require a long postoperative stay in the hospital; a new procedure has promise of less morbidity and quicker recovery. Does it? Such reasons can be generalized into two kinds: 1) A better treatment is needed than what has been available, "better" in some way such as more effective, more readily tolerated by the patient, cheaper, shorter in duration; 2) no effective treatment has been available. Therefore, justifying the trial being reported calls for citing and briefly reviewing the literature that establishes the "why" of Bradford Hill's question as it applies to your trial. Note that your review probably need not describe treatments antedating the kind which the trial will be using as the current standard or "control". If a lack of published literature relevant to the question your trial aimed to answer was the motive for the trial, you should indicate where and how thoroughly you sought published literature. Further note, as was suggested in Chapter 6, that you need not justify the importance of treating the disease, syndrome, or condition that is the target of your trial's intervention; such importance will be well known to your readers or they will not read your report.

By the close of your introduction the reader should know the question the trial set out to answer. If secondary questions were also posed, only the most important should be indicated. Whether you should go on at the end to succinctly describe the trial design and the trial's answer to the question is a matter of personal judgment. An alternative is confining a succinct description of the trial's design to the beginning of the Methods section and confining the trial's answer to the abstract (which, in most journals, will probably open the article). As will be seen below, the trial's results should probably be succinctly summarized at the beginning of the Discussion section, especially if the Results section is quite long and complex.

One use of the Introduction that is, unfortunately, rarely applied is citing previously published papers, and even abstracts, that reported data included within the data in the present report. Such previously published data may have been entirely legitimately published, as in a "preliminary brief communication", perhaps in a symposium proceedings. If such data are identified in the Introduction, you can then conveniently clarify later in the Results section or the Discussion the relation of those "partial, preliminary" data and their interpretation to the complete data in this report and the newly offered interpretation.

The Methods Section ("Patients and Methods", "Participants and Methods", "Study Design and Procedure")

In writing the Methods section you have to make decisions of two kinds: 1) what content is needed, what details of trial design, procedure, and execution; and 2) the sequence of this content. Deciding on what content is needed is easier if you decide first on the sequence. Why? Because the elements defining the sequence will help you to recall what content is needed.

A Suggested Sequence

The clearest sequence for the Methods section is the sequence in which the trial was carried out.

Trial design
Trial organization and procedure
Study participants
Interventions
Measurements
Monitoring
Data collection and assessment

This sequence leads the reader from the beginning of the trial to its end, at which point the reader will go into the Results sections to the findings of the trial.

The Content for the Methods Section

Writing the content may seem easier if you consider that the reader will be expecting answers to questions. This is why I have cast the suggestions below on content in the form of questions. These suggestions are just that; not all of these points may be relevant to a particular trial; some needed points may not be listed here; and the sequence may not be the best for some trials.

Trial design

- What was the trial objective? You have probably stated it by the close of the Introduction.
- What was the trial design? Controlled? Randomized controlled? Parallel? Cross-over? Placebo-controlled? Another design? Use as many terms as are needed to designate the design accurately and completely.
- What was the planned study population (new-intervention group and controls)?
- What study groups were defined? How?
- What group sizes were planned and what relevant variables (such as "detectable difference", power, alpha level) were assumed for the sample-size calculations?

Trial organization and procedure

- Who conducted the trial and where? Was the setting a community? A primary-care facility? A tertiary-care facility? Where were the data collected and analyzed, and by whom? Who funded the trial?
- Who reviewed the protocol for adequacy and ethicality and approved it? When?

- What were the procedures for randomization? For stratification? For masking?
- What procedure was selected for decisions on altering conduct of the trial or stopping it? Who was to be responsible?

Study participants

- Where or what was the source of the participants who were to represent the study population? How were participants enlisted? By advertising? By referral? Some other method?
- What were the criteria for including or excluding participants? Diagnostic criteria, stage criteria, capacities for participation, age or sex or ethnic inclusion and exclusion, concomitant treatments.
- How were participants assigned within the study? If by "random assignment", what was the randomization method?
- What prognostic variables and other potentially important covariables were ascertained for participants?
- What was the basis for decisions on the participant-size of the trial?
- What procedures were followed for obtaining informed consent? For ensuring confidentiality? Documentation?
- What procedures and criteria were followed for dropping participants from the trial?

Interventions

- What, in specific detail, were the interventions for the trial participants and the control participants and the intervention schedules? If drugs, specific preparations (trade names as well as generic names; code designations; chemical names), form of administration, dosage schedules, precautions, sources? If procedures with instrumentation, what methods were used and what equipment and its source?
- Were there concomitant treatments?
- What methods were used for masking ("blinding") of treatments?

Measurements

- What was the primary outcome measure (relevant to the main question posed for the trial)?
- How was the primary outcome measured? If not by a widely known and accepted method, validated how (references; validation for the trial)? What limits defined for clinical importance?
- What were the secondary outcome measures? (with the same questions as for the primary outcome)
- What measures to ensure safety? To detect potential adverse effects?
- What equipment was used? Manufacturer?
- What methods were used for masking of observers of outcome measures?

- Were independent laboratory determinations used as a check on the reliability of the trial's data?

Monitoring

- Who was responsible for monitoring the progression of the trial and where?
- Were any decisions made to alter the trial conduct or stopping the trial? What were they? Why?

Data collection and assessment

- Where were data collected?
- What statistical procedures were used for data analysis? Methods? Programs? References?
- Were subgroup analyses exploratory or based on a preceding hypothesis?
- For multivariate analyses, how were the variables selected?
- What procedures were applied to support the adequacy and reliability of the data, such as independent data assessments?
- From what source are data obtained in the trial available? And the detailed protocol?

More detailed lists of potential topics for the Methods section of a clinical-trial report can be found in Figure 102.3, "Topics to Include in a Materials and Methods Section", of the comprehensive text on clinical trials by Spilker (1), Table 25–1, "Content Suggestions for the Study Publication" in Clinical Trials by Meinert (2), Table 1, "Checklist of Information for Inclusion in Reports of Clinical Trials" of the Asilomar Working Group recommendations (3), and the table in the CONSORT statement (4). Note that the CONSORT statement is specifically aimed at the reporting of randomized controlled trials. A useful checklist of content expected by critical readers in a report of a drug trial is Table 2 in a paper by Cho and Bero (5). An especially clear and helpful source of broader application is Chapter 1, "Asking Questions and Finding Answers: Reporting Research Designs and Activities", in Lang and Secic's guide to reporting statistics (6).

The Results Section

You may recall from Chapter 6 the third question Bradford Hill suggested a reader would wish to have answered in reading a report of research: "What answer did you get?" That seems like too simple a question for the reader of a clinical-trial report, but it is close to the better question, "What were the results of the trial?"

Many clinicians reading your report will be looking only for the findings that answer the question posed for the trial. "Is the new drug more efficacious than the current standard drug?" "Are the side effects fewer and less serious?" But the most critical readers of your report will wish to know, first, whether the trial worked out as projected in the protocol and described in the Methods section. If it did not, the value of the trial's findings may have been weakened. For example, if the randomization process did not, by chance, lead to participants' having the same or closely similar characteristics (for example, age, sex, comorbidities, ethnicities) in the control and in the new-treatment group or groups, the interpretation of the findings may be made more difficult or uncertain. Here are some of the questions critical readers will probably expect to have answered first in the Results section.

- How many participants started the protocol in each study group and completed it?
- How many participants withdrew from the trial before completing their participation? Why did they withdraw?
- Were any participants dropped from the trial before completing participation? Why? How many participants were lost to follow-up?
- What were the estimates of adherence or compliance?
- Did the trial deviate from the original protocol in any way? How and why? Was the trial completed as planned? What was the total duration of the trial?
- What were the demographics and clinical characteristics of the participants in each trial group?
- Did the groups differ in such characteristics to possibly important degrees? What were those differences?
- What are the indicators of data quality that may have been gathered, such as interrater concordances?

Some of these questions can probably be answered with descriptive text, but most critical readers would probably expect that the most important of these questions be dealt with by your presenting the data in one or more tables.

With these results on how the trial proceeded to a completion, you can turn to presenting the findings relevant to judging drug efficacies and safeties and comparing treatment groups on these points. There are no rigid rules on how to do this, but keep in mind that the judgments on how the new drug or treatment differs from the present standard treatment (control) depend on knowing first how the standard-treatment, or control, group fared. In a relatively simple trial, perhaps all of the data on efficacy can be given in only one table. In this case, the standard-treatment or control group can be placed first and followed by the new-drug or treatment group. Data in more complex trials may have to be presented in more than one table.

Whether the trial findings are presented only in text or in text and tables, readers will expect answers to a number of questions bearing on efficacy and safety.

- What are the efficacy and safety data and how are they summarized for each trial group?
- What are differences for these data between or among trial groups—differences in absolute numbers and not just in percentages? What are the explicit statistical assessments of these differences?
- What are the distributions of these outcome measures (such as, for example, by standard deviations) and what are the ranges for the estimates of the outcome effects (such as confidence intervals)? If you are giving p values, these should be exact values, not simply, for example, "<0.05".
- What effects, if any, did potentially confounding variables have on the outcome measures?
- Were there adverse effects in any of the groups? What were their frequencies and differences between or among trial groups?
- How did dropouts affect the conclusions?

If there were subgroup analyses or many outcome measures, the presentation should, in general, move from the most important outcome measure or measures to the least important. Likewise, subgroup presentations and analyses should follow the main group presentation and analyses.

More detailed lists of potential topics for the Results section of a clinical-trial report can be found in the sources cited above (1–4) with reference to reporting methods.

The next step is into the Discussion.

The Discussion

The best opening for the Discussion section depends in large part on the complexity of the trial and its results. In a report of a simple trial, the conclusion that can be drawn from the findings is probably already quite clear to the reader by the end of the Results section and need not be restated. In reporting a complex trial, the Results section may be of such length and complexity that the reader may not reach the Discussion section with a clear view of the main conclusion. Hence, it is fair to the reader of a long report to state succinctly at the beginning of the Discussion section what you have concluded about, at least, the main efficacy outcome measure and adverse-effect findings along with, if necessary, your assessment of the strength of the conclusions. Similar attention may be needed for any subgroup analyses, with particular attention to conservative assessments of the findings in subgroup exploratory analyses. Do not, however, restate the rationale for the trial that was already given in the Introduction. What comes next?

The main evidence for the final answer to the question posed for the trial certainly comes from the findings you report in the Results section. But you will recall from Chapter 6 and Table 6.1 that there may be evidence supporting your answer in already reported trials. Such supporting evidence should be presented early in the Discussion. But perhaps some already reported trials came to differing conclusions. This is what is called in Chapters 5 and 6 "counterevidence". You should not ignore it and not mention it if it exists and you aware of it. If you do, you can be reasonably sure that a peer reviewer reading your report in manuscript is highly likely to call such an omission to the attention of the editor. Previously reported trials may have come to a different conclusion for quite sound reasons: a different sex-distribution, different ages of participants, different doses, different dosage schedules, different duration of treatment, different ethnic composition. But even if you cannot identify differences of this kind that appear to account for a different conclusion, you are ethically bound to not bury such "counterevidence" in uncited obscurity; some reader of your report may be able to account for the differences.

The other aspect of "counterevidence" that may need your attention is that of possible sources of bias in your study design and execution. Between designing the trial and preparing your report, you may have become aware of decisions or other actions that could have led to findings shifted in a direction you did not anticipate at the outset. If you have come to see unanticipated sources of possible bias, you should discuss them and share with readers their possible implications for your findings. You do owe your readers adequate self-criticisms of your own work.

Has the subject of your trial been considered in any metaanalyses? How do your findings compare with the findings in published relevant meta-analyses? Do they agree? Do they disagree and, if so, in what way? Can you account for the disagreement?

Most important for many readers, especially those in clinical practice, may be your view on how widely applicable are your findings. Can they be generalized from your population sample to all clinical practice? Are they confidently applicable only to patients of the same ethnic group or age range represented by your participants? Do the adverse effects reported suggest a need to exclude particular kinds of patients from treatment with the new drug? Any limits to generalizability of the results can then be discussed as suggesting kinds of additional research needed.

The once frequently used closing "Conclusions" section of research reports has tended to give way to confining a succinct summary of findings to the abstract appearing on a paper's title page. If, however, a clinical-trial report has dealt with a large and complex trial, some readers who have gone through the entire report carefully may be pleased to find a closing summing-up at the end of the Discussion a helpful view of what the trial has produced. Such a summing-up is properly labeled "Conclusions". Note, however, that you should check on whether the journal to which you are planning to submit the report accepts the use of "Conclusions"; look at some recent issues.

Additional Possible Content

The references you have cited will, of course, be placed in the "References" section at the end of the paper. But there may be need to place other material between the end of the Discussion and the beginning of the References section.

Acknowledgments

One frequently needed section is an "Acknowledgments". Granting agencies may expect you to acknowledge their support with specific citation of the grant. In reports of trials with commercial support, this may be the journal's specified location for statements of commercial funding or of financial holdings by investigators that could be construed as potential conflicts of interest. You may wish to publicly thank some colleagues for their help in reviewing drafts of your report; be sure, however, that you have their written permission to acknowledge their help. "Acknowledgments" of this kind may imply approval of your report that those readers have in fact not given. You may wish to give public thanks for technical help of a useful kind despite its not justifying authorship.

Appendixes

As mentioned in Chapter 6, one or more appendixes can be a convenient place for a detailed description of a method specifically developed for the trial, for a trial questionnaire, or other kinds of content that would interfere with ready and rapid reading of the report if placed in its main body.

OBSERVATIONAL STUDIES: CASE-CONTROL STUDIES AND COHORT STUDIES

The principles set forth in Chapter 6 that should guide an author in preparing any kind of research report and many of the more specific principles for reporting clinical trials discussed above also apply to reports of case-control and cohort studies. If you are working on a report on an observational study, you should review in these two chapters the sections that discuss the needs that are common to all research papers. Introductions should make clear why the study was launched, with relevant citations, and exactly what question or hypothesis was framed for the study. Results sections should make clear the successes and any failures of the research design and conduct and should present findings in a descending scale of importance. Discussions should briefly recapitulate the answer that comes from the findings and the strength of that answer; they should also present supporting evidence from previous research and deal with any counterevidence. Discussions should close with assessments of generalizability of the findings and with implications for further research.

Just as critical readers of trials reports will have many questions about the research design, the research protocol, participant selection and assignment, specific procedures, and data collection and analysis, the critical readers of observational studies will have many similar, if not identical questions. Here are the likely major questions to be answered in the Methods and Results sections.

- What was the intended population for the study?
- How were study and control groups defined? Specific criteria: diagnostic criteria, variables definitions?
- For a case-control study, what was the source of case materials? For a cohort study, was the study one with active participants (recruited or assigned) or passive participants (persons monitored for an ongoing database)? Were the samples representative of the populations they were intended to represent?
- In a case-control study, were there unanticipated voids in available data? What was their effect, if any, on the conclusions?
- In a cohort study, what were the dropouts, if any, and what was the possible effect on the conclusions?
- Were assessors of variables, especially qualitative variables, masked ("blinded") against the group assignment of cases or participants?
- Were all "outcome" variables defined by adequate criteria *a priori*? What were they?
- How homogeneous were the compared groups for variables other than those that were the specific subject of the study?
- Were any biases detected in case or participant selection or in variables assessments that had not been anticipated when the study was designed or launched? What were they and what are their implications?

Adequate attention to these questions in your Methods and Results sections (as appropriate) will strengthen the view of readers that you have conducted a properly designed, executed, and analyzed study.

OBSERVATIONAL STUDIES OF DIAGNOSTIC TESTS

Standards for methodological reporting of assessments of diagnostic tests have been available for at least two decades but, as pointed out by Reid and coauthors (7), have not been widely and rigorously applied. Critical readers of reports of diagnostic-test research will have many questions they will expect to have answered. Some of these are indicated here.

- What, in detail, was the spectrum of patients studied, including such details as age and sex distributions and perhaps other variables such as ethnicity? Were there any criteria for exclusion of subjects?

- What was the definition of the disease, syndrome, or other morbid state studied for which the test was applied? What about comorbidities? Were there any exclusion criteria related to the disease or morbid-state stage?
- Was the study group categorized by subgroups? If so, were the data analyzed for differences in findings among the subgroups?
- Were there any possibilities for workup bias, as in referring of only patients with positive findings in the studied test for a standard-reference ("gold standard") test?
- What were the safeguards against observer and reviewer bias? Were judgments based on blinded assessments?
- Have the data been presented adequately with regard to evidence of reliability of findings, for example, with confidence intervals for sensitivity and specificity indices or other measures?
- Have indeterminate findings been included in the presented data and their related analyses?
- Have test and observer reliabilities been adequately documented and considered?

The various functions of the Discussion section presented in Chapter 6 should, of course, be considered in preparing reports of research on diagnostic tests: assessment of the validity of the report's own findings, of supporting evidence, of counterevidence; discussion of generalizability and implications of the findings.

CONCLUSION

The value of your report of a clinical trial, a case-control study, a cohort study, or of an assessment of a diagnostic test will depend greatly on whether it includes the information that its most critical readers will expect to find in it. The general principles discussed in Chapter 6 do apply, but much more specific information will be needed in the Methods and Results sections. These needs are suggested by questions set forth in this chapter. Some of them apply only to clinical trials but many are relevant to all three types of reports.

REFERENCES

1. Spilker B. Preparing articles for publication. In: Spilker B. Guide to clinical trials. New York (NY): Raven Press; 1991: Chapter 102.
2. Meinert CL, Tonascia S. Clinical trials: design, conduct, and analysis. New York: Oxford University Press; 1986.
3. The Asilomar Working Group on Recommendations for Reporting of Clinical Trials in the Biomedical Literature. Checklist of information for inclusion in reports of clinical trials. Ann Intern Med 1996;124:741–3.

4. Begg C, Cho M, Eastwood S, Horton R, Moher D, Olkin I, Pitkin R, Rennie D, Schulz KF, Simel D, Stroup DF. Improving the quality of reporting of randomized controlled trials: the CONSORT statement. JAMA 1996;276:637–9.

5. Cho MK, Bero LA. Instruments for assessing the quality of drug studies published in the medical literature. JAMA 1994;272:101–4.

6. Lang TA, Secic M. How to report statistics in medicine: annotated guidelines for authors, editors, and reviewers. Philadelphia (PA): American College of Physicians; 1997.

7. Reid MC, Lachs MS, Feinstein AR. Use of methodological standards in diagnostic text research. JAMA 1995;274:645–51.

CHAPTER 8

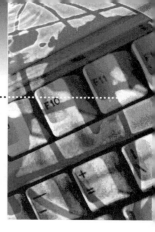

The Research Paper: Reporting Laboratory Research

All well-written papers reporting laboratory research observe the principles for scientific reporting that are developed in their general form in Chapter 6 and specifically for clinical research reports in Chapter 7. But reports of laboratory research may need to have quite different overall formats. They certainly have to present quite different kinds of details about materials, methods, and procedures.

FORMATS

Most reports of laboratory research published in journals have formats identical with, or closely similar to, the "IMRAD" format (**I**ntroduction [usually not labeled as such], **M**ethods, **R**esults, **a**nd **D**iscussion; Acknowledgments, References) discussed in Chapter 6. You can verify whether this is true in the journal for which you are writing your report by looking at recent issues. Some reports may have a simpler format, for example, those identified as "Letters", or "Brief Communications", or "Preliminary Reports". A journal's information-for-authors page(s) is likely to identify such special categories of reports and specify the formats and allowed lengths.

Some journals specify little detail about acceptable formats and leave it to authors to scan issues of the journal for a view of acceptable formats; the weekly journal *Science* is a good example. Some other journals have requirements for format that differ noticeably from the IMRAD style. Such a journal is *Cell,* which asks that the section on materials and methods be placed at the end of the paper's text (following "Results and Discussion" and preceding "References") and identified as "Experimental Procedures".

CONTENT

The principles discussed in Chapter 6 apply as much to laboratory reports as to reports of clinical studies.

The Introduction (opening paragraph or paragraphs, even if not headed Introduction) must make clear the scientific reason or reasons why the research was planned and carried out, with relevant citations. It must make clear the question or questions it was to answer or the hypothesis to be tested. The Results section must present the findings relevant to the aims for the research in the Introduction and statistically assess their strength as evidence. The Discussion section should assess any uncertainties about the validity and strength of the study's findings, discuss supporting evidence and any apparently conflicting evidence, and resolve any uncertainties as to the final conclusion. It may properly close with attention to the findings' generalizability and their implications. What about the Methods section ("Materials and Methods", "Experimental Procedures")?

Methods Section

That the Methods section anticipates and answers in adequate detail readers' questions about what was done and why is as critically important in papers reporting laboratory research as in clinical-trials reports, but for a reason in addition to giving methodologic evidence supporting the validity of the findings. Such detail is needed in trials reports mainly to give critical readers what they need to know to be able to judge whether the findings can be trusted and applied in treatment; replication of the trial may be conceptually possible but practically impossible. But in papers reporting laboratory research, detail is needed to enable other investigators to replicate, if they wish, the reported research and findings. Replication may be vital to eventual acceptance of the findings.

What kinds of content may be needed in the Methods section? Here are some examples.

- Description of experiment design, if it was not a standard design readily recognized or described succinctly by a standard term
- Specific descriptions of experimental materials and methods
  Animals: Species (strain if necessary), physiologic or pathologic state (such as pregnancy, castrated, rearing method and so on), nutritional state; supplier.
  Animal diets: Maintenance; treatment diets; constituents; sources.
  Drugs and other interventional agents: Generic and trade names; chemical names if nonstandard drugs; suppliers.
  Drug administration schedules, forms, doses.

Procedures for other kinds of interventions, for example, surgical procedures; references if standard; detailed description if not.

Tissues and tissue cultures: Source, prior treatment, supplier.

Cell lines, DNA: All details needed for unequivocal identification; supplier.

Immune sera: Adequate description; supplier.

Bacterial cultures, viruses: Identified with standard taxonomic nomenclature; source.

Reagents: Detailed chemical identification; supplier.

- Statements on availability of materials not commercially available: distribution by the author or some other noncommercial source.
- Identification of equipment used (with specifications if appropriate); supplier.
- Ethical approval of the research; safeguards for humane treatment.

If standard statistical methods were used for data analysis, they probably need be identified only by name in the presentation of results ("Chi-square, $p = 0.027$"); unusual methods should be identified in the Methods section with citation of references.

The content suggested immediately above is simply representative. Journals in particular medical sciences are likely to indicate in their information-for-authors page(s) the specific information on materials and methods they will expect to find. These sources should be consulted.

Other Considerations

Some kinds of laboratory research generate data of such dimensions and detail that they cannot be practically presented in a published formal paper. Examples are nucleic acid and protein sequences and x-ray crystallographic coordinates. Access to such data may be critically important to some readers. Either the Results section or an appendix to the main text should indicate where such data are held, in what form, and how they can be accessed.

As with other kinds of research reports, an Acknowledgments section may be needed to indicate grant and other kinds of financial support, indebtedness to colleagues for materials or review of the paper, and other matters not reported in the paper itself. Appendixes may be needed for methodological detail.

CONCLUSION

Reports of laboratory research should be prepared with attention to the principles applicable to all research reports: statement of motive for the research and of the question investigated or hypothesis tested; description of experimental materials,
continued

Conclusion continued.

methods, and procedure sufficient to validate the findings and enable replication; assessment of findings in the light of supporting evidence and apparent counterevidence; generalizability of findings; their implications.

CHAPTER 9

The Review Article and The Metaanalysis

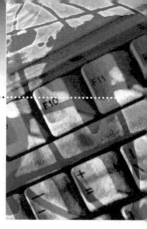

Our medical literature is so large that no one, clinician or investigator, can keep up with more than small fractions of it. We must rely heavily on synoptic papers: review articles, metaanalyses, scientific editorials, and other kinds of summaries. The review, metaanalysis, or scientific editorial carefully conceived to answer an important question, based on critical assessment of the literature, and written with a logical structure is a valuable document. It spares clinicians the burden of searching and sifting the literature for reliable guidance in practice. It tells investigators where their research field stands on a particular problem and may suggest what directions new research should take.

The other kind of synoptic paper that may be useful for clinicians is the case-series analysis based on a critical review of case records in the author's practice or institution as well as on a critical review of the literature. Case-series papers are discussed in Chapter 10.

THE REVIEW ARTICLE

The review appears to differ greatly in structure from the research paper, but a thoughtfully conceived and clearly organized review is also built as a critical argument. Most of the overt structure, often indicated by subheadings that divide parts of the text, usually has to represent the sequence determined by the subject of the review.

Reviews are of two general kinds: descriptive (sometimes called "narrative" reviews) and systematic reviews. This section is concerned mainly with descriptive reviews. The following section on metaanalyses takes up the most rigorous type of systematic review, which calls for systematic assessments of quantitative data, most often of drug trials.

The Introduction

A potentially useful review answers a question or closely related questions: What do we know and not know about acute myelocytic leukemia? How should we treat constipation? What are the adverse effects of cimetidine, and what should be done about them clinically? The question should be made clear at the beginning of the review; the title may not be able to reflect fully the review's scope. The stated or implied question usually should not come first; an opening more helpful for the reader is a clear indication as to why now is the time to raise the question for review. Thus, a review of adverse effects of oligocycline (a fictitious drug) might start with opening sentences like these:

> Oligocycline has been available in the United States as a prescription drug for over several decades. Because of its efficacy, it is now among the most frequently prescribed drugs. The variety of adverse effects reported since it was introduced is substantially greater than when the drug was approved by the FDA.

Such an opening points to what the review has aimed to answer—what is the range of adverse effects one might expect to find patients experiencing—and thus justifies your reading the review if you prescribe oligocycline.

If the subject of your review has already been covered by one or more recent reviews, you may need to indicate why your review is needed. Perhaps they drew on only the English-language literature, perhaps they ignored important age groups of patients, perhaps they were insufficiently critical of research reports, perhaps new recently reported research leads to a different conclusion.

Methods

A conclusive and useful review article is likely to emerge from the process of reviewing the relevant literature and deciding what it means for the question only if the process is deliberate and thorough. (For a detailed tabular summary of the process, see "The Stages of Research Review" in Chapter 1 of *The Integrative Research Review: A Systematic Approach* (1) by Cooper.) The topic of the review must be defined and limited before the review is written. In a properly designed review, these definitions (such as diagnostic criteria) and limits (such as age limits on cases) are decided on before the literature search and selection of relevant papers that must be digested. A review on acute myelocytic leukemia should tell the reader what definition (diagnostic criteria) the author used for this disease. The reader needs this definition to be assured that he or she shares the author's concept of the disease.

The reader also needs to know how the author decided on the relevance of the reviewed papers for the review (2, 3) and the validity of their data and conclusions. In a review on adverse effects of cimetidine, the drug will not have to be defined, but the reader should be told what criteria have been applied in critically assessing case reports for possible judgments, for example, "possible adverse effect", "probable adverse effect", and "proved adverse effect". These definitions and limitations are most logically placed immediately after the Introduction, in a Methods section, which serves a function like that of the Materials and Methods section in a research paper. Some editors may find this location to be too unorthodox and will suggest that this content be appended at the end of the review.

The Methods section in a review should fully describe the literature search (2–4): the bibliographic indexes and databases searched, limits on years and languages, search terms. A discussion of the search terms may be critically important if there is a chance of disagreement on the diagnostic criteria given for the disease under review. Supposedly synonymous terms for diseases do not necessarily have the same meaning among different readers, and differing terms may in fact refer to the same entity. Reviewers who have gone into literature more than 5 to 10 years old may have to explain how they related present definitions and terms to the older definitions and terms.

Reviews based on papers reporting quantitative data must specify how the data from different studies were integrated for generalizable conclusions (2); this methodologic information is indispensable in a metaanalytic review (5) and is discussed later in this chapter.

The Body of the Review: Sequence of Sections

The sequence of topics (to be represented by sections of text) is usually determined by how the reader will want to look at the overall subject of the review. A descriptive review of a disease will probably follow the conventional sequence found in textbooks; the body of the review is likely to have these main sections.

ETIOLOGY
PATHOGENESIS
MANIFESTATIONS
   Clinical
   Roentgenographic
   Laboratory
DIAGNOSIS
TREATMENT
PROGNOSIS

This sequence has a logical basis. It is a chronologic sequence well known in clinical concept and experience: A disease has a cause (or causes); it develops before it becomes clinically manifest; the patient becomes aware of the disease, and evidences of it are detected by the clinician in history-taking, examination, and special studies; diagnosis also calls for differentiating the patient's disease from other possible diseases; diagnosis leads to treatment; the clinician has to estimate the probable outcome of treatment.

Other sequences are useful for other kinds of topics. Topics might be presented in order from the general to the particular, or from the components of a system to its integrated structure. A review of adverse effects of a drug might use a sequence proceeding from cellular effects to whole-body or systemic effects.

EFFECTS ON CELLULAR METABOLISM
EFFECTS ON MEMBRANE STRUCTURE AND FUNCTION
EFFECTS ON MYOCARDIAL CONTRACTILITY
HEMODYNAMIC EFFECTS
    Blood pressure effects
    Congestive heart failure
SYSTEMIC EFFECTS
    Fever
    Dehydration

For another kind of topic the best sequence might run from the most frequent and important problems to the rare, as in a review of hypercalcemia.

METASTATIC MALIGNANCY
PRIMARY HYPERPARATHYROIDISM (and so on to rare causes)
IDIOPATHIC HYPERCALCEMIA OF INFANCY

Whatever kind of sequence is used, the sequence should be made clear by subheadings that correspond to an outline (see Chapter 12).

The Body of the Review: Elements of Critical Argument

As much as the author of a research report, the author of a review is obliged to present all the elements of critical argument needed to support the conclusions reached. If the Methods section suggested above as an early section of the review describes the literature search used in finding papers for assessment, this information on the thoroughness of the literature review helps to support the credibility of what is concluded in the review.

The author of a carefully prepared review critically assesses the evidence—the papers read—long before beginning to write. Papers not meeting critical standards are rejected as not-useful evidence. Most of these decisions need not be defended in the review. Sage authors of reviews do not promise the reader a "complete review of the world's literature". Certainly all papers widely known to readers of the review and likely to be regarded by them as having sound data and valid conclusions must be assessed in the review; the author must make clear the basis for any disagreement with their content.

In a thorough and careful review of a topic, the author may have identified certain issues and problems as unresolved and needing further study. These points can be regarded as "implications of evidence not wholly rejected" (Graves and Hodge's phrase used in their description of "critical argument"; see Chapter 5). If they have to do with issues pertinent to the entire subject of the review, they may be best dealt with in a closing section of the review, perhaps designated Discussion. The reader will be able to leave the review with a view of what is not known about the subject (6), to accompany the view earlier in the review of what is known. The Discussion could also deal with implications of the points concluded in the body of the review. For example, a drug may be judged to have efficacy superior to that of what had been the preceding standard treatment. But the drug is conspicuously more expensive. Should physicians switch to the new and more expensive drug? What is the author's opinion on the balance of costs (retail prices, adverse effects) and benefits (better efficacy, simpler dose schedule)?

A Conclusion

Most review articles are much longer than research reports and are likely to cover many subtopics. Hence their readers may get to the end of a review and wonder "What does all of this add up to?" A closing summing-up of your judgments in the body of the review will be useful to many readers. This summation could, of course, be in an abstract of the review on its title page if the journal accepts that kind of format. Abstracts of reviews are discussed in Chapter 13.

THE METAANALYSIS

Older reviews dealing with questions of the efficacy of a drug or some other kind of intervention with an outcome that can be measured were almost invariably built on an author's informal assessment of the soundness of findings in the relevant research he or she reviewed. Say, for example, that a drug's efficacy had been studied in 10 clinical trials, six of which reported desirable outcomes and four of which reported efficacies no better than what had been the standard drug for the disease treated. What would the author decide to conclude for his or her review? The resulting conclusion could be an opinion that might differ among three or four authors preparing reviews on the same topic, an opinion biased by personal experience or shaped by private judgments on the severity of adverse effects. More and more this kind of hidden assessment of evidence (private "eye-balling") has become unacceptable. Light and Pillemer (7) have summarized the objections to traditional reviews. They are usually based on subjective judgments on what studies to include and what studies to exclude. They too often render opinions based on "vote-counting" (as in the example suggested above). The author's process of assessing data in a large number of studies is unsystematic and thus prone to considerable error. Thus, more and more, readers are expecting visible and rigorous assessment of quantitative data from a number of clinical trials that are the foundation of reviews (8), especially those dealing with drug efficacies. Assessments of this kind are what is carried out in the process called metaanalysis, and a review article built on this process is likely to carry the term "metaanalysis" in its title or subtitle.

Although metaanalysis (often spelled "meta-analysis") has been a growing, increasingly visible method of systematic review in medicine for over 50 years (9), it still faces a number of criticisms. These criticisms (5, 9) focus mainly on questions of methodologic procedure. If you are the author of a metaanalysis, you can cut the risk of adverse judgments on the validity and value of your review by taking pains to be highly explicit about your procedure and careful in presentation (10, 11) of your findings. The section below on "Content" suggests questions of potential critical readers about your metaanalysis that your review should aim to answer.

Format

Formats for metaanalyses have not yet been rigidly standardized. But metaanalyses are indeed a variety of research and can be helpfully formatted with a closely similar, if not identical, structure. It probably need not be pointed out here that the title and abstract for a metaanalysis should make unequivocally clear that you are reporting a metaanalysis. The abstract should, as for abstracts of other kinds of research, represent as well as possible within the allowed length all the main elements of your paper: motivation for the analysis, main elements of methods, main findings, and implications.

A metaanalysis should open with an introductory section, proceed with a detailed description of methods and procedure, present the findings (main question first, then secondary questions such as subgroup findings), and close with a discussion bearing on possible weaknesses of the metaanalysis and weighing supporting evidence and counterevidence from any other metaanalyses on the same question before proceeding to a final conclusion. What content should these sections offer?

Content

At the outset, readers should be given a clear view of why the metaanalysis was launched. Were no metaanalyses on the topic available, only descriptive ("narrative") reviews? What were the judgments rendered in those reviews?

Were previous metaanalyses flawed? If so, why? Have new clinical-trials reports become available and should be incorporated into a fresh look at the topic they represent? This introduction should close with having made clear what question the metaanalysis was designed to answer and whether subgroup questions were also to be answered.

Methods

The most critically important section of a metaanalytic review is its Methods section. If you can answer in advance all of the questions that critical readers are likely to raise about how you proceeded, you raise the odds that, if your analysis was properly and carefully conducted, it will be judged to be a valid and useful review. While most of these questions are properly dealt with in a Methods section, some are properly answered in a Results section. What are the questions likely to be raised about your metaanalysis?

- Did you have a formal working protocol? It need not be reproduced as part of your presentation, but your explicit answers to many of the questions below will probably indicate that you did have a definite protocol. Was the condition at which the intervention was aimed explicitly defined: disease definition, stages, and other potential variables? Were the patients of interest explicitly defined: age, sex, ethnicity, other possible variables? Was the intervention of interest explicitly defined?
- How did you conduct your literature search? What databases? With what search strategies? What search terms? Identification through titles? Abstracts? Keyword indexing? Papers in all languages, or only those in English? Through how many years? To avoid missing clinical-trials reports that might have been inadequately indexed for bibliographic databases, did you carry out manual searches through journals that could be expected to report relevant clinical trials? What journals? Through how many years?
- Did you search for unpublished trials? How? Through what routes? Grant listings? Personal inquiries to identifiable investigators? Inquiries to drug companies?
- How did you decide what trials to include or exclude? What were the specific criteria? Have you identified excluded trials with reasons for exclusion? (The paper by Wilson and Henry [10] suggests criteria for quality assessment of randomized controlled trials, cohort studies, and case-control studies.)
- How were the validities of the findings in included trials judged? Were trials graded for quality of evidence? By what system? Were judgments "blinded"? How?
- How were data extracted from the trials reports? Were there parallel efforts carried out to minimize possible biases ("inter-pair variation") in judgments on how to treat the available data?

- Were included trials explicitly categorized as to study design, population samples and their sizes, their heterogeneity, intervention details (doses, schedules, duration, and so on), definitions of outcomes?
- What outcomes were explicitly considered?
- Have you detailed your statistical procedures? Tests of homogeneity? Of systematic differences among trials? What did you do about missing data?

Results

Some of the questions about the design and conduct of the analysis can be answered at the opening of the Results section.

- What were the results of parallel judgments on inclusion–exclusion, on data extraction?
- Have you presented concise descriptive summary data on each trial considered, which indicate the care taken in analysis of trials reports?

You can then go on to report the results of the analysis, including the results of sensitivity analyses for preanalysis selected variables and variables emerging in the analysis. For those readers not familiar with metaanalysis, a clear graphic presentation of individual trial findings and your summation of the pooled analysis of outcome measures is indispensable. Confidence intervals are a valuable part of such graphic presentations. Wilson and Henry (10) make a number of suggestions for appropriate graphic summaries. The central conclusion will be made more clear to most readers if it is represented by a graphic presentation of the cumulative values of the outcome measure, for example, the odds ratio, than simply by a graphic presentation of the value for each trial considered and a summary statement.

Discussion

The discussion section of a metaanalytical review has much the same functions as the Discussion in any other kind of research paper.

- Summarizing the main findings, those bearing on the main question posed in the introduction.
- Assessing possible weaknesses in your analysis (for example, such as publication bias, difficulties in finding unpublished trial-reports, defective "blinding", and so on).
- Weighing your findings against those in other metaanalyses (if any) of the same question.
- Resolving or explaining conflicting judgments.
- Suggesting clinical implications of your analysis, including generalizability of your findings.
- Suggesting further research: new trials, alternative analysis methods.

CONCLUSION

The confidence of readers in the judgments you express in a review article of the traditional type or a metaanalysis will depend, at least for critical readers, on the rigor with which you reviewed the relevant literature and treated the data you found. The rigor of your review will be judged in large part on the quality of the literature review you carried out and on how clearly you describe how you selected reports for integration into your judgments. Metaanalytic reports call for especially detailed descriptions of methods and procedures; these should be presented in a formal Methods section.

REFERENCES

1. Cooper HM. The integrative research review: a systematic approach. Beverly Hills (CA): Sage Publications; 1984:12–4.
2. Mulrow CD. The medical review article: state of the science. Ann Intern Med 1987;106:485–8.
3. Cooper HM. The integrative research review: a systematic approach. Beverly Hills (CA): Sage Publications; 1984:115–6.
4. Huth EJ. Needed: review articles with more scientific rigor. Ann Intern Med 1987;106:470–1.
5. L'Abbé KA, Detsky AS, O'Rourke K. Meta-analysis in clinical research. Ann Intern Med 1987;106:224–33.
6. Morgan P. An insider's guide for medical authors and editors. Philadelphia (PA): ISI Press; 1986:62.
7. Light RJ, Pillemer DB. Summing up: the science of reviewing research. Cambridge (MA): Harvard University Press; 1984.
8. Cook DB, Mulrow C, Haynes RB. Systematic reviews: synthesis of best evidence for clinical decisions. Ann Intern Med 1997;126:376–80.
9. Sacks HS, Reitman D, Pagano D, Kupelnick BA. Meta-analysis: an update. Mt Sinai J Med 1996;63:216–24.
10. Wilson A, Henry A. Meta-analysis: Part 2: Assessing the quality of published meta-analyses. Med J Aust 1992;156:173–87.
11. Meade MO, Richardson WS. Selecting and appraising studies for a systematic review. Ann Intern Med 1997;127:531–7.

CHAPTER 10

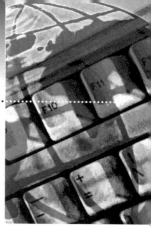

The Case Report and the Case-Series Analysis

THE CASE REPORT

In the 19th century, clinical teaching gradually shifted from lectures accounting for disease by theories and classifications more speculative than factually verified to bedside analysis of cases. Pathology increasingly based on histologic methods could demonstrate more clearly how structural changes could cause symptoms and signs. Biochemistry brought methods for detecting evidence of disease long before the eye could see it. With these new capacities for case analysis, the professor and students now could see a patient and add to the facts elicited by history-taking and physical examination such observations as protein in the urine or unusual cells in a blood smear. They could more fruitfully explain the condition of the patient and predict what treatment, if any, might alter the course of the disease.

With these changes in clinical teaching, the case report became a staple in the menu of clinical literature. The findings in a single case were usually not adequate, however, to explain and predict clinical events. Previously described cases with features in common had to be drawn on. The kind of paper that described and interpreted individual cases thus was labeled "a case report with review of the literature".

Since World War 2, great growth in clinical investigation and clinical pharmacology has generated a still rising flood of competing papers. Reports of single cases have become less and less acceptable for publication in major journals, mainly because of their tending to carry little or no important new information. Four kinds of case reports may still occasionally merit publication.

- The unique, or nearly unique, case that appears to represent a previously undescribed syndrome or disease.
- The case with an unexpected association of two or more diseases or disorders that may represent a previously unsuspected causal relation.

- The case representing a new and clinically important variation from an expected pattern: the "outlier" case.
- The case with an unexpected evolution that suggests a possible therapeutic or an important adverse drug effect.

The kinds of evidence needed to support conclusions in case reports differ among these varieties. The sections below point out how these differences may call for differing structures to place them properly in the sequence of an argument that adequately supports the report's conclusion.

Authors considering preparing a case report must be aware of the great difficulty or impossibility of publishing case reports in front-rank journals. Single-case reports of potentially clear clinical value are sometimes accepted by good journals if they are in the concise format of a letter-to-the-editor; a review of letters-to-the-editor through the issues of the past six months may indicate whether the journal does accept brief case reports in this format. Chapter 11 discusses the qualities needed in a letter-to-the-editor.

TYPES OF CASE REPORTS

The Unique Case

A sharp-eyed and well-informed clinician sees a patient with disease manifestations so extraordinary that they cannot be accounted for by known diseases or syndromes. In coming to this judgment the clinician initially relies on personal experience and recall of relevant medical literature. The judgment may be wrong; the clinician may not know enough to be sure that the case does not represent a previously described disease. For most cases of this kind, the best the clinician can do to establish that the case is unique is to search through bibliographic indexes to the clinical literature for previously described cases with identical or similar manifestations. Failure to find such cases may mean that the newly observed case represents a disease or syndrome not described before, but caution is in order. The failure may mean only that the search was not carried far enough or that the disease or syndrome was seen in the past but described in terms we do not use today. Previous observers may have lacked the ability of today's clinician, better equipped conceptually and technically for closer observation, to identify those features that are now apparent. All of these possibilities may have to be considered in the report's Discussion. But even if the Discussion can conclude that the case is unique, a claim such as "discovery of a new syndrome" or "the first report" ought to be eschewed and that distinction conferred not by one's self but by posterity.

The apparently unique case may have some features that give a clue to a specific chemical disorder, perhaps the result of a genetically determined defect in enzyme function. Investigation may identify the defect and establish that the case is unique. Papers describing such cases may need a format like that of research papers.

The Case of an Unexpected Association

Two uncommon diseases or disorders are found in one patient. The rarity of each suggests that their occurrence together may reflect some causal relation. The pathogenetic mechanism known or suspected for each may be similar (for example, an immunologic mechanism) and this implies that both may have developed from a single primary defect in the patient. Such case reports may be hard to get accepted for publication even if a review of the literature fails to turn up a similar case. The association may be coincidence. Further study might find a pathogenetic basis for the association through research; then the case report will have to have some elements of a research report. The best evidence the clinician is likely to be able to put forth against coincidental, rather than causal, association is statistical evidence on the odds of a coincidence; this line of argument can usually be developed in the Discussion.

The Case of Important Variation

An adult develops a disease or disorder previously seen only in children. Internists should know its diagnosis must now be included as a possibility for adults; the case report will change a clinical concept. Or a bacterium previously not known to be a pathogen is shown to be the cause of a case of endocarditis. The bacterium is unlikely to be found through routine culture methods. The clinician should know about this new pathogen so that appropriate culture methods can be requested. But such cases should be considered seriously for case reports only if they are likely to really change concept or practice.

The Case of Unexpected Events

Clinical medicine is not an exact science, but we do know much about how many diseases evolve and what effects of drugs can be expected. Clinicians can predict with some confidence what will happen in many cases they see. The unexpected event may be a clue to useful new information. Unexpected improvement in one or more signs or symptoms may be a clue to an unexpected, heretofore unknown beneficial effect of a drug. Unexpected deterioration of a patient's condition or an unexpected laboratory finding may be the clue to an unknown adverse drug effect. Again, unless the suspected causal association can be shown directly—by therapeutic trials in groups of patients, by rechallenge reproducing the beneficial, or the adverse, effect—the case report may be hard to get published. Critical readers of such case reports will at least expect that the postulated causal association be supported by excluding alternative explanations. The author must be sure that all data needed to consider possible alternative explanations are available before work on the report is begun.

Minor Case Reports

Some other varieties of case reports are unlikely to get published in front-rank journals.

The Everyone-Should-Remember Case

Uncommon features turn up in a case of a not uncommon disease. But what clinician will read the report, walk around for the next 10 years with it in his head, and then recall the fact to apply it? A report of the case will be particularly useless if its other presenting features were typical.

The Grand-Rounds Case

An atypical or unusually complex case lends itself to a virtuosic analysis of diagnostic possibilities or a staggeringly encyclopedic recall of relevant literature. But there is, in essence, nothing new about the case. All that can be said about it has been said before, not only in case reports and reviews but also in textbooks and from the lecture stand.

The I-Am-a-Clever-Chap Case

The lucky clinician stumbled onto a valuable clue to diagnosis in the case by accident. Or a new technical device just came on the market and gave the diagnostic answer. Good luck is not synonymous with new thought.

The Variations-on-a-Well-Known-Theme Case

A patient suffers an adverse effect from a drug that is the tenth variant of a widely used class of drugs. The adverse effect has been described for the first nine drugs. Who did not expect the adverse effect to turn up sooner or later with any new drug of this class?

The Goodness!-Book-of-Medical-World-Records Case

A woman of age 104 develops fungal endocarditis. The last GBMWR similar case was in a man of age 94. The fact of an additional 10 years does not add 10%, or even 1%, to what we need to know for clinical work about fungal endocarditis.

Case reports of these varieties all fail to change, improve, or enlarge how we think about disease—how we interpret signs and symptoms, how we make diagnoses, how we plan treatment. Any one of us may learn something from such cases, but this possibility does not justify their publication. The question the editor faces with reports of such cases is whether they bring enough new information to warrant giving them space. Will they change concept? Will they change practice?

STRUCTURE OF THE CASE REPORT

Even though research papers usually include far more detail than case reports, they are in some ways the easier kind of paper to write. The sequence in a research paper is usually that of a story: what happened one step after another, up to and including analysis of findings. Case reports may have to have a more complex structure than research reports. The case description itself is a story, but one or more elements of the whole story developed in the report may have to be out of the chronologic sequence.

Reports of single cases do not arise out of searches for cases unusual enough to merit reporting. The usual sequence runs through 6 or 7 steps. The clinician

- Becomes aware of unusual case features.
- Checks memory, colleagues, textbooks, other sources.
- May get additional case data.
- Tentatively concludes that the case is unique or has unexpected features.
- Decides to write a case report.
- Formally reviews the medical literature.
- Decides whether the case is unique or is adequately unexpected to justify a report.

A case report with a format built on this sequence would be boringly long. The reader would not want to hear all the details of the author's wanderings in mind and body up to the point of writing the paper. The reader needs only five elements in the paper.

- A statement of why the case is worth reading about
- An account of the case, with all relevant data
- Discussion of evidence that the case is unique or unexpected
- Possible alternative explanations for case features
- Conclusion, with implications

Although in the early years of medical journalism case reports were often written entirely in narrative style and sequence, they long ago evolved into the present and more efficient conventional format summarized below.

Introduction

The reader caught by the case report's title needs to know right away what there is about the case that justifies the report. Therefore, the Introduction has to compress into one paragraph or two a concise summary of how the case came to the author's attention, its main features worth reporting, in brief what literature search or other studies were carried out, and why the case is unique or unexpected. Details on the literature search can be presented in the Discussion, where you must assess the strength of the evidence for your conclusion.

Case Description

Usually the clearest way to "tell the story" is to describe the case in a chronologic sequence, starting with the first evidence of the problem that is the focus of the report. The narrative sequence may have to be interrupted with a "flashback". If, for example, the striking feature of the case was discovered when the author first saw the patient but events in the past turned out to be important, a jump back in time may be needed to summarize them adequately. The text that follows such flashbacks must make clear that the story is returning to the present time of the case narrative.

All relevant, but only truly relevant, data should be included. Dates and times that data were collected should be specified as needed for clear sequence and adequate interpretation. A long case description that must include a large number of data can often be presented more clearly if most of the detail is set up in a table with a chronologic structure rather than strung out in the text.

Steer clear of stereotypic rhetoric of the kind too often heard in oral bedside presentations; prefer accurate use of terms actually used by the patient. An especially perceptive discussion of this problem is the paper, "The Language of Medical Case Histories", by Donnelly (1).

Variations in Format

In most case reports, the Case Description can be followed immediately by the Discussion (see below). Occasionally other elements have to be added at this point. If the case details suggested that the syndrome could be an inherited disorder and the patient's family was studied for evidence of genetic abnormalities, a section on this family study may have to be added after the Case Description, particularly if the family study turned up evidence confirming a genetic disorder. If the initial case observations led to special detailed laboratory studies, the author may have to insert Materials and Methods and Results sections at this point, as in a research report.

Discussion and Conclusions

You will justify reporting the case in your Introduction, but your argument that the case is unique or unexpected belongs in the Discussion. The features of the case that justify the report are in the case description, but other evidence to support the argument is needed. Such additional evidence may be, in part, drawn from extensive case records in the author's institution. The Mayo Clinic, for example, has such large numbers of well-indexed and detailed case reports that a search of those records can produce convincing evidence that an apparently new syndrome had not been seen there before. Some drug companies keep large, detailed files that are particularly useful in searching for evidence of previously recorded cases of adverse drug effects. Most of the additional evidence is likely to have to come from a thorough search of the medical literature through one of the bibliographic services. But you cannot simply say that "a search of the literature failed to turn up any similar cases". The extent of the search should be summarized: the indexes searched, the search terms used, whether only English-language papers were reviewed, the dates of the literature covered. This information, rarely given in case reports, will help to convince the reader that you have weighed carefully the question of the case's value. The details of the search will also indicate what literature you have not searched; do not forget that in an honest critical argument in science you do not conceal any weaknesses in your evidence. And future students of the problem will be greatly helped by knowing what additional searches of the literature they may find helpful.

Clearly the needs for full and fair argument also apply to other aspects of some case reports. How credible is the evidence in the case description? If the report is of liver injury thought to be due to a drug, is the observed change in serum enzymes adequate evidence of liver injury, or could there be causes in the liver other than the drug? If the evidence for liver injury is abnormalities in histologic sections obtained by liver biopsy, are the findings specific for drug injury or could there be other causes? Counter- or contradictory evidence must be dealt with. If a case is thought to be unique but a review of the literature turns up cases with similarities, this potential counterevidence must be presented fully and assessed.

Useful discussions of the kinds of evidence needed in case reports on adverse drug effects and drug–drug interactions can be found in many sources. A notably concise comment on case reports of adverse drug effects can be found in *Guide to Clinical Trials* (2) by Spilker.

As with research papers, a Conclusions section may not be needed at the end of the Discussion if the journal for which the report is being prepared places abstracts or summaries on the title pages of articles. If a formal Conclusions section is not allowed, a concluding paragraph at the end of the Discussion can suggest possibilities for further study or point to implications for clinical practice.

THE CASE-SERIES ANALYSIS

A hybrid kind of paper is the so-called "case series", a paper based on retrospective study of case records, usually cases collected in one institution or in an individual practice. The cases may be described in short case reports that are followed by such generalizations as can be drawn from these cases and, perhaps, from similar case reports in the literature. In this format the paper has much of the character of the single-case report. Case-series papers are likely to have value mainly in reporting a spectrum of manifestations in a group of patients with clearly defined diagnoses or having experienced a particular intervention such as a specific surgical procedure. The spectrum can be one of adverse effects, postoperative morbidities, or other variables that lend themselves to qualitative description. The problems of selection bias and hetereogeneity of disease stage and the lack of control data tend to limit the value of case-series reports.

Some papers based on analysis of a series of cases are written only after authors define questions they hope to be able to answer from their case data and cases in the literature. If the case review is carried out with enough intellectual rigor (specific questions or hypotheses are posed, entities are defined precisely, control or contrast case-data are sought, data are tested statistically), the format of a research paper (see Chapter 6) is the right structure. A third option in format for the case series is that of the review article. In this approach the cases reviewed at the author's institution are treated as a unit, "my series", as if the cases and their data had already been described in a published paper. The cases are not presented in separate reports, however; rather, the data are combined, usually in tables, along with the data from published case material. The sequence of topics is chosen by one of the criteria discussed for the body of reviews in the first part of this chapter. In the review format, the paper must include a Methods section to state the definitions and limits used in selecting the author's cases, so the case material can be judged critically, as in other kinds of critical reviews.

CONCLUSION

The case report, a format much less frequently used today than in the past, has to be prepared with as much attention to the elements of critical argument as in other kinds of papers. The format, however, may not follow the sequence of critical argument as closely as research papers do; the various kinds of case reports may call for variations in format. The case-series analysis may use the format of the single-case report, the research paper, or the review.

REFERENCES

1. Donnelly WJ. The language of medical case histories. Ann Intern Med 1997;127:1045–8.
2. Spilker B. Guide to clinical trials. New York (NY): Raven Press; 1991:46–7.

CHAPTER 11

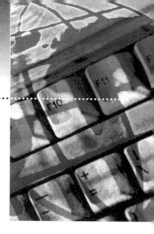

The Editorial, the Book Review, and the Letter-to-the-Editor

Because of their brevity and lack of overt format, editorials are often regarded as an informal kind of paper. In writing them, perhaps the author may not feel that he or she need pay the close attention to their intellectual structure that is needed in writing research reports or review articles. That point seems even stronger in considering book reviews and letters-to-the-editor. Yet in fact, careful attention to what elements are needed for critical argument (see Chapter 5) helps to ensure that the editorial, the book review, or the letter-to-the-editor will be an effective document.

THE EDITORIAL

At one time the term *editorial* indicated that the editorial was indeed a message from the journal's editor. Today the editorial in professional journals usually serves other functions. Many editorials are concise, critical reviews of scientific topics, especially topics that represent recent important developments. An editorial may comment on an original paper published in the same issue. The commentary editorial may critically assess the paper for its scientific validity, may differently interpret its data. It may put the paper's contribution into perspective with other recently reported findings that could not have been taken into account when the paper was written. It may speculate on what the paper implies for future concepts or practice. Some editorials take political positions; if they cite documentary evidence, they may also have some of the character of a review article.

Structure of the Editorial

Writing an editorial is in some ways more demanding than writing a research paper. The well-known usual format for research papers is a mold into which data and interpretations are set easily; at first glance the editorial has no format. The research paper usually runs to more than two printed pages, and an occasional slackening in its thought may not be noticed; the editorial is short, and flawed ideas and sequence can stand out. So the task is to fit what you have to say into a tight space and give it a clear and logical sequence.

The task is easier if you keep in mind the steps of critical argument. The editorialist has to settle on the issue, the problem, the question; has to pose one or more possible answers; has to weigh the evidence supporting these answers; has to assess counterevidence; and has to conclude with an answer. The answer might seem to be that there is no answer and that more information is needed, but that is itself an answer! Even such an answer is reached in a well-reasoned editorial through critical argument.

Table 11.1 illustrates how the structure and sequence of an editorial relate to the elements of critical argument. The length of an editorial and the number of its paragraphs depend on how complex a problem it considers, the amount of evidence it examines, and the number of possible answers. Some editorials might consist of only one paragraph and yet carry the main elements of argument in their natural sequence.

The opening paragraph states the first element of argument: the problem or question. Most readers will need more than a simple statement of the problem. Experts on the subject will know what new events or new knowledge led to awareness that a problem needs an answer, but most editorials are not written for experts. The question of how much background to include in the lead-in to the statement of the problem is probably best answered as it is for the Introduction to a research paper. The editorialist should assume that readers know less than he does about the topic of the editorial but are well informed on the larger subject field within which the topic lies. The author of an editorial on the usefulness of exercise in lowering the future risk of stroke should assume that the reader knows less than experts experienced with critically analyzing the physiological benefits of exercise but is well informed in general on the problem of stroke in elderly persons and knows that exercise in general has beneficial effects. The editorialist can immediately open with a brief summary of how little has been known about exercise and stroke prevention. This stance will guarantee an adequate, if brief, lead-in, while avoiding a long-winded and patronizing ramble to the main point to be made by the end of the introductory paragraph.

Although the middle paragraphs of an editorial carry the evidence considered in the argument, they differ from one of the counterpart sections of a research paper, the Results, in not presenting detailed data. They resemble more the paragraphs in a review article in that the evidence is likely to consist of statements supported by citations to published papers. Usually there is not enough space in an editorial to examine "the credibility of evi-

TABLE 11.1. A typical editorial as critical argument

Paragraphs	Elements of critical argument
Introductory paragraph	
Too many persons cannot afford good medical care; we need national health insurance.	Statement of the problem; tentative answer
Middle paragraphs	
National health insurance would spread costs among industry and the wealthy.	Evidence in support
Other countries have successful national health insurance.	Evidence in support
Our country cannot afford such insurance in the face of competing demands for defense spending.	Counterevidence
Closing paragraph	
Health is more important than military spending. We should work politically to get top priority for national health insurance.	Assessment of all evidence; final answer

dence"; the reader can assume that the "credibility" of papers selected for citation in the editorial was "examined" by the editorialist while reading the papers considered as possible references.

The closing paragraph should carry a clear final answer to the question posed in the opening paragraph. If the answer is that there is no answer, so be it. But then the editorialist may wish to suggest possible routes to new evidence that may dispose of the no-answer answer.

A Variant of The Editorial: The Position Paper

Some journals have a section for opinion papers that the editor prefers not to publish as editorials. The papers may be too long. They may take positions the editor does not wish to seem to support by giving them the authority implied in an editorial. Examples of such sections include "Sounding Board" of *The New England Journal of Medicine* and "Perspective" of the *Annals of Internal Medicine*. Well-written papers of this kind usually have the same structure as a clear and logical editorial, although they may differ widely in their use of documented reasoning and rhetorical heat. The points made above about editorials apply as well to position papers.

THE BOOK REVIEW AND THE LETTER-TO-THE-EDITOR

Short papers such as book reviews and letters-to-the-editor need as much care in writing as longer papers. There is no room for wasted words and wasted motion. The author must be sure that all that needs to be said is said, but no more. A wrong sequence of ideas will stand out as clearly as a misspelled word. Careful planning before the first draft is started should go into deciding what is to be said and how it should be arranged.

The Book Review

Book reviews are usually invited by a journal editor, who restricts invitations to reviewers believed to be qualified to render critical judgments. In spite of this practice, anyone who scans the book review sections of clinical journals is likely to be struck by the indifferent quality of most of the reviews. A dismaying fraction of reviews read like extracts from the dust jacket or the table of contents followed by some remarks about paper and price. The reader is often unsure whether the reviewer has read the book. Such reviews assess a book as if it were sitting alone on a table in the middle of the Sahara. We do not learn whether the book is the first of its kind and, if it is, whether it is needed. We are not told whether it is better or worse than similar books if they exist, or for whom it may be valuable. These faults likely stem in part from reviewers' concluding from the short length usually allowed (and specified with invitations) that they need only read or sample the book, jot down a few notes on content as they go, start at the top of the sheet of paper, and write through to the bottom, briefly summarizing the book's content, writing without thinking in advance about why the review is needed and what its structure should be.

A well-thought-out, thorough, and carefully written book review has no less structure (Table 11.2) than an editorial. The review opens with a question, usually implied but sometimes stated; it moves to the evidence and counterevidence; and it closes with the answer. The review must develop each step fully within the length allowed by the editor; even the one-paragraph review should proceed in these steps. Thus, in preparing to write, the reviewer should start by considering what question is going to be answered: Is this book needed? Is the book better than others of its kind? Why did I enjoy the book? For whom is the book written and is it right for that audience? Development of the evidence and counterevidence will make up the middle sentences of a one-paragraph review and the middle paragraphs of a longer review. The conclusion, with the answer, may be no longer than a sentence if the reviewer is willing to take a stand.

Most readers of book reviews expect to find the book assessed. An occasional review presents instead an essay of reflections touched off by the book. Such an essay can bring many readers great pleasure if the author has

TABLE 11.2. A book review as critical argument	
Examples of points made	**Elements of critical argument**
Introductory paragraph	Question
Five major textbooks of pathology are available.	
Is this new one better? Were more needed? What need does this book meet?	
Body of review	Evidence
Text has unusual sequence of topics reflecting newer developments. Text is detailed and critical. Text reflects wide experience.	
Wide range of illustrations, from electron micrographs to fine color photographs of gross lesions.	
Scanty use of references; inadequate index.	Counterevidence
Concluding paragraph	
In the balance, the virtues outweigh the defects.	Assessment of conflicting evidence
The most up-to-date general text book of pathology; recommended.	Answer

a rich enough view of life, personal or professional, and the skill to get that view down on paper. The author of the essay is obliged, nevertheless, to make clear to readers early on that the essay is moving from the book to other matters and that they should not expect to find an assessment of the book at the end.

The Letter-to-the-Editor

Why should a manual on writing papers for professional journals have a chapter on writing letters-to-the-editor? People dash off letters all the time; anyone can write a letter. Yes, but not everyone can get a letter published in a professional journal. Getting a letter published can have valuable consequences. Letters of substance in a major journal like *The Lancet* are indexed in the National Library of Medicine's MEDLINE and *Index Medicus*. Pharmaceutical manufacturers and publishers of pharmaceutical newsletters scan letter sections for reports of adverse drug effects. A letter briefly reporting an unusual case may start the author on a fruitful exchange of correspondence with others around the world interested in the same problem. The competition to get letters published is less intense than that with formal reports, but not many journals publish letters-to-the-editor. With this competition, letters should be drafted carefully.

Before you write a letter, read closely the journal's requirements. They may be stated at the beginning of the letters section in the journal, on the information-for-authors pages, or in both places. If the journal does not set a limit on the length of acceptable letters, the letter writer may be able to estimate the allowable length by scanning the journal's letters section. Most journals do not publish figures or tables with letters. The number of references allowed may be limited.

Most letters are miniature equivalents of research reports, case reports, reviews, or editorials. In writing a comment on a paper that has been published in the journal, that paper should be cited near the beginning of the letter to make clear why the letter was written. The style for letters may call for identifying the paper commented on by giving its authors and title in the text of the letter; other journals may prefer a citation in the text and its reference at the end.

Letter writers should take as much care with their drafts as they would with the much longer text of a paper. Of two letters with the same message, the long, windy, and foggy one is more likely to get rejected; the short, concise, and clear letter is more likely to get accepted. Be especially careful about keeping the letter's tone proper for a scientific journal. Avoid personal attacks or slurs on the authors of a paper you are criticizing and, of course, on the editors of the journal that published the paper. It is wise to hold letters for a week or two before sending them off so that you can tone them down if, on rereading, they are seen as angry, emotional complaints rather than objective analysis.

Before the final draft is typed, count the number of words in the text to make sure the letter does not exceed the allowed length. Like manuscripts of formal papers (see Chapter 20), the letter should be typed double-spaced; some journals will return a single-spaced letter for retyping or simply decide against publishing it.

Permission to publish, with an indication that it covers all authors of the letter, should be included with the submitted letter. Some letters received in editorial offices do not make clear whether they are only for the editor or are submitted for possible publication.

CONCLUSION

An editorial has little room in which to deliver its message. The structure must be well worked out, with the right sequence of the elements of critical argument, lest the very brevity of the editorial expose all too clearly any flaws in logic.

Book reviews and letters-to-the-editor are short forms of papers, but they should be written with as much attention to structure and sequence as formal scientific

continued

Conclusion continued.

papers. The book review should be built on the elements and sequence of critical argument: the question posed, the evidence considered, and the answer. A letter-to-the-editor may have the structure, in miniature, of a research report, a case report, a review, or an editorial. As much care in writing is needed as for papers with longer formats. The journal's requirements for letters should be followed. Structure and prose style should be revised for clarity and brevity, and the final version should be prepared in an acceptable form.

PART 3

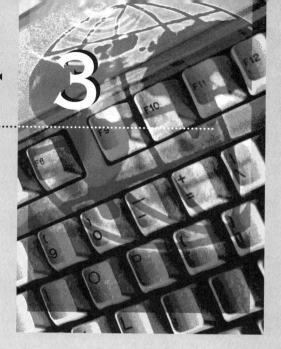

Writing and Revising

CHAPTER 12

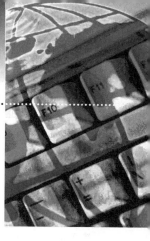

The First Draft: Text

You are ready to write. If you took the steps suggested in Chapter 2, you have decided on your paper's message, defined its audience, and selected the journal to which you will send the paper. You have completed your search or re-search of the literature. You have decided on authorship, looked up the manuscript requirements of the journal, and put together all the raw materials for your paper. You have decided on the best format.

Everyone who does a lot of writing sooner or later finds a way to get into the work of writing. And writing is work, even for professionals like novelists and playwrights. Many experienced writers in science use a methodical approach akin to that suggested below; they have found that building up a paper early in systematic steps can cut down sharply on the later work in revising first and later drafts. You will need more than one draft; all writers who want to write accurately and clearly revise again and again.

GETTING STARTED

The Research Paper: The Title

The method of writing a paper suggested here is the reverse of summarizing it (see Table 12.1). All journal papers carry titles, and most include abstracts. A title is a highly condensed version of the abstract; an abstract is a highly condensed version of the full text. The title may not tell what the abstract concludes, but it at least conveys what the abstract covers. As pointed out in Chapter 13, the author must make sure in writing an abstract that every main element of the paper is represented. In preparing the title, the careful author makes sure that the title carries the irreducible number of terms needed to accurately describe the content of the paper.

TABLE 12.1.   Writing a paper as the reverse of summarizing it

Summarizing	Writing
Read the full text, jotting down the main paper's point of each paragraph.	Write out an informative title that states the message.
List these points as a kind of outline.	Draft an abstract limited to 150 or 200 words that gives what will be the main point of each section. In an outline state main points, add minor points and other details.
From these points draft an abstract that represents the main point of each section.	
Write a title that succinctly states the paper's message (informative title) or indicates the paper's subject.	Expand the outline into a first draft of text.

Approach the first draft of your paper by first writing a title. Do not worry whether it will be the final title; you will probably revise it several times before you finish revising the whole paper. As discussed in Chapter 13, titles are of two types, indicative and informative. An indicative title tells what the paper is about; an informative title tells briefly in sentence form the message of the paper. For a start in writing, an informative title is more helpful because writing it forces you to come to an unequivocal decision on the paper's main message. You may change the title later to the indicative type (which is more widely used than the informative type), but that change may be made in a later draft.

The Research Paper: The Abstract

Once you have drafted the title, you can move to writing at least a preliminary version of the abstract you will need. As also described in Chapter 13, abstracts are either informative—giving a concise summary of the content of a paper—or indicative—indicating what the paper is about. Abstracts of research reports should certainly be of the informative type, and even abstracts of some review articles can be too. Adhering carefully to the need to have an abstract that concisely represents the main content of each section of a paper will force you to develop at least a preliminary view of what each section should carry. Be sure to represent each eventual section of the paper (Introduction, Methods, and so on) by at least one sentence. Using the structured-abstract format (see Chapter 13) when it is appropriate can help you focus on the main needed elements even if the journal for which you are writing the paper does not use structured abstracts. You need not fuss about trying to write a perfect abstract at this point; you will have plenty of time to polish the abstract later.

The Research Paper: The Outline

With preliminary versions of the title and the abstract in hand you can proceed to draft an outline that can represent more details of the eventual paper than can be represented in an abstract. Do not worry about whether you can prepare a full formal outline with the elements under the main headings being either all phrases or all sentences. Jot down your thoughts as they come. If your first outline is a hybrid, you will not have hampered progress, nor will you have to turn it in to your high-school English teacher. Your first outline might run like this.

INTRODUCTION
– present multidrug regimens and cytolysane good (40% survival at 1 year)
– we need better regimens
– new agent, nohistine, hits at critical point in cell cycle
– have substituted nohistine for plustocine in the standard multidrug regimen
– our controlled clinical trial compared this new multidrug regimen with cytolysane

PATIENTS AND METHODS
– standard NCI protocol
– 10 cooperating oncology clinics
– metastatic breast cancer
– criteria for case selection
– standard lab, x-ray, and scan studies
– randomization to new regimen or to cytolysane
– new regimen: drugs, doses, schedules
– cytolysane: doses, schedules
– follow-up: studies and schedules lab methods
– data analysis: statistical methods

RESULTS
– effects of randomization—good homogeneity between the two groups (except for age, but 90% in each group over 50)—Table 1
– cytolysane (Table 2): survival 40% at 1 year
– new regimen (Table 2): survival 55% at 1 year
– adverse effects (Table 3): nausea and vomiting, hematologic, alopecia, other

DISCUSSION
– difference in 1-year survival real advance
– similar results reported last year by ECCS (see Eur. Cancer Chemoth. Rep.)

– higher adverse-effects rate of cytolysane disturbing
– but recommend cytolysane for general clinical use
– modifying the schedule we used may reduce adverse effects

The outline is not a formal outline; it looks sloppy—none of the usual "I, A, 1" structure, a mixture of phrases, half sentences, full sentences, abbreviations. So what? Your writing is under way!

At this point, you can choose one of three options.

- Clean up this outline, putting all lines into parallel form (for example, converting all entries under each section heading into sentences) and assigning the usual Roman numerals I, II, and so on, to the headings, and A, B, and so on, to the entries. Then begin to write.
- Start writing from the present outline.
- Put the rough outline aside for a few days and then patch some more details into it, perhaps adding mention of more tables (or graphs or illustrations) that will accompany the text and making notations of other papers to be cited. After this patching, sit down to write the first draft.

I like the third option ("Put the . . . outline aside . . . then patch . . . more details into it . . ."). If you choose the third option, here is a point at which you might add some section subheadings into the outline. Some authors find especially difficult the organizing of a "Materials and Methods" section. A review of "The Materials and Methods Section" in Chapter 6 may suggest such subheadings as "Study Design", "Trial Participants", "Drug Schedules", and so on. These can help you to organize your content for the first full draft. Similarly, you might be helped in organizing the Results section by drafting some subheadings that will indicate the probable sequence of its content. Chapter 7 may help you develop your initial choices of subheadings for all of the sections of your research paper, including the Discussion.

Perhaps you will prefer the first or second option.

THE REVIEW ARTICLE AND THE METAANALYSIS

If you are about to start writing a review article, you probably wrote a tentative outline of it before you started the search for relevant literature. Chapter 9 describes some typical kinds of structure for review articles and may be helpful in your developing this initial outline. With this step you defined and limited the scope of the review and selected the terms to be used in the literature search. You also defined the categories of notations ("histopathology", "epidemiology", "differential diagnosis") to enter on your file cards as you digested the papers you selected from the search. Before you start the first draft of the text, prepare a second outline, fleshing it out with phrases or sentences on specific data and conclusions you found in the literature. You may also wish to patch in some notes on papers to be cited and tables you have already sketched out. Then you will be ready to write the first draft.

A metaanalysis serves much the same function as a review article but with its more rigorous approach and research methodology, it must be, in structure, essentially a research paper rather than a narrative summary and digest of literature as is a review article. Hence, the opening section of this chapter on developing a title, an abstract, and then an outline is a better guide on how to start writing the metaanalysis.

THE CASE REPORT

The scheme described for starting to write a research report can also be used for a case report, with the outline built on the formats discussed in Chapter 10.

THE EDITORIAL

As an editorialist, you can proceed much the same way as with a review article: Decide on the message; draft an outline with attention to the sequence of argument summarized in Chapter 11; read new articles you have found and review the reprints already in your file; then redraft the outline, fleshing it out with short summary phrases or sentences for each intended paragraph.

WRITING THE TEXT OF THE FIRST DRAFT

Each author works out his or her own way to write. With a well-prepared outline and the materials recommended in Chapter 4 (preliminary tables and graphs, photographs, references), you should be able to start a first draft at the beginning and write through to the end. But almost certainly you will not try it at one sitting. Even professional writers rarely write for more than two or three hours at a stretch. Pick the time of the day you prefer. Turn on the phone-recording machine. Write in a place where you like to work and lock the door!

Use the writing medium you feel comfortable with. If you type fairly quickly and can run a word-processing program, you can save quite a bit of money and time in keyboarding the paper yourself. Some authors, the born talkers, like to dictate for transcription by someone else. You may prefer paper and ballpoint pen: paper, to be able to scan back now and then to see how the flow of ideas is running (harder to do with a dictating machine or with jumping through 24-line screens on a monitor); ballpoint pen because it gives a sharp, good-contrast line, not a weak, fuzzy line like that from a pencil.

Temporary Forms Of Citations

A few practical suggestions put to use in your first draft may help you later.

The first has to do with reference citations in the first draft. You will be citing papers in the text to be identified later in the reference list (or "bibliography" or "literature cited") at the end of the paper. Most clinical journals in medicine use the citation-sequence system ("Vancouver style") in which the references in the reference list are numbered in the order in which they are first cited in the text (see Chapter 19). Some journals, especially in the basic medical sciences, use the name–year date system ("the Harvard system") in which the paper cited is identified by author name and year of publication. A passage in a journal using the citation-sequence system would read thus.

> Most of the acute injuries to the first metatarsal–phalangeal joint in ballet dancers (1) have led, in the patients we have seen, to destruction of the articular cartilages.

The paper cited with "(1)" is a paper written in 1890 by Adams and Giselle; the reference to it is reference number 1 in the references list at the end of the present paper. In the name–year system the authors' names and the paper's year of publication are used instead of the reference number.

> Most of the acute injuries to the first metatarsal–phalangeal joint in ballet dancers (Adams and Giselle, 1890) have led, in the patients we have seen, to destruction of the articular cartilages.

Even if the journal for which you are preparing your paper uses the citation-sequence system, use the name-year system for the citations in the first and other early drafts. If you assign numbers to references at this early stage, those numbers will have to be changed in successive drafts if you add or delete references or change the sequence of citations. The numbers can be assigned to the references later; replace the name-and-date citations when you have finished revising your paper and the final version is prepared.

Note that some bibliographic management programs for computers (see "Managing References" in Chapter 4) enable you to insert a "reference marker" at an appropriate citation point in a text being written with a word-processing program. When you get to the final version of the manuscript the program will enable you to automatically apply the desired citation format in the text and prepare the references in the proper reference format. Such programs can be a real timesaver in preparing the final version of a paper.

If you are not using a bibliographic program with these features and you or your typist is using a word-processing program with a "find-and-replace" function, you can later speed up the finding of citations for replacement of name-year citations with reference numbers. In the first draft, place at the beginning of each citation a character not used elsewhere in the text, for example, an asterisk (*).

> Most of the acute injuries to the first metatarsal-phalangeal joint in ballet dancers *(Adams and Giselle, 1890) have led, as in the patients we reported recently *(Copland and del Tredici, 1985), to destruction of the articular cartilages.

You, or your typist, will be able to use the asterisk as the character to be searched for in using the "find-and-replace" function; this function will move you rapidly through the text to each citation when you have to revise citations in successive drafts, including the final version. The asterisk will, of course, have to be removed from the final version as it is completed.

Line Numbering to Facilitate Identification of Text

When coauthors, especially coauthors in two or more locations, have to exchange criticisms of intermediate drafts, they may have to refer to many different locations in the text. "Fred, I think you better take out those 2 sentences of lines 5 through 11 in paragraph 1 on page 7". You turn to page 7 and wonder whether he means lines 5 through 11 in the top paragraph which began on the preceding page or lines 5 through 11 in the first full paragraph. In either case you have to count down the lines to get to the part of the text he is referring to.

If your word-processing program has a line-numbering function, it can automatically place line numbers in the left margin at the beginning of successive lines. The function may offer the option of numbering lines continuously through the entire text or starting numbering on each page.

> 123   in this kind of case, we find that total extirpation offers the
> 124   best chance for complete relief from pain and the smallest

125 number of potential postoperative complications. This is not,
126 however, the experience of the group at the

    1 and in this kind of case, we find that total extirpation offers the
    2 best chance for complete relief from pain and the smallest
    3 number of potential postoperative complications. This is not,
    4 however, the experience of the group at the

Continuous line numbering through all pages offers the easiest device for quick reference to a part of the text. You may prefer the renumbering on each page if each section of the paper is maintained as a separate file in your computer.

Identifying Drafts

As you go on from the first draft and revise the paper in successive drafts, you must be sure that you do not mix up pages from different drafts. Therefore it is wise to mark each page of a draft with a brief note of the number of the draft, the page number, and the date. If the drafts are being prepared with a word-processing program, such notes can be easily and automatically placed on each page with its headers-and-footers function. Such headers for the second draft might look like this at the top of a page in the Materials and Methods section.

[Nohistine Regimen, 2nd draft]   [14 July 88]
    and the patients were alternately assigned to the nohistine group or the cytolysane group and . . .

If you work on the first and successive drafts of the text from beginning to end, you can number the pages successively. If you write sections out of order (see below, "Writer's Block") or the various sections are worked on by different coauthors and the text is produced with a word-processing program, you may wish to maintain each section as a separate file with its own sequence of page numbers. The sections will, of course, eventually be assembled in their right order and the pages numbered from the beginning.

WRITER'S BLOCK

What if you sit down to write and cannot get started? You chew your nails, you stare out the window, you get up for a coffee, you decide to shop for groceries. You have "writer's block". A diagnosis is not much help without treatment. Fortunately, the syndrome is treatable. Professional writers usually work out a treatment—they, too, often find writing painful. You can find a treatment that suits you.

Two good discussions of writer's block (1, 2) point out that blocks come basically from three related causes. Writing is your work laid out plain for you and others to see. You dislike judgment by others of your work and, hence, of you. You are burdened by your own internal self-criticism (Freud's "super-ego") developed unconsciously to try to spare yourself the pain of being harshly judged by others and even punished. Different solutions are available, some of which are akin to what is suggested earlier in this chapter, building from a title to an outline.

One solution is called "nonstops (kitchen-sinking it)", a method (1) in which you repeatedly sit down and write nonstop for a fixed but short time, say 15 minutes, about any aspect of your topic. These bits can be revised and pieced together for a first draft that may be crude but is a start.

Another solution (2) is called "satisficing". You satisfy yourself by sacrificing the ideal of a flawless first draft. You make up your mind to get a first draft down on paper no matter how defective it will look.

Some authors start on the first draft by writing sections on the material they already know best: Materials and Methods, Results. They had to prepare a research protocol, perhaps for a grant proposal, when they designed their study; the protocol may be readily expanded (or condensed) to text for Materials and Methods. They have preliminary tables of data with statistical analyses, which is why they decided they were ready to write; the Results will be little more than a text summary of those data.

Keep this in mind: a first draft is a first draft is a first draft; it will not go to the journal, the journal's peer reviewers, or the printer. Do not fear criticism; learn to welcome criticism of a first draft, a second draft, a fifth draft. Embrace the fact that a first draft will have intellectual faults and flaws in prose style. You will be able to correct these later.

WHAT NEXT?

The first draft should not be the final draft. A first draft is just a first draft. A few fine writers publish what they write in the first draft, but most go through many drafts. A close acquaintance of Dr Karl Menninger, the eminent psychiatrist who wrote some classics in psychiatry for the general reader, told me that each of his books went through 10 manuscript versions. Most of the persons I know in academic medicine who have published many research papers always go through at least four drafts and usually five.

CONCLUSION

Just as the full text of a paper can be condensed into an abstract and then into a title, so can a paper be developed in the reverse direction. An informative title, one that
states the paper's main message, can be expanded first to an abstract, which can be
expanded to an outline from which the first draft can be written. Difficulties in getting
started in writing the first draft, or writer's block, can be overcome; a first draft is only
a first draft, and subsequent drafts will take care of its inevitable defects.

REFERENCES

1. Mack K, Skjei E. Overcoming writing blocks. Los Angeles (CA): JP Tarcher; 1979. Distributed by St Martin's Press, New York.
2. Flower L. Understanding your own writing process. In: Flower L. Problem-solving strategies for writing. 2nd ed. San Diego (CA): Harcourt Brace Jovanovich; 1985:21–42.

CHAPTER 13

The First Draft: Titles and Abstracts

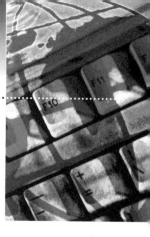

A properly constructed title and abstract will raise the odds that your paper will be read when it first appears in the journal and that it will be retrieved from a bibliographic database like MEDLINE by searchers looking for papers on its topic. The second value in taking care to write a good title and a good abstract is that these steps will help you at least a little bit in focusing on what your paper will say when you sit down to write the first draft.

TITLES

Types of Titles

Titles are of two kinds: indicative or informative. An indicative title tells what the paper is about: "A New Multidrug Regimen for Treatment of Metastatic Breast Cancer". The content of the paper may be made a bit more clear by adding a subtitle: "A Cooperative-Group Trial Comparing It with Cytolysane". Note that this indicative title and subtitle do not tell the reader the main message of the paper but only on what the paper is reporting.

A title of the informative kind can be more helpful for a start in writing. The informative title tells briefly in sentence form the message of the paper: "A New Multidrug Regimen for Treatment of Metastatic Breast Cancer Produces Greater Survival at One Year than Cytolysane". Yes, this informative title is too long, and some journals might not accept it. But note that it contains words representing most of the elements that will have to be expanded into a full paper. The Introduction of the paper will have to tell the reader why "A New . . . Regimen . . ." is needed. The Materials and Methods section will have to give us the details of the ". . . Multidrug Regimen . . ." and of the comparison treatment with ". . . Cytolysane"; it will also have to give the methods for detecting and diagnostically defining ". . . Metastatic Breast Cancer . . .". The Results section will have to give us the data on ". . . Survival at One Year . . ."

with the ". . . New Multidrug Regimen . . ." and with ". . . Cytolysane" and will have to give the statistical assessment of ". . . Greater Survival . . . Than . . .".

Note that some journals do not allow the use of informative titles and insist on indicative titles. A journal's information-for-authors pages may tell you whether both types of titles are acceptable. If it does not, you can scan the contents pages of recent issues where you may get a clue that both types are. The other approach is to write to or telephone the journal's editorial office and ask about the journal's policy on titles.

Sequence of Title Terms

The position of terms within a title may influence whether a reader scanning the journal's content page jumps quickly to look at the paper. In general, a title should begin with its most important term or terms.

> Metastatic Breast Cancer Treated with a New Multidrug Regimen or with Cytolysane: A Cooperative-Group Trial [This title puts the name of the disease and the new aspect of the paper right up front. Isn't it stronger than the title below?]
> A Cooperative-Group Trial of Cytolysane and a New Multidrug Regimen for the Treatment of Metastatic Breast Cancer [The most important terms are at a greater distance from the beginning.]

These examples illustrate only two possible sequences of terms that are needed.

Clinical papers, in general, are more likely to need titles that include terms like "randomized controlled trial" that help to indicate the reported research was rigorously designed to give a clear answer. Titles of reports of laboratory research may be simpler because readers are likely to assume that appropriate laboratory methods have been used for the reported research.

A need to identify the kinds of participants in reported clinical research may depend on whether the research was undertaken to answer previously not settled questions, such as the efficacy in women of a drug that has been studied before only in men. Ethnic groups may also be desirably identified in some titles.

Title Structures

Titles are almost invariably structured in one of three ways.

- A single continuous title

  > Metastatic Breast Cancer Treated with a New Multidrug Regimen or with Cytolysane in a Cooperative-Group Randomized Controlled Trial

- A title with subordinate terms following a colon

  Metastatic Breast Cancer Treated with a New Multidrug Regimen or with Cytolysane: A Cooperative-Group Trial

- A title and subtitle

  Metastatic Breast Cancer Treated with a New Multidrug Regimen or with Cytolysane [title]
  A Cooperative-Group Randomized Controlled Trial [subtitle]

A look through some recent issues of a journal will suggest to you what kinds of structures may be allowed by the journal. Some journals may not allow the third type. The value of the second type is that it offers possibilities for writing shorter titles while keeping the most important terms in the title at its beginning.

Abbreviations in Titles

Abbreviations should not, in general, be used in titles. But there are exceptions likely to be acceptable.

- Widely and frequently used abbreviations will probably be acceptable: DNA, AIDS, NIH, and others of this kind.
- Some scientific symbols such as pH (the symbol for the negative logarithm of the hydrogen ion concentration; it can be considered to be an abbreviated form of the term "hydrogen potential"), °C for "degree Celsius", and others of this kind.
- Abbreviations that replace a long multiterm name, for example, MOPP, the abbreviation for the four-drug regimen consisting of mechlorethamine, oncovin, procarbazine, and prednisone.

With this third kind of use, the author is usually expected to define the abbreviation as early in the paper as possible (unless the abbreviation is well established and widely used by the paper's audience).

Revision of Titles

If you drafted a title as an aid in beginning to write the first draft, you need not feel compelled to stick with this initial version of a title all the way through to the final version of the paper. Some of your coauthors may see the need for a rearrangement of the title or the addition or subtraction of some terms.

Keep in mind that before the final version of the title is written, you will have to check with the journal's information-for-authors pages on its requirements for titles.

THE ABSTRACT

Why is the recommendation here to prepare an abstract as part of the process of writing the first draft? As noted above, organizing at least a preliminary version of an abstract can help you organize your plan for the entire first draft. You will, of course, have to check with the journal's information-for-author pages about its requirements for abstracts and look at some examples of abstracts in recent issues for further guidance before you prepare a final version of the abstract.

Abstract Types

Informative Abstracts

Abstracts are also of two kinds: informative and indicative. For the research paper or case report you will need an informative abstract that, like the informative title, summarizes what the paper actually says. You need not try to write a polished final abstract when you start to write the first draft. The abstract, like the text of the paper, will probably have to be revised many times. In writing the first draft of the abstract, keep to the usual format for research papers. Keep in mind that an informative abstract should represent, if possible within the allowed length of abstracts, each section of the paper by at least one sentence, as in this preliminary abstract.

> Present multidrug chemotherapy regimens for treatment of metastatic breast cancer and single-drug treatment with cytolysane improve survival to 40% at 1 year. A new multidrug regimen that includes nohistine was compared in a clinical trial with cytolysane. Ten cooperating oncology centers using a standard protocol compared the 2 regimens in 320 women, with random assignment of patients to cytolysane or the new multidrug regimen. The 2 groups were found to be adequately homogeneous with regard to histologic classification and extent of bone and pulmonary metastases. The survival rates at 1 year were 40% for cytolysane and 55% for the new regimen, a statistically significant difference. Adverse effects with the new regimen were more prolonged. These findings are similar to those recently reported from the ECCS group and suggest that the new regimen with nohistine should replace use of cytolysane.

Notice how sentences and parts of sentences in this preliminary abstract represent eventual main points in all the sections of the paper.

Introduction	Present multidrug chemotherapy regimens for treatment of metastatic breast cancer and single-drug treatment with cytolysane improve survival to 40% at 1 year. A new multidrug regimen that includes nohistine was compared in a clinical trial with cytolysane.
Materials and Methods	A new multidrug regimen that includes no-

histine was compared in a clinical trial with cytolysane. Ten cooperating oncology centers using a standard protocol compared the 2 regimens in 320 women, with random assignment of patients to cytolysane or the new multidrug regimen.

Results   The 2 groups were found to be adequately homogeneous with regard to histologic classification and extent of bone and pulmonary metastases. The survival rates at 1 year were 40% for cytolysane and 55% for the new regimen, a statistically significant difference. Adverse effects with the new regimen were more prolonged.

Discussion and Conclusion   These findings are similar to those recently reported from the ECCS group and suggest that the new regimen with nohistine should replace treatment with cytolysane.

Note that many journals (for example, *Annals of Internal Medicine, British Medical Journal, Journal of General Internal Medicine,* and others) are now requesting structured abstracts (1, 2) for papers reporting prospective trials and for review papers. The journals of the American Medical Association also accept structured abstracts for consensus papers (3). Structured abstracts do not differ greatly in content from traditional single-paragraph abstracts but include headings that reflect the main elements of the papers thus represented; each section of these abstracts usually carries more explicit detail. Here is a typical sequence of headings for an abstract of a research report.

Background
Objective
Design
Setting
Participants
Measurements
Results
Conclusions

For an example see Figure 13.1.

Headings for a structured abstract of a review article will differ. Here is the sequence of headings for such an abstract recommended for the journals of the American Medical Association (3). This example also represents appropriate headings for an abstract of a metaanalysis. Note the similarities it has with headings for research-report abstracts.

Objective
Data Sources
Study Selection

Background: Protein S is an important regulatory protein of the coagulation cascade. The risk for venous thrombosis with associated protein S deficiency has been uncertain because all previous risk estimates used phenotypic evaluation alone, which can be ambiguous.

Objective: To quantitate the risk for thrombosis associated with a characterized S gene mutation that causes G295ÆVal substitution and protein S deficiency.

Design: Retrospective study of a single extended family.

Setting: University hospital referral center.

Participants: A 122-member protein S-deficiency family, in which 44 members had a recently characterized gene defect.

Measurements: Comprehensive history of thrombosis, history of exposure to acquired risk factors for thrombosis, levels of total and free protein S antigen, and genotype for the mutation causing the Gly295→Val substitution.

Results: Kaplan-Meier analysis of thrombosis-free survival showed that the probability of remaining free of thrombosis at 30 years of age is 0.5 (95% CI, 0.33 to 0.66) for carriers of the Gly295→Val mutation compared with 0.97 (CI, 0.93 to 1.0) for normal family members ($P<0.001$). In a multivariate Cox regression model that included smoking and obesity, the mutation was a strong independent risk factor for thrombosis (hazard ratio, 11.5 [CI, 4.33 to 30.6]; $P<0.001$). For free (but not total) protein s antigen levels, the distributions of persons with and without the mutation did not overlap.

Conclusions: Protein S deficiency, as defined by the presence of a causative gene mutation or a reduced level of free protein S antigen, is a strong independent risk factor for venous thrombosis in a clinically affected family.

FIGURE 13.1.   Example of a structured abstract representing a research paper. Simulated from *Annals of Internal Medicine* 1998 Jan 1;128:8–14 with the permission of the copyright holder, American College of Physicians.

> Data Extraction
> Data Synthesis
> Conclusions

While such headings may be appropriate for systematic reviews (including metaanalyses), they may be inappropriate for a descriptive ("narrative") review. Recent issues of the journal for which you are preparing the review can suggest its preference for traditional-form abstracts for descriptive reviews or structured abstracts and what headings they should have.

Structured abstracts are carried in MEDLINE, and additional examples can be found in that database by searching for references and abstracts from the journals promoting their use. Even if you do not use this structure for the final version of your abstract, this approach can be helpful in that it forces you to represent all important elements of your paper in the abstract; you will be able to revise it later to the older format.

Indicative Abstracts

The other type of abstract is the indicative abstract, an abstract that simply indicates what the paper is about and does not "abstract" (summarize) what it actually says. This type is frequently used for abstracts of articles like reviews containing a large amount of detail that is not readily boiled down to a few main points. The following abstract illustrates this type.

> This review covers the many different adverse effects that have been reported for the drugs most widely used in the treatment of breast cancer. It considers them as generalized systemic effects and by body systems. An attempt has been made to assess their degree of life-threatening severity and to suggest how patients can be monitored for their early detection.

In general, for review articles informative abstracts are to be preferred over indicative abstracts when the detail needed for an informative abstract can be carried within allowed length. This is especially true for metaanalyses, which are in one sense review articles, but which in fact are properly considered research that uses organized systematic searches for relevant literature and quantitative analytical techniques applied for data analysis. Details on these two points are important in judging the probable value of the metaanalysis and because they must be specified in the methods section should also be represented in the abstract.

Abbreviations in Abstracts

As with titles, abbreviations should be avoided as much as possible in abstracts. The rules suggested above for abbreviations in titles can be applied in abstracts. What abbreviations are allowable in a particular journal will depend in part on what abbreviations are readily understood by most of the journal's readers. The journal's information-for-authors pages may indicate what abbreviations it considers to be standard and widely understood in its field.

Length of Abstracts

A journal may specify in its information-for-author pages the maximum length of abstracts it will allow. If such a limit is stated, you should observe it. If an allowable length is not stated, consider keeping your abstract to within the limit of 250 words. This recommendation comes from the fact that the National Library of Medicine truncates abstracts in its MEDLINE database at 250 words. If an abstract that MEDLINE includes is shorter, it will appear in its entirety. If its length exceeds 250 words, its will be cut off at that limit. If this happens, what may be the most important part of the abstract—its conclusion—will not appear.

CONCLUSION

Both titles and abstracts should represent as well as possible within allowed lengths all of the major content of a paper. Informative titles and abstracts tell the reader in brief what the paper has to say. Indicative abstracts, used mainly for long review articles, simply tell the reader what the paper is about. Carefully considering what to put into a title and into an abstract can help an author decide on how to focus the content of the paper before even the first draft is written. Both the title and abstract cam, of course, be revised as much as needed before the final draft of the paper is reached.

REFERENCES

1. Ad hoc working group for critical appraisal of the medical literature. A proposal for more informative abstracts of clinical articles. Ann Intern Med 1987;106:598–604.
2. Mulrow CD, Thacker SB, Pugh JA. A proposal for more informative abstracts of review articles. Ann Intern Med 1988;108:613–5.
3. Iverson C. Chapter 2: Manuscript Preparation. In: Iverson C, and others. American Medical Association manual of style. 9th ed. Baltimore (MD): Williams & Wilkins; 1998:19–23.

CHAPTER 14

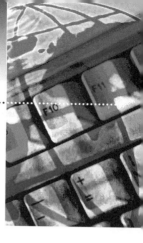

The First Draft: Tables

When you were preparing to write your paper, some of the materials at hand probably included tables of data. If the paper is to report clinical or laboratory research, an epidemiologic study, or a drug trial, you gathered analyzed numerical data in tables for a synopsis of your findings before you began to write. If your paper is to be a review article, you may have compiled tables to help you pull together concise summaries of what you had read. At some point between the first draft and the final version, you must decide which tables you really need, which tables you should replace by graphs, and which tables you should discard in favor of simply summarizing the data in the text. The first draft should, however, include tables that you believe at that point should be used, or at least notations for those tables. You may change your mind later, but it is easier to delete tables before you get to the final version of the paper than to add them then.

DECIDING ON USE OF TABLES

Uses for Tables

Tables serve four main kinds of needs.

- Presenting precise numeric values rather than just proportions or trends.
- Presenting large numbers of related data.
- Summarizing information made clearer in a tabular form than in running text ("list tables").
- Presenting complex information more clearly than in running text or a figure.

These needs are discussed in more detail below.

Decide as you work on your first draft what components of your paper will be more effectively and efficiently presented in one or more tables than in text. The tables you propose may be at hand—as indicated above—or you may have to prepare them. They need not necessarily appear as part of the first draft, but it should at least carry indications of your decision about tables at this point even if they are only notations of them in the text at appropriate points.

If you are going to use tables, do not delay in finding out what numbers of tables the journal may allow for text of a particular length. The journal may state in its information-for-authors pages its limit on the number of allowed tables. If it does not, look at papers in some recent issues, estimate the number of text words (excluding references), count the tables and illustrations (single or multipart figures), and calculate the number of tables and illustrations per thousand words of text. Then estimate in words what the final length of your text is likely to be and round the estimate down to the nearest thousand. Multiply the calculated limit of numbers of tables and illustrations per thousand by the estimate of your text length in thousands, and you have the maximum number of tables you can probably use, assuming you are using only tables and no illustrations.

If a typical paper in the journal has an estimated text length of 3300 words accompanied by 4 tables, the ratio of tables to text is 4/3.3 thousand or 1.2 tables per one thousand words of text. If your paper has a text of about 4800 words, round this figure down to 4000. Then $4 \times 1.2 = 4.8$ tables; in round numbers, 5 tables.

A useful general rule is no more than 1 table (or illustration) per 1000 words of text. Because the average page of text in a manuscript with double-spaced text and with 1-inch (or 3-centimeter) margins usually runs to between 200 and 250 words, the rule can be stated roughly as no more than 1 table (or illustration) per 4 pages of manuscript text. Some journals may accept a larger number of tables in relation to text length, but many will not because of the resulting difficulties in avoiding confusing page layouts.

Thus the first step in deciding on use of tables is figuring the maximum number the journal will probably accept in relation to the length of the paper. If you estimate that five tables and illustrations would be acceptable, and you will need one illustration, you will be able to use no more than four tables. But will you really need the maximum number the journal might accommodate? Peer reviewers and editors are likely to point out tables with so few data that they can be dropped in favor of giving the data in the text. Tables are more expensive to compose than text, so editors are prone to ask authors to eliminate tables. What if you have too many tables for the length of your text? What if you wish to reduce the odds that you will have to delete tables in a last-minute revision asked for by the editor? Which tables, then, can you eliminate and which should you keep?

Obviously the length of your paper in its final version and hence the number of tables it could include may differ from your estimate about the first draft. But it is safer to try to make a good estimate early on than to get stuck late in the writing process with too many tables for too short a paper.

Tables of Numerical Data

If you have read a short version of your paper at a research meeting, you may have shown some slides with simplified structures that made them easy for an audience to read rapidly. That would have been good judgment; a simple table can economically summarize and emphasize data for the desired effect on an audience. Such a table is illustrated in Figure 14.1. Do not use this kind of table in your paper; its content can be easily summarized in the text.

> Of the 3 patients with negative penicillin skin-tests, 1 was positive to noxicillin. Of the 7 patients positive for penicillin, 2 were positive for noxicillin. The difference in noxicillin positivity between the 2 penicillin groups is not statistically significant, Fisher's exact test ($P>0.05$).

If you persist in using a large number of such simple tables in your paper, you give the editor the impression that you have spent little time in thinking about how to translate your meeting talk into a journal paper.

Some tables should be dropped, not to be replaced by text statements but by illustrations. These are tables with data more important for their known or potential relationships than their precise values.

- *Data on two related variables:* a dependent variable whose values are determined by an independent variable, such as maximum systolic blood pressure after different doses of epinephrine, or maximum blood levels of alcohol after different doses of whiskey.
- *Data on one or more variables changing through time,* such as clinical data like temperature, blood pressure, leukocyte counts for a patient during a hospital stay.

Table 1. Skin reactions to noxicillin

Patient	Penicillin	Noxicillin
1	0	0
2	+	0
3	+	0
4	+	+
5	0	0
6	+	0
7	+	+
8	+	0
9	0	+
10	+	0

FIGURE 14.1.   A table put together to summarize data for the authors before they began to write their paper; the table was also used as a slide for a talk. The findings are readily summarized in words in the text; the table should not be used in the paper.

- *Data important to the reader for the extent of their differences and how these differences might be related to unknown factors,* such as differences in mortality rates for stomach cancer in the individual states of the United States.

Data of these kinds can usually be presented more effectively in one or more types of illustrations: graphs, charts of patients' clinical courses; epidemiologic maps; and other types.

Use tables when the reader will want exact values for numerical data. In a study that included measurements of serum electrolytes (sodium, potassium, chloride, calcium, phosphate, magnesium) and acid–base variables (pH, CO_2, bicarbonate), some readers may be interested in carrying out their own calculations of relations among the data. You could not meet these possible needs in the text without providing a long stretch of text crowded with numbers and hard to read.

The rules for use of tables with numerical data can be summarized thus.

- Do not use tables when the data can be summarized in the text with a few sentences.
- Do not use tables when the relations of data to each other or to a time sequence can be shown more clearly in a graph than described in the text.
- Do use tables when readers will want the exact values of more data than can be summarized in a few sentences of text.

Tables Instead of Text

In some papers, descriptive information (which can be summary statements, data, or both) may be more efficiently presented in a table than in the paper's main text. Perhaps the most frequent uses of tables in place of text are summarizing research reports in a review article or case information in a case-series analysis.

Full description of 5, 10, or more cases in the usual format of case reports can take up many pages of text. Even though each case may have its own nuances of clinical variation, the cases are likely to have many features in common, and each case description reads a good bit like the next. An efficient solution may be a large table that gives for each case only the essential numerical data (age, weight, temperature, and laboratory-test values) and brief descriptive phrases for symptoms, physical findings, roentgenographic findings, and so on. You might retain a full case report or two in the text to give the clinical "flavor" of the disease or syndrome. In constructing large case-summary tables, you will have to be very careful to find out what size tables may be acceptable to the journal.

If your paper is to be synoptic (a "teaching" article, a review), you can emphasize important points by listing in small tables the main features of a disease or syndrome, symptoms and signs of adverse effects, and differential diagnoses. Such "list" tables often include the frequency or percentage of occurrence for each item; these additional data help to make clear the relative importance of the listed items. The sequence in such tables should have a readily grasped logic: descending order of frequency; grouping by body systems; chronologic order, or some other clear basis.

Relations of Tables

When you have decided which tables are needed and which can be discarded, check the relation of the remaining tables to the text to be sure that their sequence is correctly tied into the text sequence; then number the tables accordingly. Next consider the tables as a sequence, with appropriate relations to one another. In many clinical papers the title of the first table may adequately identify the main subject of the paper, with shorter titles for the following tables. The first table, for example, in a review of 25 cases of puncture wound of the heart, might be titled "Puncture Wound of the Heart: Clinical Features". The second table might then be simply "Operative Findings and Postoperative Course". A look at the tables by themselves in the proposed sequence will help you judge whether the tables are understandable on their own (and they should be) and how well their titles are related to one another.

PARTS OF A TABLE

Editors and printers identify the parts of a table by terms that should be known by authors. These terms often turn up in correspondence or phone calls (especially from manuscript editors) about revision of papers (Figure 14.2).

- The *title* briefly describes the content of the table and includes the table number.
- The *field* is the space carrying numerical data and descriptive terms or phrases that together carry the table's message; the content of the field is arranged in horizontal *rows* and vertical *columns*.
- Each *column heading* identifies the kind of data and descriptions lined up vertically in the column beneath it.
- Each *row heading* identifies the kind of data and descriptions aligned in the horizontal row to its right.
- The *footnotes* explain details of content of the table.
- The column headings for the field are also known collectively as the *box heading;* the column heading for the row headings beneath it is called the *box heading for the stub* ("stub" is a term for the group of row headings).

Title ---

Table 1. Tired Author Syndrome: Case Features at Admission

Column

Patient*	Age (yr)	Sex	Weight (kg)	Height (m)	Temperature† (°C)	Chief Complaint
1	27	F	50.2	1.73	37.0	Double vision
2	31	M	65.7	2.01	36.4	Poor memory
3	42	M	75.3	1.94	37.2	Cramp, right hand
4	57	M	68.8	1.92	36.4	Poor appetite
5	61	F	63.5	1.81	37.1	Restlessness

Column Headings

Row Headings

Field

Row

Footnote:
* Patient 1 was seen at the University Hospital;
Patients 2–5 were seen at the General Hospital.
† Temperature of Patient 1 was measured rectally;
the other temperatures were measured orally.

FIGURE 14.2. A fictitious case-summary table illustrating the usual parts of a table and their names. Knowing the names of the parts can help an author in discussions with a journal's manuscript editor about revisions of a table.

Journal Style and Specifications for Tables

Journals rarely describe the details of style to be used in their tables, but these details can usually be quickly deduced from tables in recent issues. The size of acceptable tables is likewise rarely specified, so you will probably have to scan tables in a recent issue to work out estimates.

A useful rule for the width of a single-column table in a journal with a double-column page is that the width should not exceed more than 60 characters (and equivalent spaces) in a row (with its row heading). The width of a table running the full width of a page should not exceed 120 characters and spaces, including row headings. If you must use an even wider table, the journal may be willing to accommodate it on facing pages, but before you prepare and submit such a table, consider whether its data could be divided between two tables. For example, a very large table summarizing cases might be divided into one table for clinical features and a second table for laboratory-test data. If you must use a wide table that will span two facing pages, the reader may have trouble following each row across from the left-hand page to the right-hand page. Each row will be scanned more readily if the row headings at the left-hand end of the rows are repeated at the right-hand end of the rows (the right-hand edge of the field).

Another solution for some wide tables is reorienting the table so that columns and their headings become rows with row headings and the rows become columns. Such a change could be made, for example, with a table of data on 20 different laboratory tests for two patients. The data would usually be arranged so that the data on the tests for each patient form a 20-item row and the data for each test form a 2-item column. This arrangement would produce a very wide but very flat table; it would probably not fit on a single page. If the data are rearranged so that they form 2 columns, 1 for each patient, and 20 rows (each row giving the data on a test for the two patients), then the wide table becomes a tall, narrow table that will fit into a single column of a double-column page. A good test to apply to your table's format is to compare the number of column headings to the number of row headings. If the ratio is greater than 2:1, consider reorienting your table.

Logical Structures for Tables

Each of your tables should be readily understood without referring to the text; an adequate title will help to ensure that understanding. Needed even more is a logical structure for the data in the field that can be deduced from the column headings and row headings. Consider a table summarizing data from several cases. Most readers will expect to find the data arranged in a sequence of columns read from left to right that corresponds to how the data were collected in the clinical course. In such a table the rows might be logically arranged so that "Patient 1" (the first row) is the youngest patient and "Patient 6" (the sixth row) is the oldest. Another sequence of rows might progress from the "mildest cases" at the top to the "severest cases" at the bottom. In a table reporting data from a drug trial, the left-hand column might include pretreatment data and the right-hand column, post-treatment data. The rows would probably be arranged so that the top part of the table carries data from the "placebo group" and the bottom part data from the "drug group".

BUILDING A TABLE

Title

The title of a table should be specific enough to enable the reader to understand the table without referring to the text. The title should, however, avoid stating the information carried by the column and row headings. Consider a table summarizing in three groups of columns the admission diagnosis and roentgenographic and autopsy findings in 20 fatal cases of pulmonary embolism. Its column headings identify the nature of the findings as "Admission Diagnosis", "Chest Film", and "Autopsy", and its row headings run down from "Patient 1" to "Patient 20". The table title can be simply "Cases of Fatal Pulmonary Embolism" rather than "Twenty Cases of Fatal Pulmonary Embolism: Admission Diagnosis, Chest Film, and Autopsy Findings". If the reader needs details that the title cannot carry without being too long and that are not in column or row headings, these details can be carried in footnotes. Footnotes may specify, for example, drugs, dosage, and administrative procedure in a table with data from a drug trial.

Column Headings

Each column heading for numerical data should include the unit of measure for the data. That unit should apply to all data under the heading. Another unit of measure (and corresponding data) should not be used farther down in the column. Rather than forcing the reader to take note of a second kind of unit in a single column, restructure the table to accommodate the second kind of unit and its accompanying data in another column.

If groups of columns logically belong together, label them with a grouped-column heading and place a heading straddle-rule over the column headings to which it applies.

Patient	Admission laboratory data		
	Hemoglobin g/L	Serum glucose mmol/L	Serum albumin g/L

The straddle rule will eliminate any uncertainty about which column headings are included under the grouped-column heading.

Row Headings

If groups of rows are logically related, indicate such groupings and subgroupings with appropriate headings and indentations that will make clear their relations with each other.

Placebo groups
    Men
    Women
Drug treatment groups
    Men
    Women

If the row headings designate numerical data, give the unit of measurement immediately after headings (within parenthesis marks or after a comma, according to the journal's style).

Blood glucose, mmol/L
Blood glucose (mmol/L)

The Field

The columns should be centered under their headings, and numerical data should be centered on expressed or implied decimals.

	Patient 1	Patient 2
Serum glucose (mmol/L)	4.05	5.45
Serum creatinine (μmol/L)	105	97
Serum uric acid (mmol/L)	0.12	0.24

Intersections of columns and rows should not be left blank. If the appropriate datum at such an intersection is "none", indicate this fact with a zero.

Contraceptive	Healthy	Thrombophlebitis	Pulmonary embolism	Total cases
Oral	120	10	3	133
None	129	3	0	132

If an intersection does not have a datum, the absence should be indicated by three ellipsis dots (. . .) or an abbreviated notation explained in a footnote, such as ND for "Not done" or NA for "Not available" or "Not applicable".

Large numbers that need not be given with a high degree of accuracy can be expressed in smaller numbers with the appropriate multiplying column heading.

Tuberculosis cases (thousands)		Tuberculosis cases
120	rather	120 000
1.5	than	1 500

Do not use such headings as "$\times 10^3$" for thousands or "$\times 10^6$" for millions; these may be ambiguous as to whether the data below should be multiplied by such a factor or already have been multiplied by the factor.

Do not mix units in a single column of data (see related comment above under "Column Headings"). If, for example, a column gives data on duration of an effect on symptoms and some of the data are in days and some in weeks, change the weeks to equivalent totals of days so that the single column-heading "days" can apply to all data in the column.

Avoid pseudo-precision in giving percentages. Journals differ in what denominators they will accept as an adequate basis for a percentage. One rule used by some clinical journals is to allow percentages only for fractions with denominators greater than 50. The field of a table following this rule might carry data expressing cases with particular findings as a fraction of total cases examined, with percentages being given for the reader's convenience only for fractions with denominators greater than 50.

100 (98%)	47/58 (81%)	31/76 (41%)
32/46	12/25	7/10

Percentages given for compared fractions with small denominators are likely to imply statistically significant differences; if such differences are assessed statistically, the assessment must be based, of course, on the absolute numbers, not on the percentages. If the presence of data with and without percentages seems confusing, omit the percentages. If percentages are given for small numbers, confidence intervals provided for the percentages will, obviously, indicate their low precision.

If data in the field have been assessed statistically, indicate by footnotes the exact meaning of indicated assessments and the test applied. For example, "12.1 ± 0.3" could indicate a mean of 12.1 with a standard error of the mean of 0.3 or a standard deviation of 0.3 for the distribution of the values represented by the mean. Two means in a table assessed for statistical significance of the difference between them should each be tagged with the same footnote sign referring to a footnote explaining the test used and the conclusion drawn from it.

Group	Cases n	Serum calcium* mmol/L
Group 1	27	2.42 ± 0.13
Group 2	33	2.91 ± 0.05

* Plus-minus values (±) are standard errors of the mean. Difference between means assessed by Student's t-test, $P < 0.05$.

Make sure that all data in a table agree completely and exactly with their presentation anywhere else in the paper (title, abstract, text, or another table). Make sure, too, that all the data in a table are internally consistent—for example, that percentages that should add to 100% do add up correctly. Check all addition, subtraction, and any other mathematical operations implied in the table.

To save space, editors often allow some abbreviations to be used in tables that they would not allow in text. All abbreviations in tables (but not standard symbols for units of measurement) must be explained in footnotes, even if they are abbreviations explained in the text.

Dates

Shorthand forms for dates such as 5/15/99 can be understood differently in different regions. In Europe 4/11/87 means 4 November 1987; in the United States it usually means 11 April 1987. Use the form, number of day [space] abbreviated month [space] abbreviated year, to avoid misunderstanding: 4 Nov 82. Months can be indicated in a uniform style with 3-letter abbreviations (Jun for June, Jul for July, Sep for September) or the full 3-letter name (May for May).

Footnotes

As already discussed, footnotes can be used to explain abbreviations, define study conditions, state statistical assessments, acknowledge the source of the table (if it has been adapted from a published table), and in other ways make a table entirely understandable by itself. Some journals prefer to have elements in the table that are explained in footnotes tagged with superscript numbers corresponding to numbers of the footnotes, but superscript numbers can be confused with powers (squared, cubed) and reference numbers. Other journals prefer either a conventional sequence of footnote signs (*, †, ‡, §, //, ¶, #, **, ‡‡) or superscript lowercase letters in alphabetic sequence ([a], [b], [c], and so on).

Formatting of a Table for the Manuscript

All parts of a table should be double-spaced, including column headings and footnotes. Double-spacing is needed to give the copy editor enough room for marks to indicate publication style to the printer and for the compositor to insert typesetting codes.

Journals differ in use of horizontal lines (rules) and vertical lines in tables. In general, avoid rules and lines in the table except for a rule under the column headings to separate them clearly from the field (and straddle rules for grouped-column headings); the journal's manuscript editor can add rules and lines if they are needed for the journal's style. Word-processing programs are often used to produce tables, but their convention may apply both horizontal and vertical lines to enclose data within "boxes". This kind of table structure may be unacceptable to a journal, so the person keyboarding a table might advantageously avoid table-building through the "table" part of such a program and build it with careful use of tabs while paying attention to a need to center a vertical column of numerical values on the decimal point.

Place each table on a separate page. If a table cannot be completed on a single sheet, it can be continued onto a second sheet, with the title-number designation repeated, followed by "continued". If the table is extended down onto the second sheet, column headings, too, should be repeated to avoid any uncertainties about column alignments; if the extension is to the right on a facing sheet of paper, repeat the row headings.

Wide tables that will not fit onto a page with the normal vertical ("portrait") orientation may readily fit onto a page or pages with the horizontal ("landscape") orientation. If this solution is inadequate, a shift to a smaller font size may be needed.

ADDITIONAL GUIDANCE

Further detail on styles for tables and how to prepare tables can be found in Chapter 31, "Accessories to Text: Tables, Figures, and Indexes" of the Council of Biology Editors style manual (1) and in style manuals described in Appendix E.

CONCLUSION

The number of tables that can be used in a paper may be limited by a journal to minimize difficulties with page layouts and hold down costs of composition. You may avoid having to revise your paper to remove tables before you get to the final version by consulting the journal's information-for-authors pages for the limit or by examining papers in recent issues and estimating the ratio of tables per thousand words of text. Then with an estimate of the probable length of your first draft, you may be able to decide right away in working on it how many tables the paper will probably be able to carry.

Tables should not be used for numerical data if the data can be readily summarized in the text or their relationship needs to be made clear in a graph. Tables (tabular lists) can sometimes be used to summarize or emphasize descriptive content in the text.

The structure of each table should be carefully thought out for a logical internal sequence. The sequences of the column headings and the row headings should each have a clear logical basis for the sequence. Tables should relate to each other logically in sequence and title.

Great care should be taken with proper use of units and clear presentation of the data in the field of the table. It is important to be sure that data stated in both tables and text agree with each other.

REFERENCE

1. Style Manual Committee, Council of Biology Editors. Scientific style and format: the CBE manual for authors, editors, and publishers. 6th ed. New York (NY): Cambridge University Press; 1994.

CHAPTER 15

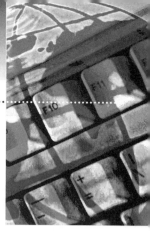

The First Draft: Illustrations

Before you began to write the first draft, you pulled together the materials you needed to start work on it. These may have included, for example, photographs, roentgenograms, scans, electrocardiographic tracings, graphs of experimental data. Some time before you prepare the final version of the paper (see Chapter 20), you must decide which illustrations to use or whether to use any at all. You should make these decisions as far in advance of the final version as possible. At least preliminary decisions should be made as you work on the first draft. You may need the services of someone skilled in producing computer-generated graphs, or a professional artist, or a photographer; the consulting time needed and the time needed for the work on illustrations are usually greater than expected.

DECIDING ON USE OF ILLUSTRATIONS

Illustrations should be used not just because they are available but for one or more of three needs.

- Evidence
- Efficiency
- Emphasis

The editor of the journal may not agree that all of the illustrations in the submitted manuscript serve one or more of these needs. If you can anticipate how the editor is likely to judge their usefulness, you may save some time, effort, and money by not having to discard illustrations and in revising the paper to rewrite the text related to them.

Evidence

Illustrations should be used in research papers only when they carry evidence needed to support a conclusion. If a paper is about a new species of *Legionella* as a pathogen in a case of pneumonia, a chest roentgenogram showing typical findings of pneumonia should not be used just because the film is available. The reader can be expected to take your word for a not-unusual roentgenographic diagnosis. But if the paper is about newly discovered structural details of a bacterium's flagellum, an electron micrograph of it is the main part of the paper's evidence.

Efficiency

An illustration may be far more efficient in presenting the evidence for a conclusion than a long statement in text. A family tree, for example, can quickly make clear that a newly identified syndrome appears in members of the family as a mendelian autosomal dominant trait; a written description of the same evidence would run on for many lines of text and probably would not make the point as efficiently. Numerical data make the same point whether presented in a table or a graph, but if the point is the relation of two variables, the reader will see it more quickly in a graph.

Emphasis

Emphasis is the reason least likely to be accepted by the editor for use of illustrations. A simple bar graph comparing deaths from lung cancer in men and women between ages 50 and 70 might effectively emphasize a big difference in mortality, but the same point could be stated just as efficiently, or more efficiently, in the text. Unless the difference in mortality is the main conclusion of the paper and the editor agrees that this point merits visual emphasis, you will probably be asked to drop the bar graph. The emphasis needed in a lecture to make sure that a point is caught by the audience is less likely to be needed in a paper. A slide in a lecture can help to drive home a point that might be forgotten by the audience as you move on to other points. The lecture cannot be replayed in the head; the text of a paper can be scanned again if the reader has missed a point.

WHEN NOT TO USE ILLUSTRATIONS

After reviewing the illustrations you have planned to use, you will retain those that seem justified by needs of evidence, efficiency, or emphasis. You will discard the rest, but you may still have too many. You can not be sure that the editor will let you use your final selection if the paper is accepted. Editors must hold down numbers of tables and illustrations because of their cost in production and potential difficulties in layout.

Check the journal's information-for-authors pages again for limits on illustrations. If you cannot find a limit, you can estimate a probably safe limit by scanning recent issues of the journal or using the procedure given in Chapter 14 for estimating the number of tables the journal may be willing to accommodate for a paper of a certain length. A usually safe maximum for the total number of illustrations and tables (any combination of the two) is 1 per 1000 words of text. If the total you are planning to use exceeds the journal's specified limit or your calculated limit, you have two possible solutions.

- Discard tables or illustrations in favor of equivalent statements in text.
- Combine two or more illustrations into a single, multipart illustration (or do the same with two or more tables). The illustrations to be combined should be related in subject; if they are graphs, they should also be similar in proportion and scale of lines and lettering. Finally, do not use illustrations that duplicate data presented in tables.

When you are not sure about whether to use an illustration, consider applying the rule that can be usefully applied to all parts of a paper: "When in doubt, leave it out".

PREPARING ILLUSTRATIONS

Unless you are competent in computer graphics, in drawing graphs manually, in photography, you are likely to need the services of others with these skills. They will be aware of the technical details needed for illustrations that will make their points and be technically acceptable to the journal. Incompetently prepared illustrations may lead the editor and manuscript reviewers to wonder about the competence of the author and perhaps even about the soundness of the text. Illustrators and photographers do need guidance from authors about what points the illustrations must make. Obviously, authors also have to provide both the raw materials for the illustrations—for example, numerical data, tracings, roentgenograms—and the journal's specifications.

If you plan to prepare your own illustrations you will find helpful various principles discussed in the books on illustration described in Appendix E. A notably valuable and comprehensive source is *Preparing Scientific Illustrations* (1). An authoritative guide to graphic presentations of numerical data with complex relationships is *Visualizing Data* (2). Many of the better computer programs for statistical analysis can generate good-quality graphics.

Line Illustrations

A wide variety of illustrations can be prepared with black lines inked on white paper. The simplest are graphs showing the relations of two variables, for example, a graph showing diastolic blood pressure for a large number of persons plotted against their ages. Many types of graphs and diagrams can represent clearly even complex data and relations; the possibilities are illustrated in detailed guides to graphic illustration; see Appendix E for some recommendations. The most complex line illustrations are drawings used instead of photographs to depict subjects like surgical procedures and anatomic views. Such drawings take a lot of a professional illustrator's time and are much more expensive than photographic equivalents.

Graphs and Diagrams

The illustrator needs the actual values for the numerical data to be shown, not just a freehand sketch of the graph or diagram you envision. Just as for a table, the units in which the data are expressed will have to be given. An independent variable is usually shown on the horizontal (x) axis, the dependent variable on the vertical (y) axis. If a graph is to show a line fitted to the data points, you should calculate enough values of y for values of x to enable the illustrator to place the line precisely. Be sure to specify that the graph or diagram is to be used for publication. Slide illustrations for a paper to be presented orally usually have to be more simplified than may be desirable for illustration in a published paper. A copy of the journal and a copy of its information-for-authors pages may help the illustrator in deciding how to proceed.

Computer graphics-methods can be used to produce a wide variety of graphs, but care must be taken to produce copy of adequate quality; see "Computer Graphics" below.

Electrocardiographic and Other Kinds of Tracings

Tracings recorded against a clean white background or an even-toned gray background may be copied photographically to yield the photographic equivalent of a line drawing (black lines against a white background). If some parts of the tracing lines are very thin, the photographer may not be able to reproduce the fine detail. Occasionally, tracings are better reproduced as a facsimile drawn on clean white paper that is then photographed. When this method is used, check closely on the drawn reproduction to be sure that it preserves exactly the characteristics of the original tracing.

Flow Charts

Diagrams can be used to illustrate relations of connected units—for example, a sequence of procedures such as in a diagnostic algorithm, or a "table" of organizational titles and responsibilities. For such diagrams the illustrator will probably want to have at least your rough sketch of what has to be shown and certainly will need exact terms and titles. You should type or print neatly any text to be used in the diagram to avoid misspellings by the illustrator. Some computer programs can construct charts of this type.

Family Pedigrees

Diagrams showing relationships among family members and generations should use well-established conventions, which are illustrated in text books on human genetics and genetically determined diseases. Generations are numbered with Roman numerals, the oldest generation represented being designated by roman numeral I. The symbols for members of a generation are usually arranged on a single line, with the symbol for the most senior placed at the left and numbered 1 (with the roman numeral for the generation, for example I-1) and the symbol for the most junior at the right (for example, I-5). Women and girls are represented by circles, men and boys by squares.

Molecular Graphics

The rapid growth of molecular biology and genetics has brought forth a wide variety of needs for graphic presentation of base sequences in DNA, diagrams of restriction sites, and other related graphics. Good sources with examples of such graphics are journals such as *Nature Genetics* and *Cell*. Another helpful source is Chapter 5 in the Briscoe book (1).

Computer Graphics

Graphs generated by laser printers are likely to be satisfactory for journal publication if careful attention is paid to the overall size of the illustration and to the size of lettering and symbols; see the section "Size and Format" below.

Graphs produced by a dot-matrix printer connected to a computer may be reproduced as line illustrations if the printer's impressions are dark enough; too often the photographs made from such copy contain too many lines, letters, numerals, or symbols that will not reproduce legibly. Your illustrator or photographer will be able to advise you on whether the copy will photograph well enough or should be prepared in a hand-lettered, drawn, or typed version before being photographed. Many of these problems can be avoided if copy is printed out with a high-density dot-matrix printer using a program that yields high-resolution images.

Continuous-Tone Illustrations

Even if you are skilled enough to draw graphs and diagrams acceptable for publication, you are likely to need a photographer to produce satisfactory prints of clinical views, roentgenograms, and photomicrographs that cannot be accurately or economically represented by line drawings.

Patients

Written permission to reproduce photographs of patients in which the patient might be identified should be acquired when the pictures are taken. Preferably, specific permission for use of a photograph in a journal paper should be sought again when you begin to plan the paper (as discussed in Chapter 4). Parts of photographs that might identify a patient should be blacked out or cropped, if possible. Keep in mind that although a close-up of a skin lesion, for example, may show what you wish to show, you (or the editor) may decide later that a longer view may also be needed to show the lesion's location.

Roentgenograms, Scans, Echocardiograms, and Related Kinds of Images

If only a section of a diagnostic image is the subject of interest, the whole image need not be photographed or otherwise reproduced, but be sure that the field of view is large enough to include structures that show the location of the point of interest. Images should not include labels that identify patients by name or case number. If successive images were taken on different dates, verify the dates and be sure the photographic copies are in the right sequence. Left and right orientations should be indicated if they are important.

Some abnormalities illustrated in images are difficult for readers to identify because of complex details in the view or subtleties apparent only to experts. The reader may be helped in seeing important details if the photograph of the image is accompanied by a line drawing showing in simplified or outline form the location and shape of the abnormality.

Photomicrographs and Electron Micrographs

A professional photographer will use lighting and color filtration to ensure the best images but will need your guidance on what fields are to be shown and whether low-power views will be needed to orient the reader on the location of high-power views. The photographer should keep records on the powers of microscope objectives used and the relation of the photographic print to the image size. A scale applied to the illustration can show the dimensions of the subject regardless of the degree of reduction applied to the photograph for fitting it into the journal's page layout. Letters and arrows may also have to be applied to the photograph to identify specific parts, or the photograph may be accompanied by a line drawing showing the main elements in outline, with identifying letters or abbreviations.

Black-and-White or Color Illustrations

Color printing is far more expensive than black and white, and few journals will publish color illustrations without passing on the cost to the author. If you think color illustrations are needed for your paper, be sure you know the journal's policy on, and charges for, use of color.

Color transparencies (slides) and color negatives (negatives for color prints) are usually preferred by journals over color prints. Because of the problems that might result from loss in the mail of transparencies and color negatives (as with pictures of a patient who subsequently died), you should ask the photographer to take duplicate exposures at the photographic session. Duplicating transparencies and negatives from their originals usually leads to degrading of color quality and image sharpness.

When do you really need color illustrations? Many medical illustrations can make their points as effectively in black and white. Some exceptions are illustrations of some skin lesions (like faint rashes), subtle histologic-stain colors, and multicolor scan images. If photographs you wish to use are in the form of color transparencies or color prints (and the subject cannot be rephotographed for black-and-white prints), ask your photographer to produce black-and-white copies. With appropriate filtering techniques you may get black-and-white equivalents that are almost as effective as the color originals.

SIZE AND FORMAT

Proportions

An illustration will usually fit within the layout of a journal's page if it has the proportions of a horizontal rectangle, with a longer horizontal than vertical axis. If the details of the illustration (letters, lines, and symbols of a line illustration and features of interest in a continuous-tone illustration) are not too small, and if the journal uses a double-column page format, the illustration may be printed as a single-column figure. If the detail is small, the illustration will be printed with a width roughly two-thirds of the page width or at the full width.

Square-format illustrations should usually have details scaled large enough to enable the journal to use the illustration as a single-column figure on a double-column page. Vertical-rectangle illustrations (vertical axis longer than horizontal axis) may have to be used for specific needs. One example is having to show together the changes of many variables over time. An illustration of the vertical-rectangle type may be acceptable if its detail is large enough to allow for reduction of the illustration to the width of a single column (on a double-column page). This point should be kept in mind by the illustrator or photographer doing your work. If you are drawing your own illustrations, pay careful attention to the sizes of letters and widths of lines and to how small or how large they will be after the illustration is reduced in size for printing (see "Details of Line Illustrations" below).

Some illustrations that might seem to need the format of a vertical rectangle at first thought, may be—with some reflection and ingenuity—reformatted to the square or a horizontal rectangle. An example is a chest roentgenogram. The original film of a chest roentgenogram, for example, has the proportions of a vertical rectangle. Do you really have to show all of the film? Could the feature of interest be shown more clearly if the illustration based on the film shows only a part of the entire field of the film? Can the illustration be made up in a horizontal rectangle, or at least in a square?

Details of Line Illustrations

Because an illustration should be understandable without having to refer to the text it accompanies, all of its features should be identified on it or in its legend. Graphs of numerical data must have their horizontal and vertical axes labeled to indicate the variables plotted and their units. Unless the labeling would crowd the field of a graph, individual lines should be labeled ("control group", "treatment group"; or, to save space, "CG", "TG") with any abbreviations explained in the legend. If most of the field of a graph is too crowded for such labels, they may be grouped in one part of the field in a key. An alternative is to use standard symbols in drawing the graph that can be reproduced and explained in the legend.

In drafting line illustrations (graph, family tree, and other types), care must be taken to produce lettering that in publication will not be obtrusively bold or too small. The lettering should be of such a size that after the illustration is reduced for publication the capital letters are approximately 2.0 mm in height. If the original drawing is twice as large as the illustration will be when printed, the capital letters should be drawn 4.0 mm high; at 3 times the size, 6.0 mm high. Lines for the x and y axes and the trend lines should be no wider than the width of the lines making up the letters.

Details of Continuous-Tone Illustrations

The most effective photographs are those that show the points of importance and no more. Hence photographs should be made of only the point of interest, cropped to indicate to the editor and printer the area of interest, or submitted with removable markings showing appropriate final cropping. In the process do not forget, however, that the orientation of the subject should be apparent. A photograph, for example, of a skin cancer on the upper cheek should probably include some of the outer corner of the eye or the forward part of the ear to make clear the location.

Wax pencil is often used to mark areas for cropping, but these marks are easily wiped off or smudged. Another procedure is to paste or tape a piece of translucent paper (like tissue paper) to the top of the back of the photograph so that it can be folded over the top of the photograph to lie over its face. On this paper mark (lightly) in pencil the area of the photograph that should be shown in the published illustration. A safer procedure is to mark crop lines with a ball point pen in the white margin of the photograph (if it has white margins) but never on the photograph. You could send with the photograph a sketch on a separate piece of paper indicating desirable cropping. Probably the best method is running off a xerographic copy of the photograph and marking the cropping lines on that copy; the copy will reproduce the photograph well enough for such instructions.

Details on a photograph can be emphasized, if necessary, with pressure-sensitive letters and arrows (available in art supply stores). Such identifying letters must be explained, of course, in the legend. Dark areas are best labeled with white letters; light areas, with black letters. If the exact size of the subject of the photograph is important, a short scale line from which dimensions can be judged should be part of the photograph. If the photograph is of a skin tumor, for example, a centimeter–millimeter rule can be laid on the skin so that its edge is seen in the finished photograph. A scale for a photomicrograph will have to be applied to it.

Labeling Illustrations

Each illustration must be labeled on its back to indicate its number (for example, "Figure 2"). Additional identification should include names of authors and a short title for the paper to help prevent loss of the illustration by an editor or a manuscript reviewer. The labeling is best done by typing the needed data onto a pressure-sensitive label. If such labels are not available, write the information on the back with a soft pencil while the photograph lies face down on a hard, flat surface; do not write on the back of a photograph with more than minimal pressure lest impressions of the writing show on the front. The labeling should indicate the edge of the photograph that should be regarded as the "top"; the proper orientation of a roentgenogram, a picture of a skin lesion, or a photomicrograph will not be apparent to the printer, and even the editor may have trouble in deciding what is the "top".

Grouped Illustrations

Photographs of closely related subjects are sometimes more effectively presented as a single, multipart illustration. An example is a general view of the cut surface of a kidney sliced longitudinally accompanied by several close-up photographs of details of the cortex, a pyramid, and the pelvis. Most journals would not wish to have such a composite illustration submitted already mounted on cardboard in the arrangement you think best. The better method is to label each component as a part of a single figure—for example, Figure 1A, Figure 1B, and so on. You can then send with the figure a sketch showing the components labeled and in the arrangement you prefer. The editor may not wish to use all of the components and may think of a better arrangement.

LEGENDS

Each illustration must be accompanied by a descriptive legend. A legend must include the figure number indicating the sequence in which the illustration was cited in the text ("Figure 12", for example), the subject of the illustration ("ventral surface of the liver as seen through the laparotomy incision"), any needed technical details such as stains and magnification, and additional description needed by the reader to understand the illustration without referring to the text.

Legends should be typed on a separate page of the manuscript as indicated in Chapter 20.

SUBMITTING ILLUSTRATIONS

Consult the journal's information-for-authors pages for instructions on how to submit illustrations. Most clinical journals prefer to receive illustrations as separate photographs on glossy paper, rather than receiving the original art work—a roentgenogram, an electrocardiographic tracing, or a photograph—mounted on illustration board (see Chapter 20). To avoid injury to loose photographs, place them in special envelopes available in standard photographic print sizes. The envelope should be labeled with the authors' names and a short title for the paper.

Be sure to keep any original art work on which the illustrations are based and at least one duplicate set of all illustrations in case of loss. Mail does get mangled occasionally or even lost!

CONCLUSION

Illustrations should be used when the evidence bearing on the conclusions of a paper cannot be adequately presented in a written description or in a table. Emphasis on especially important points to be made is another fair reason for their use. Limits set by a journal on the number of illustrations it will accept must be observed; if the journal does not specify the limit, it can be estimated by examining recent issues to calculate the number of illustrations (and tables) used per 1000 words of text.

Some illustrations are best prepared by professional graphic artists and photographers; numerous details in format, lettering, and labeling call for careful attention. Their legends should be written with a view to ensuring that the illustration can be understood when it is seen by itself with its legend, without consulting the text of the paper.

REFERENCES

1. Briscoe MH. Preparing scientific illustrations: a guide to better posters, presentations, and publications. 2nd ed. New York (NY): Springer-Verlag; 1995.
2. Cleveland WS. Visualizing data. Summit (NJ): Hobart Press; 1993.

CHAPTER 16

Revising Content and Structure

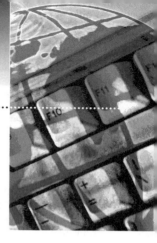

Most experienced authors expect to work through no less than two drafts of a paper before the final version. Indeed, the more experienced you become, the more you continue to see defects that need to be corrected, even in third and fourth drafts. Some authors revise the content and structure of a paper and its prose style at the same time, but it is more efficient to concentrate on content and structure first. Why polish the prose style of text you may discard later?

STEPS IN REVISION

Table 16.1 lists a sequence you might like to follow in revising your paper. This sequence need not be followed fully in some circumstances. Short papers, like "brief reports" and editorials, book reviews, and letters-to-the-editor, might be readily written and revised in three drafts. If you have coauthors, one or more may not be able to respond quickly with suggestions for revising the second, or a later, draft because of a trip abroad or an illness. You should insist with coauthors, however, on a definite schedule for revision and hold them to it.

Most first drafts are not good enough for review by coauthors or colleagues. You should revise the first draft's content and structure before you ask someone else, even a coauthor, to take time to read it. Unless you have a rapidly approaching deadline, put the first draft aside for a week or two before you look at it again. The labor of writing the first draft often drains the energy you need for looking critically at what you have written and for preparing the second draft.

All coauthors should be expected to read at least one of the early drafts

TABLE 16.1. A sequence for revising content and structure

Write the first draft.
   Hold the first draft 1 or 2 weeks, then revise its content for sequence and structure.
Work on the second draft.
   Distribute copies to coauthors and to colleagues willing to offer thorough criticism.
   Read this draft and make notes on revisions needed. Changes may include new
     decisions on tables and illustrations.
   Get written recommendations for revision from coauthors and other colleagues.
Work on the third draft: same procedure as for the second.
Work on later drafts.
   Confine readings to coauthors.
   Continue to concentrate on structure and sequence of content.
   When satisfied with content, move to revising for prose structure and style.

and recommend revisions of content and structure or indicate their approval of that draft. If a coauthor has had only a small part in the work leading up to the first draft, he or she may be excused from reading every draft. All coauthors must be expected, however, to read and approve the final version that will be submitted to the journal; see "Criteria for Authorship" near the beginning of Chapter 4 and "Principle 2" in Appendix A. Any coauthors who foresee an obstacle to reading the final version should authorize the author who will submit the paper to submit it without his or her final approval. An author in that position should give the submitting author a written and signed statement of approval of the last draft read. If the journal to which the paper will be sent expects to receive with the paper the signatures of all authors (on a form by which they affirm that the paper is submitted in its final version with the approval and consent of authors), the submitting author can include the written statement authorizing submission without a review of the final version.

THE GREAT VALUE OF EXTERNAL CRITICISM

Familiarity with the content of a paper often dulls the eye. After you have worked on the first draft and on revising it, you can easily fail to see defects that can be seen by others. If you have coauthors, they may readily pick up those defects. But if they have been closely associated with the research being reported, they may also fail to pick up defects, especially defects in evidence and interpretation. Sharper critics of your paper than your coauthors may be colleagues aware of, but not familiar with, the research you are reporting, the case you are describing, or the literature you are reviewing. Someone who does not understand every detail in a paper may be better able than the authors to see what is not clear, is out of sequence, deviates from the subject or—

what is most important—is lacking as needed evidence. Pick some honest friends to serve as preliminary "peer reviewers" and give you a close reading of the paper and all possible criticisms, not "friends" who will simply pat you on the back and tell you how good your paper is.

Keep in mind that you may wish to acknowledge in the paper the help you have gotten from reviewers who are not coauthors. If you do, you should ask their permission to acknowledge their help. They may have some unexpressed reservations about the paper or the reported work and be concerned that an acknowledgment of their help could be interpreted as their having given the paper a final approval.

AIMS IN REVISION

By the time you finish writing the first draft, you have been laboring so long in the work it represents that nausea may sweep over you when you sit down to revise. You may feel that you have done your job, that this is what you have to say, and that the reader is going to be impressed with your paper. But you have not finished your work until you have gone as far as you can to make sure:

- That you have said all that has to be said, and no more than is needed, for your message;
- That all elements of your paper are in the right sequence and every detail is clear to other readers.

Your job now is to shift from being solely a researcher or a reviewer of the literature toward being as sharp a critic of your paper as the editor of the journal to which you will send it and as those who are likely to read it for the editor, including the peer reviewers.

Editors and reviewers consider many and various questions in sizing up a paper. You can criticize your own paper just as sharply if you consider the same questions in reading your first and subsequent drafts. Many of these questions apply to any kind of paper.

The Title

Is the title accurate, succinct, and effective? Not all elements of the paper need be represented in the title, only those that make up the main message. For a paper that reports a double-blind trial of penicillamine for treatment of rheumatoid arthritis in which gold-salt therapy was the contrast (control) treatment, the title might simply be "Penicillamine Treatment of Rheumatoid Arthritis". But note that a hasty bibliographic searcher looking for papers with content about gold therapy would be more likely to pay attention to your paper if its title were "Penicillamine or Gold Therapy for the Treatment of Rheumatoid

Arthritis". The structure of the study could be described in a subtitle, "A Double-Blind Randomized Controlled Trial", if the journal allows subtitles.

Although well-edited journals do not allow most unexplained abbreviations in titles, the occasional use of abbreviations in online bibliographic searches now justifies including widely known abbreviations in titles after the full terms they represent, for example, "Peripheral Neuropathy from Infection with the Human Immunodeficiency Virus (HIV)".

Titles are more effective, more likely to catch the scanner's eye, when they begin with a key word; avoid nonspecific openings like "A Study of . . .", "An Investigation into . . .", "A Review of . . .", or "A Case Report of . . .". If the journal does not use subtitles, it may accept titles with subordinate elements after a colon: "Aspirin for Treatment of Headache: A Double-Blind Randomized Controlled Trial with Placebo Control".

The Abstract

Does the abstract represent the most important content of all the main sections of the paper, within the length allowed by the journal? If you worked up to your first draft by preparing an abstract before the outline, the abstract may contain all that it should. Be sure that the abstract summarizes the Introduction, the central text of the paper, and its conclusions. If the paper is reporting research, the central text to be represented includes the study design, experimental subjects (animals, human volunteers, patients), methods, results, and interpretations (Discussion). The abstract of a case report should briefly characterize the patient as well as the unusual features of the case. A review article usually has to be represented by an indicative abstract, one that tells what the review is about, rather than an informative abstract, one that represents the content in highly condensed form. The abstract of a metaanalysis should take the form used for research papers. If you did not check in the journal's information-for-authors pages on whether it accepts or expects structured abstracts before you started work on the first draft, now is the time to check on that point.

The Introduction

Does the Introduction make clear the basis for the main question considered, or the hypothesis tested, in the paper? Is that question or hypothesis made clear by the end of the Introduction? Research is undertaken because a question has to be answered. Is a new antibiotic a better treatment for pneumonia? Is a certain drug the cause of some cases of congenital blindness? Can bedsores be prevented by twice-daily massage of vulnerable areas of skin? The Introduction should describe what knowledge and lack of knowledge, or new information, led to the posing of these questions: the recent treatment of pneumonia up to the availability of the new antibiotic; unusual numbers of cases of congenital blindness being reported; dissatisfaction with present treatment of bed-sores. But the Introduction should not explain what is already known to readers who can understand all the terms in the title: pneumonia, congenital blindness, or bedsores need not be defined for most readers in one of the health care professions or their textbook descriptions summarized.

When your readers have come to the end of the Introduction, they should know from a research report the "why" of the research and the "what" it sought to answer, from a review article or metaanalysis what questions were posed for it, or from a case report why the case is worth reporting. The opening paragraph of an editorial or a book review should just as clearly indicate where you are going to carry the reader in the rest of the paper.

The Main Text

Is all of the rest of the text in the right sequence? Even though you wrote your first draft from an outline, you may have strayed from the outlined sequence in your rush to get the first draft written. Or the sequence may have been defective.

Because most research papers are cast in the conventional format of Introduction, Materials and Methods, Results, and Discussion, they are less likely to have a defective sequence than papers in less rigid formats. But the careful author of a research paper will make sure that the sequence is right in each of its sections. The description of the study (Materials and Methods) should usually follow the sequence in which the research was actually planned and carried out. The Results section should usually proceed from the findings or comparisons directly related to the main message of the paper to any subordinate findings. The Discussion should proceed from the apparent answer to the question posed in the Introduction to considering, as necessary, the validity of the evidence supporting this main conclusion—first your evidence, evidence from other studies—to considering counter-evidence, and on to resolving any conflicts in evidence. If lesser conclusions also have to be developed, they should follow the same sequence. But the main conclusion should be taken up first, with lesser conclusions following. Any implications of the study's conclusions, such as needs for further research or changes in diagnosis or treatment, should come at the end of the Discussion. As indicated already, the structure of a metaanalysis should be closely akin to that of a research report.

Papers without a formal structure as obvious as that of the research paper or metaanalysis are more likely to show defects in sequence. If you are writing a traditional-style descriptive review article, a case report, an editorial, or a book review, you may wish to reread the appropriate chapters from among Chapters 9 to 11 before you look at your first draft for possible problems in sequence.

Is all of the text really needed or can some be discarded? Does any of the text repeat information found elsewhere in the paper? Most first drafts, and even many finished papers, are overwritten. Introductions explain more than most readers attracted by a paper's title need to know. Results sections present data that have little or nothing to do with the message of the paper. Discussions open with a restatement of points made in the Introduction. Or they run on with speculations about the study's findings that go far beyond hypotheses that can be tested in the near future. In shorter papers like editorials and book reviews, authors may succumb to airing pet peeves that break the line of argument.

Does your first draft have paragraphs that can be dropped? You may be reluctant to leave out any text when you have sweated so hard in getting through the first draft, but remember that the reader will not thank you for unneeded text. The reader will thank you for a paper that gets to the point, sticks to it, and presents only content directly relevant to that point. If you decide to delete some text, you might wish to hold it in a separate file for possible later retrieval.

Is any needed content missing? Although many papers are overwritten, at least in early drafts, some needed content may be forgotten in writing the first draft. The outline was defective, or your writing was interrupted and then resumed without your looking at the preceding text. Such gaps will probably jump to your attention when you read the first draft through.

Have you applied the proper conventions for scientific reporting? Accurate scientific writing must use the generally accepted conventions for scientific papers, for example, correct symbols for metric units, proper microbiological nomenclature, unequivocal statistical statements, other conventions expected by journal editors and readers in your field.

Do data in the text agree with data in the tables? If you wrote the first draft with the tables before you, data in the text and the tables should agree. Your coauthors are likely to pick up discrepancies and know which figures are correct, but other reviewers may not know which of a pair of discrepant data is correct.

Have you cited unnecessary references? Have you omitted needed references? Careful reviewers of your second draft may note redundant or unneeded references. Cite only the references needed to support key statements in the text. If you must refer to a textbook description of a disease so that you do not have to describe the disease, refer to one or two complete and reliable sources; do not give an additional four or five to show that you are familiar with all of the related literature. Be sure, too, that all statements needing support with references cite them. The Materials and Methods section of a research paper, for example, should include enough detail to enable another investigator to repeat your study, but methods previously described need be represented only by cited references.

Can you omit any of the tables or illustrations? As you read the first draft, you may see that some of the data you collected have little to do with the point of the paper. Be no less willing to drop unneeded tables than unneeded text. Illustrations should be limited to those that will show what cannot be conveyed in text. If a case report, for example, mentions an electrocardiographic tracing that confirms a diagnosis of acute myocardial infarction, do not illustrate the tracing. The reader should be willing to take your word that the tracing was diagnostic.

THE MECHANICS OF REVISION

You have read your first draft with these questions in mind. You have written notes in the margin on what to do in the second draft, notes such as "delete", "move to discussion", "cut 2 references", "combine Tables 1 and 2". You are ready to prepare the second draft. This is the time to consider some practical steps that may simplify preparing the second and subsequent drafts.

Additional Copies

If your drafts are being keyboarded for you by someone else, you should consider asking for two or three copies of your first draft. You may need one copy to cut up for pasting of some paragraphs or parts of paragraphs in new locations for better sequence. Revising does not always call for complete rewriting of text, and each paragraph that can be moved intact is less writing for you and clearer copy for whoever is keyboarding the manuscript. You should retain one copy of the first draft as a safeguard against accidentally losing one or more paragraphs in your cut-and-paste work. And sometimes parts of your first draft may prove to be better than their counterparts in the fourth draft.

If you are reworking the manuscript yourself with a word processor you may not have to make additional paper copies at this stage because paragraphs and other segments of text are readily moved with the block-move function. Be careful, however, to keep backup files of each draft.

Draft Numbers and Dates

Unless you dated each page and identified the number of the draft as it was completed, you may subsequently mix up similar pages of different drafts. See "Identifying Drafts" near the end of Chapter 12. With word-processing programs such notations can easily be made as headers or footers that will clearly identify on every page of a draft its sequence among drafts and its date.

Revision by Coauthors

If your coauthors believe entire paragraphs or pages need to be revised for content or sequence, they should prepare new drafts of those pages so that they leave no question as to the changes they recommend. Their new pages should carry their initials and dates of revision to distinguish them clearly from your drafts.

CONCLUSION

The first task in revision is reworking the first and subsequent drafts to be sure that the paper says no more than it must say, that it says all that it should say, and that all of its content is in the right sequence. Revision along these lines should continue until every coauthor or other reviewer agrees that the content and its sequence cannot be improved. Probably at least three drafts will be needed; a long and complex paper may have to go through many more drafts. Once you and your coauthors or colleague-reviewers are satisfied with the content of the paper, you can begin to revise it in details of prose structure and style.

CHAPTER 17

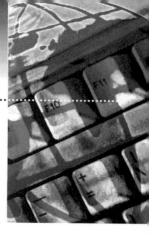

Revising Prose
Structure and Style

Whether a scientific paper gets published depends far more on what it says—the content and its sequence—than on the prose in which it is said. If the editor sees the paper as important for the journal's audience, minor defects in style are not likely to block its getting into print. But the paper with a less important message may sit in the editor's mind between acceptance and rejection. If the paper is cast in turgid and unclear prose, these qualities may tilt the balance to rejection. So as you bring your paper to the final version, you must look closely at how it says what it has to say. You must revise for the inevitable faults in the structure and style of your prose.

Revising prose is hard work. Few of us can write first drafts in fluent and clear prose. The problems in content and its sequence get worked over in early drafts. The time comes when you must make sure that what you have to say is said with the five qualities of good scientific prose: fluency, clarity, accuracy, economy, and grace.

FLUENCY

Fluent prose runs along as the reader expects it to run; the reader is not jarred by defects that interrupt the line of thought. Fluency depends in part on sentence structures and other details in style. It also depends on the connections between paragraphs and the sequence of thought within paragraphs (Table 17.1).

CLARITY

Clarity is the second quality of good scientific prose. The devices that produce fluency can also foster clarity (see Table 17.1). But other details in prose style affect clarity. The English essayist George Orwell made the point

TABLE 17.1. The five qualities of good scientific prose

Fluency
   Forward-moving sequence of thought
      Elements of critical argument in the right sequence (see Chapters 5 to 11)
      Narrative sequence in the right order (see Chapters 5, 6, and 7)
   Paragraphs connected
   Forward-moving line of thought in each paragraph
   No slowing or interruptions from obvious devices of style; from unclear, sluggish,
      excessively long sentences; or from graceless terms
Clarity
   Clear structure and movement of content; see "Forward-moving sequence of thought"
      under "Fluency" above
   Clear connections of paragraphs
   Intent of each paragraph clear at its outset; each paragraph limited to that intent; no
      paragraph unclear because it includes more than needed for that intent
   Clear use of modifiers
   Unambiguous antecedents for pronouns
   Right choices of verb tenses for the sequences of actions
Accuracy
   Correct choice of words and terms
   No misspelled words
   Right verb tenses for discontinuity or continuity of action
Economy
   No unneeded words or phrases
   Verbs rather than abstract nouns
   No unneeded clauses
Grace
   The qualities of fluency, clarity, accuracy, and economy
   Correct sex references
   Humane terms and phrases
   Standard formal usage

in a memorable epigram (1): "Good prose is like a window pane". What you have to say should not be obscured by how you say it. Another Englishman, T E Lawrence (2), put it this way: "Prose is bad when people stop to look at it". Errors or crudities in your prose are like blobs of mud on Orwell's window pane; they come between the reader and the message. Obvious devices in prose style have the same effect; the reader pauses, eye caught by the device and mind diverted from the message.

ACCURACY

Accuracy is the third and perhaps most valuable quality of good scientific prose. Accuracy depends in part on clarity but needs more. Fastidious attention to accuracy extends beyond verifying calculations and the other steps taken to validate evidence. You must be sure that the words you choose are the right and best words for the intended meaning. You must be sure that you do not convey a wrong meaning through misspelled words.

ECONOMY

Economy is the fourth quality of good scientific prose. Journal publication is expensive; editors have to make efficient use of their pages. The hard-working professional has little time to read; economical prose is usually much clearer than wordy prose. Cast out all words not needed, words that slow the reader.

GRACE

What is graceful prose? The man or woman you call "graceful" goes beyond politeness to act with an eye to the needs and comfort of others, striving to make easier and more pleasant even the minor contacts of daily life. The qualities of graceful prose include fluency, clarity, accuracy, and economy; graceful prose does not irritate or bore readers and thus distract them from the message. Graceful prose guides readers along a line of thought; paragraphs are linked so that the reader does not start a new paragraph wondering why it follows to the one just finished. Graceful prose does not try to impress the reader with erudition, status, or clever stunts in style. Graceful prose does not offend sensitive readers with inhumane statement. All that the writer of graceful prose strives to do is done to serve the reader.

YOUR ATTITUDE TOWARD REVISING PROSE STYLE

The task of revising may bring back painful memories, those restless hours with the burdens imposed by fussy English teachers. What was the need for that nitpicking about dangling participles and ambiguous antecedents? We were not convincingly told then that we are judged not only by what we say but how we say it. Samuel Wesley (3) knew it: "Style is the dress of thought." You would not go out in dirty clothes to look for a job. Nor should you write a paper that must make its way on its message alone. If how you present that message offends the reader (the editor, the peer reviewer), the message may not get into print.

Revising your prose will be hard work if you have not been in the habit of thinking about the countless details that make up style. But the more you revise your writing, the more quickly you come to see faults. Possibilities for revision are endless. Many papers that editors would regard as well-written can be tightened up further when worked over by a copy editor, shortened by at least 5 to 10%. I shall never forget having struggled to condense a letter-to-the-editor for *The Lancet* from 500 words to 250 words only to find that the copy editor cut it down to 225 without dropping any of its message. Training yourself in how to revise calls for becoming aware of what defects to expect to find, looking for them, and learning how to correct them.

A SCHEME FOR REVISING PROSE STYLE

In revising early drafts for better content and its sequence, you first worked on the big defects: missing content, unneeded content, wrong sequence. In later stages of revision you take care of smaller problems such as unneeded citations and errors in numerical data.

Revising your paper to improve its prose structure and style should also start with the larger elements of prose (paragraphs) and then move to dealing with the smaller elements (sentences, phrases, words). Improving paragraph divisions and linkages may call for rewriting entire sentences or for new sentences; these sentences themselves could turn out to have defects in some of their details.

1. Look at your paragraphs for length in relation to their content. Divide excessively long paragraphs at logical points for new divisions.

2. Look at how the paragraphs are connected. Consider how the closing sentence of a paragraph and the first sentence of the next might link them for a clearer sequence. Revise the sentences to make the linkage clear.

3. Check each paragraph to see whether its internal sequence moves along a clear line of thought. Does the paragraph flow readily along from sentence to sentence?

4. Look at the lengths and structures of sentences in each paragraph. Do too many have the same length and structure? Should you divide some sentences, or join some? Should some structures be inverted for variety in rhythm? For different emphasis? For movement from the known to the unknown?

5. Within each sentence are modifiers placed with what they modify? Are any modifiers not needed? Are the antecedents of pronouns unambiguous? Does each verb have the right tense to make clear the sequence of actions?

6. Have you chosen the right word at each point for what you mean to say? Does each verb have the right tense to state accurately discontinuity or continuity of action? Are any words misspelled?

7. Prune out all unneeded words. Can you tighten up your text by converting some abstract nouns to verbs? Can you replace any clauses by phrases?

8. Make sure that all sex references are accurate. Prune out slang, dehumanizing terms, unwitting ethnic slurs, and other details that make for graceless prose.

9. For the last step, read the paper aloud. You may become aware of defects such as weak paragraph links that interrupt the paper's flow. If you find yourself breathless or stumbling, you may not have gone far enough with shortening sentences or changing their structure. You may find overlooked slang or unintended rhymes. Your fifth draft may have to go into a sixth.

See Table 17.2 for a summary of this sequence.

REVISING FOR FLUENCY

Paragraph Length, Connections, and Structure

What is a paragraph? Not only a unit of thought. A word is a unit of thought; a sentence is a unit of thought. Perhaps I can define a paragraph by describing what it does for the reader. Imagine how a paper would strike you if it had no paragraphs or text headings; it would be a massive, intimidating block of words broken only into columns. Would you have the courage to start reading it? The paper has the same content whether it is cut into paragraphs or not. Why is it less intimidating when paragraphed?

Reading a paragraphed paper is like being taken on a tour of the author's garden. We come to the gate and pause while we are told what kind of garden we are about to visit—the Introduction. Then we step through the gate and pause by the tool shed to look at a map of the garden—a paragraph on study design. We step inside and pause while the author describes the tools—a paragraph on methods. At each paragraph the reader pauses while

TABLE 17.2.   A sequence for revising prose structure and style

Review and revise large elements first.
   Paragraph lengths
   Connections of paragraphs
   Internal sequence of each paragraph
Move to sentences, the elements of paragraphs.
   Sentence lengths
   Sentence varieties
Move to elements of sentences.
   Clauses and phrases
   Modifiers
   Word choices
Read the revised text aloud to catch defects you overlooked in the steps above.

the author makes a point out of the details represented by the sentences. The end of the paragraph means that the author is now moving the reader to the next paragraph to see a new point or set of closely related points developed. The indentations at the beginnings of paragraphs are polite signals for pauses and progress along the author's argument. An English student of prose style, Herbert Read (4), sums up this function of the paragraph thus: "The paragraph is a device of punctuation".

Paragraph Length

An Alice-in-Wonderland rule for paragraph length might be "Just long enough and not too long". A paragraph should come to its close when what it promised at or near its beginning has been delivered. The length of a paragraph may have been determined when its topic was laid down in the first-draft outline. But when you finish the paragraph, it runs to two pages typed double-spaced. Is this too long? Probably. No authority can give you a firm rule on paragraph length, but paragraphs of more than 25 typed lines are likely to be too long. Paragraphs of fewer than 5 or 6 lines tend to have too little development of a topic or represent what is really a fragment of either adjacent paragraph.

An excessively long paragraph often can be broken into two shorter paragraphs by finding a logical way to divide its topic into two related subtopics. A review of adverse effects of a drug includes a paragraph on cardiovascular effects; the paragraph runs on for 30 typewritten lines. Perhaps the topic "cardiovascular effects" can be divided into the subtopics "effects on the heart" and "effects on peripheral circulation". If so, break this long paragraph into paragraphs, each carrying one of the two subtopics. Breaking a long paragraph into two will probably call for more than simple division; you may have to write new opening and closing sentences to provide the right connections.

Paragraph Connections

Steady movement, a quality of fluent and graceful prose, should run through an entire paper. The stopping points at ends of paragraphs and ends of sections should not really be stops but pauses that close out units of thought and signal to the reader that a new start is about to be made. The signal comes in part from the format itself. A new section in a paper is signaled by a heading such as Materials and Methods. The start of a new paragraph is signaled by the paragraph indentation. But if you are to maintain that graceful quality of motion at the paragraph pauses, each new paragraph must seem to be linked to that preceding it.

One succinct definition (2) of the right structure for a paragraph advises that it ". . . should . . . have a start, a climax, couplings fore and aft, a finish". "Couplings fore and aft" means that the sentence closing a paragraph (the "coupling aft") should set up the basis for the starting sentence (the "coupling fore") of the following paragraph. One device for this linkage is stating in the last sentence of a paragraph a word or phrase that is central to the line of thought and can be stated again in the same or a similar form in the first sentence of the following paragraph. Note that I have linked the paragraph you are reading to the one above by this device. The paragraph above concluded that a ". . . new paragraph must seem to be linked to that preceding it". The paragraph you are reading opens with a sentence that includes the phrase "couplings fore and aft", a variation on "links" and "linkage". This device should not be so clumsy that you force the reader to see it, but it should be effective enough to show that a new paragraph is about to carry you from a point just developed in the preceding paragraph into a new but logically related point.

The "coupling fore" should not be so far down in the top half of the paragraph that the reader proceeds without a sense of linkage. Consider the sequence of paragraphs in a review on adverse effects of a drug. In your outline you arranged the sequence so that it runs from the most important adverse effects to the least important. The paragraph on the important cardiovascular adverse effects ends as shown below and is followed by a new paragraph.

> . . . and these cardiovascular effects are severe enough in some patients to make pleomycin an antibiotic not to be used in cases complicated by ischemic heart disease.
> Brown and Black (13) found two cases of occult gastrointestinal bleeding among 79 patients treated for mixed-flora bacterial pneumonias. A similar rate has been reported by White and Gray (14). A much lower rate was found in 153 cases (15) at the Cheselden Hospital . . ."

The reader goes three sentences into the second paragraph without finding out unequivocally that it is concerned with hematologic adverse effects. The opening sentence, "Brown and Black . . ." might be taken to imply a shift from cardiovascular effects to another topic, but "occult . . . bleeding" might also be read as a link into discussion of vascular effects in more detail. Why not provide a clear link?

> . . . cardiovascular effects are severe enough in some patients to make pleomycin an antibiotic not to be used in cases complicated by ischemic heart disease.
> Hematologic effects can be serious enough in patients with peptic ulcer to justify . . .

Opening the new paragraph with "Hematologic effects" (a parallel with "cardiovascular effects") provides a linkage that tells the reader you have finished discussing cardiovascular effects. After the brief mental pause signaled by the paragraph indentation, the reader knows without doubt that the author has moved into hematologic effects. The reader is not left uncertain as to where the line of the paper is moving.

Paragraph Structure

Sentences have structure and papers have structure; they need structure if readers are to grasp without too much work what they have to say. Paragraphs need structure too. The start of a paragraph should seem to be aimed toward a point; through the middle the reader should sense that the paragraph is moving to that point; at its close the point should have been reached. How you give the reader this sense of movement from a start through mid-ground to a finish depends on the subject of the paragraph.

Paragraph as Narrative

Some paragraphs need the structure of narrative. A paragraph that serves as the introduction to a research paper is like a little story. It starts at a point in the past when some question emerged and suggested need for the research. We are moved along in time with a brief review of the answers to the question that came from the research efforts of others. The paragraph then brings us up close to the present by pointing out that these answers have not adequately answered the question. It concludes at the present by briefly announcing the authors' just-completed research that is the topic in detail of the rest of the paper. This paragraph is a narrative; it tells a story that moves forward through time.

Paragraphs in the case history that makes up the central part of a case report invariably have to describe details in a narrative sequence: the complaint, the hospital stay, death or discharge. One paragraph might suffice to carry the elements of this narrative if the case history is short. More often the successive parts of the story are told in separate paragraphs. Paragraph 1 gives the initial complaint, the admission history, and examination findings; paragraph 2 summarizes the initial laboratory data; paragraph 3 summarizes the clinical course in the hospital; and paragraph 4 describes the autopsy findings, first the gross findings at the autopsy and then the histologic findings issued later. The case history carries the story in four paragraphs but each has its own narrative sequence.

Paragraph as Argument

The narrative sequence may be inappropriate when a paragraph needs the structure of argument (see Chapter 5). A paragraph in a review of adverse effects of alcohol in various organ systems discusses effects on the heart. The paragraph starts at the present, making clear that the heart and the question of adverse effects are the subject, and then moves to consider studies that have shown adverse effects. These studies are not presented in chronologic sequence but in a sequence of increasingly convincing evidence. Next the paragraph assesses studies that have not shown adverse effects, again in a sequence of increasing strength of evidence, and moves on to weigh finally the conflicting evidence. The paragraph closes, as argument should, with the answer that emerges from the evidence weighed.

In reviewing your paragraphs for possible revision, pay heed to whether each paragraph has a clear internal sequence and whether this sequence gives a sense of movement. Each paragraph should start, move along a line, and stop. The very short paragraph does not seem to start, move, and then stop. The very long paragraph may have a start, but then gets into interminable movement that gives the reader the feeling it will never come to a stop.

Revising Sentences for Fluency

Fluency within paragraphs can also depend on the structure of their sentences. Sentences with unvaried structure and unvaried length can make for monotonous reading; the irritation can become an obstacle to ready reading. You have probably read papers that run on like this passage.

> Failure in early detection of breast cancer in women has been a major clinical problem for many years. Smith and Jones (15) found that 15% of physicians do not examine the breast in routine examinations. Brown and White (16) found a similar figure in their most recent study in Canada. Roe and Doe (17) found a lower figure only for physicians having wives with a history of breast cancer. Thomas and Stephens (18) have called attention to these figures. The last authors have concluded that failure in early detection of breast cancer is mostly due to failure to examine the breast routinely.

Every sentence in this passage is a declarative sentence. Each sentence has the same sequence of subject, predicate, and object. The same or similar phrases appear in several sentences. All the sentences have almost the same length. What about this version?

> Why has failure to detect breast cancer early in women been a major clinical problem for many years? A study in the United States (15) and one in Canada (16) found that about 15% of physicians did not examine the breast in routine examinations. Only physicians whose wives had a history of breast cancer showed a lower rate (17) of failure to examine. From these findings, Thomas and Stephens (18) drew the right conclusion: To detect breast cancer early, examine the breast routinely.

This version flows more easily. The irritating and hence arresting monotony of the first version has been erased. Sentence lengths and structures differ. A question is included. Instead of a catalog of points we get a line of thought.

A second important need is for sentence structures that make for a ready flow of reading from one sentence to the next. In general, sentences should open with known information obviously related to what was stated in the preceding sentences and close with the new information. Consider the last sentence in the example just above.

> From these findings, Thomas and Stephens (18) drew the right conclusion: To detect breast cancer early, examine the breast routinely.

"From these findings" is the known information just stated in the preceding two sentences. "To detect breast cancer early, examine the breast routinely." is the new information "Thomas and Stephens drew" from the known information. Some authors might have written the last sentence as "To detect breast cancer early the breast should be examined routinely was the conclusion drawn by Thomas and Stephens (18)"; this is an inversion that violates the general rule of moving from the known to the new. For a more detailed discussion of this principle, see the paper "The Science of Scientific Writing" (5) by Gopen and Swan.

REVISING FOR CLARITY

Accuracy is the most valuable quality of good scientific prose. But your prose can be accurate without being entirely clear: all of its elements can be correct, but their message may not be readily understood. Some defects in clarity are due to sequences within sentences that do correspond to what readers are likely to expect. Other defects in clarity arise from words correct in themselves but confusingly related to each other.

Revising Sequences within Sentences

Sentence sequence is a complex topic but some general rules can be helpful. One has just been discussed above.

- The content of a sentence should, in general, move from the "known information" to the "new information".

Two other rules are closely related.

- The topic of the sentence should be made clear at, or near, its beginning (in Gopen and Swan's "topic position" [5]).
- The "new information" expected by the reader should be at, or near, the end of the sentence (the "stress position" of Gopen and Swan [5]).

A simple example illustrates these rules.

> Atherothrombotic disease occurs late in life in patients with this condition.
>   [This sentence is in a paragraph about a question of treatment for pure hypertriglyceridemia (the paragraph topic); this sentence deals with one possi-

ble complication of the condition. A clearer sequence would probably be an inversion of the example.]

In patients with this condition [the topic position], atherothrombotic disease occurs late in life [stress position; new information relevant to the topic].

The paper by Gopen and Swan (5) already cited offers a thorough and truly helpful discussion of these aspects of sentence structure.

Piled-up Modifiers

Medicine and related fields use many compound terms made up of a noun and one or more modifiers that may themselves be nouns. The meaning of many compound terms is clear because they are used widely and frequently. But other compound terms may need rewording or the adding of hyphens for clarity. The term *liver function test* could mean either a "function test" applied to testing of "liver" or a "test" applied to "liver function". The second reading is the usual one even without the help of a hyphen to tie "liver" and "function" together, as in "liver-function test". The hyphen is not needed because we understand that the single term can also be read as a combination of "liver test" and "function test", the two modifiers "liver" and "function" each applying equally to "test". A similar compound term is toxic shock syndrome. We do not pause to ask whether this is a "syndrome" of "toxic shock" or a "shock syndrome" that also is a "toxic syndrome"; we know that it is a syndrome of toxic shock. Compound terms that contain no more than two modifiers usually are clear once established.

Compound terms with more than two modifiers may be unclear to readers save those familiar with the field in which the terms developed. A fictional example (derived from a real example) is "normal Fc receptor mediated marrow mononuclear phagocyte system function". Does this term mean "normal function" of "marrow mononuclear" cells serving as a "phagocyte system" through "Fc receptor" mediation? Or does it mean "function" of the "marrow mononuclear" cells as a "phagocyte system" "mediated" by "normal Fc receptor"? Another example is "hospital nurse physician staff interaction". Does this term refer to "interaction" of "hospital nurse" with "physician staff"? Or to "hospital nurses" and "hospital physicians" interacting in the "staff"? It probably refers to "interaction" of nurses and physicians in a "hospital staff" but who except the author can be sure?

If you must use a term with more than two modifiers, consider connecting by hyphens those related in function, or dividing the term into two terms, or taking both steps. The first example in the paragraph above might be made clearer by hyphenating and rearranging some of its elements: "normal function of the Fc receptor-mediated mononuclear phagocyte system in marrow" (if I interpret the term correctly to mean that the "mononuclear phagocyte" system is in the "marrow" and its function mediated through Fc receptors is normal). Semantic tangles of this kind can be avoided by not coining terms with more than two modifiers.

Unconnected ("Dangling") Modifying Phrases

The reader's eye sees what it expects to see, even if what it sees does not exist. This is why a common defect is often overlooked by authors and fast readers: the modifying phrase unconnected to a word that should be, or could be, modified. A frequent, widespread flaw of this kind is in sentences that begin with the modifying phrase "Based on . . .".

> Based on our failure to find bacteria in the blood cultures, we concluded that the patient had fungal endocarditis.

You can test for a dangling phrase by placing the modifying phrase right after the noun or pronoun it might be supposed to modify. What is "based on our failure"? Does this sentence mean "We, based on our failure to find . . . , concluded that . . ."? Or was the patient "based on": "We concluded that the patient, based on our failure . . . , had fungal endocarditis"? Surely the endocarditis was not "based on our failure to find . . .": "We concluded that the patient had fungal endocarditis based on our failure to . . .". The modifying phrase appears to be related logically to "concluded" but the sentence cannot be read "We concluded, based on . . . , that . . .". The error in the sentence is failure to provide the truly modified but only implied word, "conclusion", the conclusion being logically derived from, and hence "based on" the "failure". A corrected version reads thus.

> Our conclusion, based on failure to find bacteria in the blood cultures, was that the patient had fungal endocarditis.

"Based" is the past participle of the infinitive *to base*. Other frequently seen variants of this defect are unconnected modifying phrases that begin with a present participle (the verb form ending in *-ing*).

> Interpreting failure to find bacteria in the blood cultures as evidence of fungal endocarditis, the plan of treatment was changed.

Who or what was "interpreting"? Surely not "the plan of treatment": "The plan of treatment, interpreting failure . . . , was changed."? The action "interpreting" can be carried out only by a person. In the example above, "interpreting" presumably modifies some unstated person or persons.

> The attending physician, interpreting failure . . . , changed the plan of treatment.

There is a general rule for detecting an unconnected, or "dangling", participial modifier. Test the clarity of a sentence that begins with a modifying phrase headed by a verb form (present or past participle) by reading the sentence with the phrase or clause placed right after the word it seems to modify. Sometimes that word cannot be found, as in the "interpreting" example above, and must be added, or the sentence must be rewritten entirely.

Misplaced Modifiers

A closely related defect is the modifier so far from the word it modifies that the connection is lost.

> At the nadir, with the highest doses thrombocyte counts were decreased in these patients to an average of 10% of initial values.

What does "at the nadir" modify? What thing was, or action occurred, "at the nadir"? Not "doses"; the sequence of the sentence indicates that the drug effect followed initiation of "the highest doses". Not "thrombocyte counts": the sentence implies that the thrombocytes were being counted throughout the course of treatment. "At the nadir" seems to tell us when "counts were decreased" to the stated level.

> With the highest doses, thrombocyte counts in these patients were decreased at their nadir to an average of 10% of initial values.

The sentence may still be unclear because of the unfamiliar term "nadir" (lowest point). A simpler version would be clearer.

> With the highest doses, the lowest thrombocyte counts in these patients were an average of 10% of initial values.

Modifiers should be kept close to what they modify.

Ambiguous Antecedents

Your meaning may be ambiguous if you do not make clear the word to which a pronoun refers, its antecedent.

> Failure of treatment with penicillin could not have been predicted because of the defective assay method used. Unfortunately, this occurs in many hospitals.

What is the "this" that occurs in many hospitals—being unable to predict, use of a defective assay method, or failure of treatment?

Similar confusion arises from using *it* as an indefinite subject and *it* as the third-person neuter pronoun in the same sentence.

> Cimetidine is highly effective in suppressing gastric acid secretion in such cases. It is unfortunate that it is not prescribed more frequently.

The indefinite subject *it* at the beginning of the second sentence and the neuter pronoun *it* referring to "cimetidine" momentarily seem to refer to the same antecedent, but they do not. Revising to drop the indefinite *it* improves clarity.

> Cimetidine is highly effective in suppressing gastric acid secretion in such cases. Unfortunately it is not prescribed often enough.

Another type of ambiguous antecedent results from the false modesty that leads authors to refer to themselves as "the authors" rather than "we".

> Smith and Jones (16) found statistically significant lowering of diastolic blood pressure by hypopressol and only minor adverse effects, whereas Brown and White (17) report that its use is frequently accompanied by episodes of cerebral ischemia. The authors conclude that the drug should be used only in carefully selected cases.

Who are "the authors" at the beginning of the second sentence, Smith and Jones, or Brown and White, or the authors of the paper containing this passage? The lack of citation numbers after "the authors" implies the authors of the passage. Why not dispel ambiguity and write, "We conclude that . . ."?

Unclear Sequences Due to Wrong Choice of Verb Tenses

Sequences of events may be unclear when verb tenses are not chosen carefully. This fault often appears in case reports. A case description, for example, starts thus.

> The patient was admitted to Erewhon General Hospital on 1 November 1978 with a bleeding duodenal ulcer.

After a description of clinical events during that admission comes a paragraph about preceding events that opens thus.

> In June 1976 the patient was admitted to Utopian County Hospital with hematemesis not diagnosed during that hospital stay.

The earlier date in the second statement should show that the event at Utopian County Hospital occurred before the event of November 1978 at Erewhon General Hospital. But the sequence of the two descriptions tends to confuse the reader; perhaps the "1976" is wrong. This confusion could have been avoided by using the past perfect tense in the second description, "had been admitted", to make clear it refers to an event antedating that described in the first sentence.

> The patient had been admitted to Utopian County Hospital in June 1976 with hematemesis . . .

Now the sequence of events is clear.

REVISING FOR ACCURACY

Accuracy is the most valuable quality of good scientific prose. Correct use of scientific nomenclature (see "Nomenclature" in Chapter 19) is the main ingredient of accurate scientific prose, but accuracy also depends on carefully choosing the right word for the right meaning.

Confused and Misused Word Pairs

Some pairs of words with closely related, but not identical, meanings are frequently misused in the medical literature. The words defined below are some of the most frequently misused pairs.

accuracy: the degree to which a measurement or statement is correct

precision: the degree of refinement to which some thing is measured, or to which a measurement is reported; *precision* applied to statements implies qualities of definitiveness, terseness, and specificity

case: an episode or example of illness, injury, or asymptomatic disease; not a patient (see comments below under "Dehumanizing Words" in "Revising for Grace")

patient: the person cared for by the physician, nurse, or other professional person

comprise: equivalent to "includes"; "The curriculum comprises six courses."

compose: equivalent to "make up"; "Six courses compose the curriculum."

dosage: the amount of medicine to be taken or given in a period, or the total amount; not the amount taken at one time

dose: the amount of medicine taken or given at one time; the sum of doses may be dosage or total dose

effect: as a noun, the result of an action; as a verb, to bring about or cause to come into being

affect: as a noun in psychiatry, the sum of feelings accompanying a mental state, or the appearance of emotion or mood; as a verb, to modify or to elicit an effect

etiology: the study or description of the causes of a disease

cause: the agent, single or multifactorial, bringing about an effect, such as inducing a disease

following: the present participle of the verb *to follow,* "to proceed behind some thing"

after: the preposition indicating relative position in time; a better choice for "She began to bleed immediately after the operation" rather than "She began to bleed immediately following the operation"

incidence: the number of cases developing in a specified unit of population per specified period

prevalence: the number of cases existing in a specified unit of population at a specified time individual: as a noun, a single person contrasted with a group; confine its use to that meaning; do not use, for example, as "We screened ten individuals to find a suitable donor."

person: a single human being; prefer to "individual" when contrast with a group is not needed, as in "We screened ten persons to find a suitable donor."

infer: to conclude or deduce from an observation or premises
imply: to suggest a conclusion to be drawn from allusion or reference

pathology: the study or description of disease; do not use for *disease, lesion, abnormality*

disease: lesion, abnormality; terms not synonymous with *pathology*

people: a group of persons, either a large group such as the inhabitants of a nation or a small not-enumerated group with characteristics held in common

persons: individual human beings, even in references to a group, as in "10 persons injured in a train wreck"

prior to, before: too often "prior" is used where a priority (a necessity in sequence) is not a consideration but only a simple sequence in time; "He fainted twice before he was reached by the ambulance team" for "He was seen twice prior to being reached by the ambulance team."

theory: working or established hypothesis suggested by experimental observations; do not use loosely for *idea, concept, hypothesis*
hypothesis: a proposition for experimental or logical testing

utilize, use: "to utilize" is to give the quality of utility to something; often pretentiously selected where "use" is adequate; "We used the only antibiotic available to us in that remote hospital." rather than "We utilized the only anibiotic . . ."

varying: as an adjective, *changing;* as a verb, causing a change
various: having dissimilar characteristics; synonymous with *differing*

which: relative pronoun used to introduce a nonrestrictive (nonessential) clause ("These diseases, which cause most of the deaths each year in the United States, are the main subject of this textbook".)

that: relative pronoun used to introduce a restrictive (necessary) clause ("This is the one lesion that is usually fatal".)

Additional examples of frequently confused and misused pairs of words can be found in style manuals; a good compilation for scientific usage is in Chapter 6 of the Council of Biology Editors style manual (6).

Spelling Errors

As you read a draft of your manuscript you will probably spot misspellings that result from typing errors. The spelling checkers in word-processing programs will catch them too. It is the words of whose spelling you are not sure that will slip by undetected by you. Unfamiliar scientific terms, such as chemical names for drugs more widely known by their generic names, must be checked in a scientific dictionary or other references such as those described in Appendix E.

Nonscientific words that sound right but look vaguely incorrect need to be checked in a standard dictionary: *fluorescent* is not "flourescent"; *principle* is not *principal* (and vice versa); *consensus* is not "concensus"; *prevalent* is not "prevelant". A spelling checker will catch misspellings like "flourescent" and "concensus" but it will not correct mixed-up usage like *principal* and *principle*.

Use caution too with singular and plural forms of Latin terms such as medium (singular) and media (plural).

Wrong Choice of Verb Tense for Completed or Continuing Actions

If the reader is to know whether an action was completed at one time or continued, you must use the right tense of verbs. Defects in tense occur frequently in referring to published papers. If a paper published years ago now has mainly historical value, an accurate statement would be, "In 1963 Smith and Jones reported that . . .". The use of the simple past tense "reported" indicates that the event was completed; this meaning is backed up by the date. The use of the simple past tense without a date ("Smith and Jones reported that . . .") implies that the intellectual content of the report may have come to the end of its useful life, even though the report probably still exists in published form. If the statement is "Smith and Jones have reported . . .", which uses the present perfect tense, it implies that although the report was published in the past it was probably published in the recent past and continues to have intellectual importance. The present perfect tense cannot be used with a date; "In 1963 Smith and Jones have reported . . ." is a contradiction because the present perfect tense indicates continuing action, in this case the continued existence of the reporting as a published paper. In referring to papers just published with messages of current importance, the present tense is appropriate: "On the other hand, Smith and Jones report that . . .".

Such nuances may sound like an editor's nitpicking, but the right tense, a simple tense or a "perfect" tense, establishes accurately that an event was an occurrence not continued or is a continuing action or state. Authors well educated in English idiom usually have no uncertainties as to the right tense. If you do not trust your ear for the right choice, turn to one of the books cited in Appendix E as a reference on English grammar or ask the advice of a colleague or other friend with a firm grasp on good idiom. This topic is also discussed in the section "Perfect and Progressive Tenses of Verbs" of Chapter 18.

REVISING FOR ECONOMY

A tightly written paper is clearer and easier to read than a wordy paper. After you have dealt with the defects discussed above, go through your text and replace long words with shorter equivalents. Strike out unneeded words and phrases. Which of these sentences do you prefer?

> We conclude that penicillin is the best antibiotic for treatment of streptococcal infections.
>
> After careful consideration of all the foregoing lines of evidence, it is apparent to us that among all the antibiotics discussed penicillin is the one that should be chosen for the treatment of infections caused by the streptococcus.

The message in the second sentence is clear enough, but most readers will prefer the shorter version. The point made by these examples could be made in other ways.

> We conclude that streptococcal infections are best treated with penicillin.
> Clearly, streptococcal infections are best treated with penicillin.
> We conclude: treat streptococcal infections with penicillin.

Each version has its virtues and faults. The best choice could depend on the place of the passage in the text, the degree of economy in the rest of the text, the tone the paper should carry. The briefest possible statement is rarely the best. Brevity carried too far can lead to unidiomatic sentences, cryptic statements, or lost meaning.

> Penicillin is best for streptococcal infections.
> Streptococcal infections? Penicillin!

Do not push to recast sentences in shorter versions and rid your prose of unneeded words and phrases at the risk of writing prose that strains for economy. Remember T E Lawrence's point (2) that prose is bad when the reader stops to look at it.

Prose carefully revised for economy but still idiomatic has advantages in papers competing for publication. The text speaks forthrightly, carries a clear message, and suggests that the author knows the subject. Many a paper gets a low priority for publication from reviewers because it lacks the tone of authority. Prose style is not all that determines a paper's tone of authority, but it can support that tone.

Verbal economy in your paper also raises the odds a bit that it will be accepted. Journal publishing is expensive; editors need to make the best use of the space they have. Of two papers with equal importance, the shorter is more likely to be accepted. Many journals specify short formats ("brief communications", "short reports", "clinical notes") to indicate to authors that their messages should be presented as economically as possible. Lean prose is a main ingredient for a concise paper.

Revising to Correct Excessive Use of Weak Verbs and Connectives

In his sharp analysis of medical prose style, Lester King (7) points out the characteristic structure of the excessively long and dull sentence: Too many words (nouns and other nonverbs) are strung together by forms of the verb *to be* or *to have* and connective words such as *and, of, with. To be* and *to have* are weak verbs, one expressing a state, not action, and the other describing only static possession. To revise sentences with this fault, reduce the number of nonverbs and increase the number of active verbs, converting, when possible, abstract nouns to verbs or verb equivalents. Consider this example.

> It is especially important that health-science schools have policies and guidelines for the education of undergraduate professional students, nurses, and house officers so that there is thoughtful consideration and discussion by the faculty of the ethical, legal, and emotional aspects of abortion.

This sentence has 40 nonverbs, including 11 connectives, and only 3 verbs, of which 2 are the weak verb *is* and 1 is the barely stronger *have.* Consider this version.

> In educating undergraduate professional students, nurses, and house officers, health-science schools need policies and guidelines to ensure that the faculty thoughtfully consider and discuss ethical, legal, and emotional aspects of abortion.

This version has only 20 nonverbs, including only 7 connectives. The verb *need,* which by itself implies importance, replaces "It is especially important that" (which contains the weak indefinite pronoun *it* and the weak verb *is*). The verb forms *educating, consider,* and *discuss* replace the abstract nouns "education", "consideration", and "discussion". The number of verbs and verb equivalents has been raised to 5.

Replacing Abstract Nouns

I have just pointed out that replacing abstract nouns with equivalent verb forms both shortens and strengthens a sentence. Abstract nouns ending in *-ion* should alert you to a possible need to revise. Many stuffy, long-winded passages can be cleaned up by replacing abstract nouns with verbs or verb equivalents. Consider this example.

> The identification and classification of the various histologic types of lymphomas are vital steps toward the introduction of new therapies and the reduction of mortality.

Here are 4 abstract nouns ending in *-ion* and 24 words linked by 1 verb, *are.* Here is one possible variant.

> Identifying and classifying the histologic types of lymphomas are vital steps toward introducing new therapies and reducing mortality.

The 4 abstract nouns have been replaced by their verb equivalents ending in *-ing.* The 2 halves of the sentence are still connected by the weak verb *are,* but the total number of words has been cut by 7. Here is another pair of examples.

> After reviewing the evidence we had to come to the conclusion that an advantage with the new treatment had not been established.

After the author resolved on trimming his text wherever and however possible, he came up with this version.

> After reviewing the evidence, we concluded that the new treatment offered no advantage.

The author did more than convert "conclusion" to "concluded" but the presence of the *-ion* word probably signaled a need to rework the sentence altogether.

Until you train yourself to spot the *-ion* nouns you can use the "find" or "find and change" program in your word-processing program to get you to sentences with abstract nouns that might be replaced with verb-form equivalents. Just ask the program to find "ion".

Cutting Out Clauses

Clauses beginning with *which* often add subordinate detail to sentences that takes up too much length for its value in meaning.

> Cancer of the breast, which is known to be a leading cause of death in women in the United States, too often escapes detection in an early stage.

The relative, nonrestrictive clause that begins "which is known . . ." can be omitted without distorting the main point. The detail provided does support the idea that early detection is needed, but dropping "which is. . ." and converting the clause to a phrase clearly subordinates this detail to the main point and cuts out eight words.

> Cancer of the breast, still a leading cause of death in women, too often escapes detection in an early stage.

The statement "known to be" is not needed; stating the fact, "still a leading cause of death", indicates that it is known. The paper is about practice in the United States and is written for an American audience; "in the United States" can be assumed. These changes shorten the sentence by almost 30%, the equivalent of shortening a 10-page manuscript by 3 pages.

Deleting Empty Phrases and Words

In lectures and conversations we often fill spaces between the true units of thought with words and phrases not really needed for meaning. These fillers gain for us time in which our brains can select and process the words truly needed to carry what we have to say. In revising prose these fillers should become throwaways. Consider this example.

> In order to get a complete history from the patient, it would appear that the inexperienced clinician needs a systematic line of inquiry.

Two empty phrases can be dropped.

> To get a complete history from the patient, the inexperienced clinician needs a systematic line of inquiry.

"In order . . ." and "it would appear that . . ." are two fillers of the conversational kind. They also serve as verbal flourishes that imply a deliberate and judicious concern with coming to the right judgment, but these flourishes added to the statement only a pose. They call for notice by the reader and draw attention away from the message. They are smudges on Orwell's window pane of thought.

Below are examples of empty phrases; shifting to shorter equivalents or deleting such phrases saves the reader time and effort. A longer list can be found in the section "Unneeded Words and Phrases" in Chapter 6 of the CBE style manual (5).

Empty Phrase	*Equivalent*
a majority of	most
a number of	many
accounted for by the fact that	because
are of the same opinion	agree
as a consequence of	because
at the present moment, at this point in time	now
by means of	by, with
despite the fact that	although
due to the fact that	because
during the course of	during, while
during the time that	while
fewer in number	fewer
for the purpose of	for
the reason that	because
give rise to	cause
has the capability of	can
if conditions are such that	if
in all cases	always, invariably
in a position to	can, may
in a satisfactory manner	satisfactorily
in an adequate manner	adequately
in close proximity to	near

in connection with	about, concerning
in (my, our) opinion it is not an unjustifiable assumption that	(I, we) think
in order to	to
in the event that	if
in view of the fact that	because
it has been reported by Jones	Jones has reported
it is clear that	clearly
it is often the case that	often
it is possible that the cause is	the cause may be
it is worth pointing out that	note that
it may, however, be noted that	but
it would appear that	apparently
lacked the ability to	could not
numbers of	many
on account of	because
on behalf of	for
on the basis of	because, by, from
on the grounds that	because
owing to the fact that	because
prior to (in time)	before
referred to as	called
subsequent to	after
take into consideration	consider
the question as to whether	whether
through the use of	by, with
was of the opinion that	believed
with a view to	to
with reference to	about (or omit)
with regard to	about, concerning (or omit)

Deleting Unneeded Adjectives and Adverbs

Close cousins to these empty phrases are single words that are not needed or that should be replaced by stronger and clearer words. In the sentence, "The usual metastatic lesions in bone are very painful", what does "usual" tell us unless the author is also discussing unusual metastatic lesions? Does "very" add enough to "painful" to keep it? Either "Metastatic lesions in bone are painful" tells us enough or we need a more exact statement, "Metastatic lesions in bone cause severe pain". Unmodified "metastatic lesions" implies "usual" or "typical" metastatic lesions. If a word serves no real need for the meaning, delete it; if another word would be more effective, substitute the better choice. The general rule has been stated neatly by Herbert Read (8):

". . . omit all epithets that may be assumed and . . . admit only those which definitely further action, interest, or meaning".

REVISING FOR GRACE

Graceful prose does not offend readers or divert their minds from the message. Graceful prose moves smoothly along a clear line of thought. In revising your text, think of serving your readers as you would serve your closest friends.

Some of the defects discussed below that lead to graceless prose are defects in accuracy or clarity. They are better seen as defects in grace because they show the author to be an insensitive scribbler or a poser.

Defects in Sex Reference

Not all nurses are women; not all physicians are men. Some patients other than those seen by gynecologists are women. Keep these points in mind as you review your text and find sentences with references to sex.

> The noncompliant patient may not intend to disregard your instructions; he may simply forget them.

Why assume that patients in general are men? Such assumptions about the sex of unidentified patients often can be dealt with by switching to plural forms.

> Noncompliant patients may not intend to disregard your instructions; they may simply forget them.

In some sentences the pronoun can be eliminated.

> The patient should choose the treatment he wants.
> Patients should choose the treatment.

Such changes should, however, be consistent in number (plural or singular) throughout the text; there should not be shifts back and forth between *they* and *he* or *she*.

Some devices that get around inaccurate references to sex strike some of us who do believe in accurate statements as offensive to the ear or damaging to established meaning. "Chairperson" and "chair" are avoidances of "man" in *chairman*. To my ear "chairperson" is as ugly as "utilization", now so often a pompous substitute for *use*. And "chair" for *chairman* adds a radically different meaning to a long-established noun of simple meaning. Better substitutes are sometimes available. The term *convenor* can substitute for *chairman; convenor* graciously suggests the person who brings a group together but it does not connote a sex.

Dehumanizing Words

I pointed out under "Revising For Accuracy" the difference in meaning between *case* and *patient*. *Case* is the instance or episode of disease; *patient* is the person needing care. Ignoring this distinction turns persons into "cases".

> Recurrent urinary tract stone was shown to be a manifestation of primary hyperparathyroidism in 2 cases who were subsequently admitted for parathyroidectomy.

"Cases" are not admitted; patients are. In writing papers, forget that you hear physicians and nurses talk about the "unusual case who came in yesterday for the 10th time" or "the noisy case in Room 315". Such slang may pass in the surgical locker room, dining room, or elevator, but it is not graceful or accurate in print.

A close cousin to the misuse of *case* for *patient* is the widespread and insensitive use of *individual* for *person*. One definition of *individual* is a single human being, but the word is most accurately used under this definition to contrast single persons with persons considered as a group.

> The need of some individuals for full-coverage medical insurance comes into political conflict with the demands of the working class for lower taxes.

With its origin in the Latin *persona,* the English term *person* connotes, beyond its definition as a single human being, the view of a single being with his or her to-be-respected uniqueness. This connotation is closely related to that of *patient,* which, linked to *patience,* suggests the picture of a person with disease or suffering waiting for care.

> The need of some persons for full-coverage medical insurance comes into . . .

Some terms applied to patients seem more appropriate for animals. The best examples are "male" and "female" applied to men and women. *Females* may economically substitute as a collective term for "women and girls", but describing a patient as "a 38-year-old female" is graceless prose.

No less dehumanizing are the syndromic tags, terms for patients such as "diabetics" and "schizophrenics". These terms may pass as acceptable for chatter in hospitals, but in print they brutally reduce persons to instances of disease instead of ill persons who need care. It is a simple task to revise your prose to refer to the "diabetic patient" or the "schizophrenic patient".

Pomposity

Some authors write papers to try to reach a higher level of distinction than their associates. This motive all too often leads authors to believe that prose filled with polysyllabic and abstract words, qualifying clauses and phrases, and long sentences makes them more learned. Authors must not forget that pompous prose can also be seen as coming from an inconsiderate windbag arrogantly wasting a reader's time.

If you must write pompous prose, here are some rules to follow.

1. Write long sentences with many nouns and connectives and a small number of weak verbs.

2. Make all of your sentences long; avoid mixing long and short sentences.

3. Use abstract nouns instead of their verb equivalents: you do not "investigate" but "carry out an investigation of."

4. Use empty phrases: Do not write "to make the diagnosis in most cases", but "in order to make the diagnosis in a large fraction of cases".

5. Imply that your views are those of a remote, lofty authority by avoiding first-person statements: Write "it is an inescapable conclusion that", not "I conclude that".

6. Use polysyllabic, vague, or voguish words: "utilize" rather than *use;* "etiology" rather than *cause;* "symptomatology" rather than *signs and symptoms;* "parameter" rather than *index, indicator,* or *variable;* "impact" rather than *effect;* "portion" rather than *part.*

Slang and Jargon

The clinical sciences have their own idioms, their ways of making concise statements. An example is a report by a surgeon.

> The patient left the operating room in good condition.

A reader not familiar with surgical idiom—like your high-school English teacher—might see a picture of a patient climbing down from the operating table, mopping up the floor, and walking out from the now-tidy operating room. But the surgeon's way of speaking is the accepted, formal, and accurate idiom in surgery. These idioms (or jargons, because they are often not readily understood by outsiders) are efficient and normal ways (9) of speaking and writing for professionals. But informal idioms, or slang, in clinical fields are not acceptable in formal writing. You can complain at the lunch table in the hospital about having a hard time "intracathing the case in Room 169", but keep such slang out of papers for publication. The list of slang terms is long: "prepped", "lab", and "temp" are examples. Avoid using slang in formal papers; its meaning may be obscure to readers not familiar with your local slang (such as readers abroad) and it breaks the otherwise formal and accustomed tone of a paper, moving the reader's attention away from the line of thought.

Some terms and phrases gradually slip from slang into acceptable jargon. "Biopsy", accepted in formal writing only as a noun meaning the process of obtaining a sample of tissue from a living patient, has come to be used in jargon as a verb: "The large thyroid nodule was biopsied 3 times". Be careful about what you accept as jargon: "nodule was biopsied" will probably pass the editor's eye, but "the patient was operated" will not. Medical dictionaries offer little help on what is slang and what is acceptable jargon, but if a term or word you are accustomed to hearing used by your colleagues is not in a medical dictionary, it is likely to be slang.

Other Details of Graceless Prose

Any detail in prose that catches the reader's eye or ear and interrupts reading even if only momentarily is a defect to be corrected. Defects like slang in a formal paper are deviations from euphony, an agreeable sound. You may be able to catch other defects by reading the text of your paper aloud after you think you have revised it adequately. You may find unintended alliteration: "The professional paper put together in haste may prove pompous when perused by your partner." You may find jingles: "The patient suffered unintended strain from unremitting pain". Such defects are often more easily heard than seen.

Eliminate modish details of style that too easily creep into one's writing from unfastidious writing and speech in other fields. The possible examples are myriad. One kind of modish trend is the substituting of "more forceful" words that in fact represent new imprecisions: an example is the use of "impact" for *effect*. In scientific writing, *impact* was long carefully reserved for the meaning of "the striking of one body against another" as in "evidence of the impact of a meteorite in the coastal plain of North Carolina in the Cretaceous period". Careful scientific writers avoid watering down the meaning of terms with specific scientific meanings through using them when a simpler older term is adequate, as with *effect* instead of "impact". Another growing imprecision in scientific writing is the use of "significant" in a sentence like "The patient showed significant improvement" where a more precise term such as *perceptible* or *detectable* or *definite* would be a more exact adjective. Such care in the use of *significant* is especially important in scientific writing where it has a specific statistical meaning.

Another modish trend is the corrupting of punctuation, usually with its origin in another field: an example is the use of the slant line where the hyphen is standard; instead of *Section of Hematology and Oncology* or *Hematology-Oncology Section*, we are served up "Hematology/Oncology Section", a legalism that corrupts the standard use in scientific writing of the slant line for fractions and "per" constructions.

USING COMPUTER PROGRAMS TO REVISE

Clues to passages that may need revising have been pointed out above. Some examples are abstract nouns ending in *-ion;* noun phrases with *of;* and modifiers like *very* that add little or no meaning. The value of a word-processing program for detecting details in style that may need revising has also been pointed out. Some special programs can provide additional help, such as calculating average length of sentences, pointing out passive verbs, spotting some grammatical errors. These programs do not help with the bigger problems in prose structure and with nuances in prose style, but they can help the novice writer learn how to spot many small defects.

CONCLUSION

The content of a paper is far more likely to determine whether it is accepted than its prose style, but style with the qualities of fluency, clarity, accuracy, economy, and grace can give readers of your paper a sense that you know what you are writing about. The first of those readers will be an editor and the peer reviewers; how the content of your paper impresses them will probably decide its fate. But do not forget that a clumsily written paper can create a bad impression that might influence the judgment of a reviewer who is on the fence about the importance of your paper. Use all the skills you can muster in revising your paper for paragraph length and structure, paragraph linkage, sentence variety, and the myriad details of word choice and use. Go through the work of revising with an efficient, thorough, and organized sequence.

REFERENCES

1. Orwell G. Why I write. In: An age like this 1920–1940; vol 1. Orwell S, Ian A, eds. The collected essays, journalism and letters of George Orwell. New York (NY): Harcourt, Brace and World; 1968:7.
2. Lawrence TE. Men in print: essays in literary criticism. [London]: Golden Cockerel Press; [1940]:44.
3. Wesley S. An epistle to a friend concerning poetry. 1700. Quoted in: The Oxford dictionary of quotations. 2nd ed. London (UK): Oxford University Press; 1953:565.
4. Read H. English prose style. New York (NY): Pantheon Books; 1952:52.
5. Gopen GD, Swan JA. The science of scientific writing. American Scient 1990; 78:550–8.
6. Style Manual Committee, Council of Biology Editors. Scientific style and format: the CBE manual for authors, editors, and publishers. 6th ed. New York (NY): Cambridge University Press; 1994.
7. King LS. Why not say it clearly: a guide to expository writing. 2nd ed. Boston (MA): Little, Brown; 1991.
8. Read H. English prose style. New York (NY): Pantheon Books; 1952:16.
9. Bross IDJ, Shapiro PA, Anderson BB. How information is carried in scientific sub-languages. Science 1972;176:1303–7.

CHAPTER 18

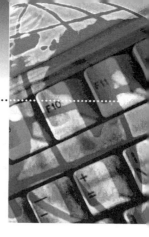

Writing English as a Foreign Language

English is not among the most difficult languages to learn to speak well enough for day-to-day needs. But learning to write scientific English with no, or next to no, flaws may be difficult for authors for whom English is a foreign language (nonanglophone authors, ESL ["English as a second language"] authors). They may be able to use English verb forms and the correct nouns well enough. But English, like all other languages, has its particular ways of making some kinds of statements and these details of English usage are readily overlooked by nonanglophone authors. Incorrect usage can be the result of trying to apply the rules of one's native language when writing English. For example, many languages do not use indefinite or definite articles (the English "a", "an", "the") before nouns. Difficulty in mastering such details can lead to writing in English that is close to correct but can confuse readers.

This chapter tries to cover the most frequently seen problems for nonanglophone authors in writing scientific English. Perhaps the best comprehensive guides to usage in English for nonanglophone authors are the *Collins COBUILD English Dictionary* (1) and the *Cambridge International Dictionary of English* (2), both described in the "Annotated Bibliography" at the end of this book.

ARTICLES: OMISSION OR INCORRECT USE

The term "articles" here refers to the short words "a", "an", and "the" that may precede nouns (terms for concrete things, such as "man", "house", "stone", or concepts, such as "strength", "theory", or actions such as "writing", "titrating") or their modifiers. Some languages do not use articles; in

English an incorrect use of an article or omission of a needed article can influence the meaning of the noun it precedes, and even that of the entire sentence.

> In five normal persons, serum calcium levels were normal.
> [In this study were there more than five normal persons, some (five) of whom had abnormal levels despite their apparent "normality"?]
> In the five normal persons, serum calcium levels were normal.
> [In this study, there were only five normal persons already identified in the paper and the serum calcium levels of all of them were normal.]
> Tumor in the lung was adenocarcinoma.
> [How many tumors in the lung? Only one or more than one, all of which were one kind or several kinds of adenocarcinoma?]
> The tumor in the lung was an adenocarcinoma.
> [There was only one tumor in the lung and it was one kind of several possible kinds of adenocarcinoma.]

Some rules can be applied to deciding on which article to use or whether to not use an article. There are two questions to consider.

- First, is the noun a proper noun, one that names one (or more) definite person, or animal, or building, or place, or other particular thing like a vehicle or planet, or is it a common noun (not a specific name)? If it is a proper noun and it is singular (name of only one thing), no article is used (with occasional exceptions).

> Our only trial subject was John Jacob Jones. [one person, John Jacob Jones.]

- If the proper noun is plural (more than one), the article to be used is usually "the".

> We sent trial questionnaires to the John Jacob Joneses in the telephone directory. [more than one John Jacob Jones. This sentence means that the questionnaire was sent to all persons in the directory with this name. If the "the" were omitted, the sentence could mean that the questionnaire was sent to some or all of the John Jacob Joneses; see the comment on the next example.]

- Note, however, that proper nouns can sometimes be used as common nouns rather than the name of a particular thing. Here an indefinite article (*a* or *an*) is correct.

> We could not find the case records of a "John Jacob Jones". [The investigators had this name in their list of once-studied patients, but they could not identify him as a particular person.]
> We sent trial questionnaires to John Jacob Joneses listed in the telephone directory. [Poor scientific usage. To how many? To two? Three? Almost all?]

- There are many exceptions. For example, the names of political institutions are usually preceded by the definite article "the" even if the proper name does not include a "the". The same is true for the names of medical journals and books.

  > Science budgets are often written down by the House of Representatives.
  > We submitted our paper to the *Journal of the American Medical Association*.
  > We consulted the *Cambridge International Dictionary of English*.

- Second, if the noun is not a proper noun (name) but a common noun (not a name), is it a count noun or an uncountable noun (sometimes called a "mass noun")? Count nouns refer to things that can be counted: cell–cells, tumor–tumors, person–persons, drug–drugs. If the count noun refers to a definite, identified or identifiable particular thing or more than one definite particular thing, it is preceded by "the" (the "definite article").

  > We chose the drug with the fewest adverse side effects. [A particular drug was chosen.]
  >   We chose the drugs with the fewest adverse side effects. [More than one drug was chosen.]

- If the count noun does not refer to a specific particular thing or particular things but to any thing of that kind, an indefinite article is needed ("a" or "an"; see further comment below).

  > We chose a drug with few side effects. [A particular drug has not been identified; the drug could have been any one of many with few side effects.]

- For more than one unspecified thing, "some" or no article is used.

  > We chose some drugs with few side effects. [More than one drug, none specifically identified.] We chose drugs with few side effects. [More than one drug, none specifically identified.]

- If "a" is the correct article, but the noun or its modifier begins with a vowel (a, e, i, o, u), the article "an" is used instead.

  > . . . a region of edema . . .   . . . an area of edema . . .   . . . an unexpected observation . . .

  But there are exceptions. When the word following the article has a long-u sound (like the pronoun "you"), the indefinite article is "a" rather than "an".

  > a united Europe   a European country [not "an united Europe" or "an European country"]

- Uncountable nouns (mass nouns) are terms representing things that may have individual components not considered countable or that are abstractions. Such nouns generally do not have plural forms and they do not, in general, take articles (a, an) before them when they do not refer to a specific particular thing or abstraction.

Always uncountable nouns and generally only singular

Fields of study (for example, physics, medicine, pathology)

> He studied medicine for four years.

Languages (for example, English, Chinese)

> He spoke only English.

Periods of life (for example, youth, senility)

> Among the early signs of senility is loss of very recent memory.

Abstract qualities (for example, truth, honesty, energy)

> Among the virtues of a true scientist is honesty.

Liquids (for example, water); gases (for example, nitrogen, helium).

> The animals needed more oxygen.

Often uncountable nouns

Natural phenomena (such as lightning)

Crop plants (for example, wheat, corn; *but* wheats, corns when referring to varieties of such plants)

Processes (such as enlargement, atrophy, dehydration).

- Some nouns can serve as count nouns or uncountable nouns. A good example is "hair".

  After radiation, the few hairs on his upper lip had all disappeared. [specifically identified hairs]
  > In her depression she refused to have her hair cut. [In French, "hair" in this sense would be the plural noun "les cheveux", "the hairs".]

Exceptions to these rules occur; they are too numerous to review here. An excellent source of rules and exceptions is *English Guides 3: Articles* (3). Another excellent source of rules is Chapter 11, "The Articles *A(N)* and *The*" in Perttunen's *The Words Between* (4). The correct use of articles can be learned gradually by compiling a list of nouns and their articles as they have been corrected by the editors of an English-language journal. Such a list can be used in reviewing drafts of later papers.

Articles are one of a grammatical class called "determiners". These are short words preceding nouns that help to indicate more specifically who or what a noun represents. The articles have been discussed above. Additional determiners include words such as "these", "those", "each", "all". Further discussion of determiners can be found in the introductory section "Grammar: Parts of Speech" of the *Cambridge International Dictionary of English* (2).

PREPOSITIONS

Prepositions can have large numbers of meanings in some languages. *The New Shorter Oxford Dictionary* (5), for example, gives 32 uses for the preposition "of". The French *Dictionnaire alphabétique & analogique de la langue Française* (6, "Le petit Robert") gives 13 uses for the French preposition "de". It is not surprising that authors for whom English is a foreign language can readily use an English preposition generally similar in use in their native language for an incorrect use in English. A good example comes from the Council of Biology Editors' style manual (7).

> Spanish *de*, English *of*: "soy de Barcelona", "I am from Barcelona", not "I am of Barcelona"

Errors of this kind are readily corrected by journal editors, and nonanglophone authors should not worry unduly about making such mistakes. As suggested above for use of articles, compilation of a list of corrected prepositions could be helpful in future writing.

Greater difficulties are the correct choices for prepositions needed for the correct form of a phrasal verb (see the section below, "Phrasal Verbs"). A preposition following a verb can change the meaning of the verb from that which it has without the preposition.

> He put the specimens into an appropriate preservative. ["put" with a meaning like "placed"]
> The patient would not put up with the adverse effects. ["put up with" with a meaning like "tolerate"]

English-language dictionaries may not list phrasal forms of verbs but their examples may illustrate the correct form.

> He became addicted to morphine. [not] He became addicted with morphine.

There are dictionaries of English phrasal verbs but they may not include phrasal verbs with special meanings in medicine.

POSITION OF VERB

The general rule for the position of the verb (the word that indicates an action or state) in an English sentence is that it should be within the central part of the sentence, not at the beginning or end.

Not It was found at the autopsy an adrenal tumor.
Not An adrenal tumor at the autopsy was found.
Rather, An adrenal tumor was found at the autopsy.

Again, there can be exceptions to the general rule. One is placing the verb to be emphasized at the end of the sentence.

The patient died before a transfusion could be arranged.   [two verbs, "died" and "arranged"]

Before a transfusion could be arranged the patient died.   [for stronger emphasis on died]

A second rule that sometimes determines where the verb should be placed is that which governs the sequence of statements within a sentence: the most understandable sequence within a sentence is one in which the sentence goes from a preceding event to a following event. That rule was applied to the last example above: the failure to be able to arrange for a transfusion was followed by the death of the patient.

Possible sequences of words in sentences are also discussed in the section "Revising Sentence Structure and Length" in Chapter 17.

MODAL MODIFIERS OF VERBS

Modals (properly called modal auxiliary verbs) are words placed before a simple form of a verb to modify the meaning of the verb. Only the main points about their use are touched on here. There are ten main modal auxiliaries.

can	may	should	will	have to
could	might	must	would	ought to

Modals can convey five kinds of special meaning when they are placed before a simple form of a verb: ability, permission, possibility or expectation, advisability or obligation, and necessity or probability.

• Ability and conditional ability: the modals *can* (*able to* for a one-time event) and *could*

We can sequence the identified gene.   We were able to sequence the gene.
We could sequence the gene if we had the additional funds.

• Permission: the modals *may, might*

Readers may receive copies of our protocol by submitting adequately detailed descriptions of its probable use.

Readers might receive copies of our protocol if the sponsoring pharmaceutical firm also consents. [This "might" form expresses a greater degree of uncertainty.]

• Possibility or expectation: the modals *can, could, may, might*

We believe we can sequence this gene given enough time.
We believe we could sequence this gene but other studies have higher priorities.
We may sequence the gene within the next six months.
Knowing this protein's structure we might find a new therapeutic agent.

• Advisability or obligation: the modals *should, ought to, have to, must*

Further studies of this new pathogen should look at new environments.
Further studies of this new pathogen ought to look at new environments if carriers are to be identified.
We have to look more closely at this new pathogen's cultural requirements.
Students were informed that they must wash their hands before leaving the laboratory.

• Necessity or probability: the modals *must* and *should*

Bacteriologists must add methionine to the culture medium if they hope to work with this new pathogen *in vitro*.
Given enough funding we should sequence this gene by the end of next year.

Additional description of the uses of the modals can be found under entries for them in dictionaries, but some of their entries may cross-refer you to another form of the modal. For example, in *The New Shorter Oxford Dictionary* (5), the entry term *should* cross-refers the reader to *shall*.

PERFECT AND PROGRESSIVE TENSES OF VERBS

Most nonanglophone authors able to write scientific papers in English probably understand the uses of most tenses of verbs well enough to be able to describe clearly past, present, and future actions and events. Errors are more likely to occur as wrong or inadequate uses of the perfect and progressive tenses.

A verb in the present perfect tense (with auxiliary verbs *has* and *have*) refers to a past event that is relevant to, or has effects in, the present. It can also express an action that began in the past and has continued to the present.

Jones and Smith have reported results (1) similar to ours.
[The verb phrase "have reported" is in the present perfect tense; Jones and Smith's results were published in the past but are still relevant to the citing paper's considerations. Compare this example with that below.]
Jones and Smith (1) reported their results in 1939.
[The verb "reported" is in the simple past tense; this is only a historical note

and use of this tense implies that their results are not notably relevant to currently valid conclusions.]

The past perfect tense (with auxiliary verb *had*) can serve a similar function but the references of the verb are all in the past: it describes an event that occurred before another past event and was relevant to the second event.

> The patient had noticed black stools for several days before she collapsed at work. [Her awareness of black stools occurred before the collapse and what she noticed was relevant to interpreting diagnostically at that past time her collapse.]

Progressive tenses, those in which the verb adds the ending *-ing*, are used mainly to express continuing action. The most frequently used forms of progressive tenses are the present perfect progressive and the past perfect progressive tenses. These combine perfect and progressive forms. They are sometimes misused for the simple perfect forms.

> We are finding additional types of tumors as apparent complications of AIDS.
> [where the authors actually meant—because their search for tumors was not continuing—"We have found additional types of tumors as apparent complications of AIDS."]

A notably clear description of the English verb tenses and their uses is "The English Verb System", an appendix in a book by Elaine Campbell (8).

PHRASAL VERBS

Phrasal verbs are composed of a simple verb followed by one or more "particles" (preposition or adverb). The combination gives a meaning to the verb that is different from the verb's meaning in its simple, nonphrasal form. The meaning depends on the preposition used. Phrasal verbs tend to be used in informal writing or speech and hence are more likely to be used correctly by authors who have learned much of their English from personal experience rather than formal study.

> The start of the clinical trial was *put off* until 100 more participants could be recruited.
> [The phrasal verb "put off" has the meaning "postponed" so the sentence means "The start of the clinical trial was *postponed* until 100 more participants could be recruited." This alternate form is a more formal way of saying what the example sentence says.]

A change in the particle can lead to a distinct change in meaning.

> His review of the literature ended with his *pointing to* the lack of adequate evidence for previous conclusions about the efficacy of the drug.
> ["pointing to" here means indicating his reason for his conclusion about the noneffficacy of the drug]

His review of the literature *pointed up* how little we know about the drug's mode of action.
["pointed up" means that he emphasized our ignorance]

Another example using "inquire" illustrates a radical change in meaning.

An important part of our selection of participants was asking them whether their personal physician routinely *inquired after* their alcohol intake. ["inquired after" = asked about alcohol intake]
The review committee *inquired into* the simultaneous use of other drugs. ["inquired into" = formally investigated, closely studied]

Many such changes in meaning are explained in the two dictionaries cited above (1, 2). Some dictionaries deal solely with phrasal verbs, for example, the *Collins COBUILD Dictionary of Phrasal Verbs* (9).

ADJECTIVES AND ADVERBS

Adjectives are words placed immediately before a noun to indicate some characteristic of the thing named by the noun.

We first examined all the obese patients. [What kind of patients? Those who were obese (an adjective meaning "fat").]

Adverbs are so named because they can be "added" to a verb to make more clear the kind of action represented by the verb. In general they are formed by adding "ly" to an adjective.

We quickly stopped the bleeding. ["quickly", formed by adding "ly" to "quick", indicates that the "stopping" was done with speed]

Another important use of adverbs is placing them before an adjective to make more clear the characteristic indicated by the adjective.

The clinically relevant questions were placed at the beginning of the history form. ["clinically", the adverb formed from the adjective "clinical", defines the kind of "relevance"]

Some nonanglophone authors have trouble with correct use of adjectives and adverbs for these functions.

The clinical relevant questions were placed . . .   [The   two   adjectives "clinical" and "relevant" mean in this use that the question was a clinical question and also a relevant question but does not make clear the kind of relevance; the form "clinically relevant" used in the example above makes clear that the "relevance" was clinical.]
He described a relatively increase in mortality.   ["increase" can be a verb but here it serves as a noun and hence should have as its modifier the adjective "relative" as in ". . . a relative increase in . . ."]

He described a relatively large increase in mortality. [Here "relatively" modifies the adjective "large" and is the correct form.]

CONFUSED ADJECTIVES

Some pairs of adjectives may seem to have the same meanings but do not and thus are readily misused.

He had little data to support his claim. ["little" means "small"; where the noun is the plural of a countable item, the correct choice is "few"]
He had few data to support his claim. ["few" means "not many"]
He had a large concentration of alcohol in his blood. ["large" means "of a great size"; the correct choice here is "high", the correct adjective meaning "of a large number"]

English-language dictionaries usually make the differences clear, especially dictionaries of synonyms (similar terms).

QUESTIONS OF GENDER

Incorrect Use of Gender for English Nouns

Some languages assign nouns to a gender category (as in French where nouns are either masculine or feminine). The gender category of a noun determines the proper form of other words used with the noun (as in French, the form of articles, adjectives, and substituting pronouns); the gender category is not necessarily related to a quality of sex of the named object. For example, in French, the gender of the feminine noun "la table", the table, does not mean that the table is female; it simply indicates that the definite article to be used with "table" is "la".

In English, nouns referring to male or female animals and human beings have masculine and feminine genders, which means mainly that the proper pronouns for referring to "masculine" nouns are "he" and "his" and for "female nouns", "she" and "her". Some nonsexual objects may be referred to idiomatically with gender-determined pronouns, but these rarely occur in scientific writing.

King George christened the new ship that was to carry the royal name. As *she* [the ship] slowly moved down the slip, the crowd broke into cheers of "Long live His Majesty".

Authors accustomed to a native language that uses gender categories for all nouns can readily make the mistake of using gender in English where it should not be used.

The drug tested in the third arm of the trial proved to have an excessive incidence of adverse effects. Although none of her adverse effects were serious, we decided to stop further study of the third arm. [In French "drogue" (5 drug) is feminine; this French author therefore unconsciously used "her" where the proper English pronoun for this sentence is the neuter pronoun "its".]

The general rule for English is to use gender references only for nouns representing the male or female sex of the animal or human being. In research reports, animals are usually referred to with plural forms, so that the problem does not arise.

Gender Bias

In recent years more and more attention has been paid in formal literature in the anglophone countries to referring to both men and women in expressions where solely male references were, for a long time, the normal style.

> Man differs conspicuously from animals in his ability to write a language.
> [now might be written]
> Men and women differ conspicuously from animals in the ability to write a language.
> [or]
> Humans differ conspicuously from animals in the ability to write a language.

Indifference to this aspect of modern English style is most likely to be found in cultures with rigid divisions of men's and women's acceptable conduct.

It can be difficult to get adequate guidance on this aspect of English style. One kind of source is the style manual of a scientific organization; an example is the section 6.7, "Bias-Free Usage", in the Council of Biology Editors's style manual (7). Another good source is the section "Guidelines to Reduce Bias in Language" in the style manual of the American Psychological Association (10). Useful suggestions may be offered by anglophone authors familiar with the scientific field the author is writing about.

FALSE PLURALS AND FALSE SINGULARS

Some English nouns appear to be plural but are usually grammatically singular.

> The news about the drug trial were an obstacle to allowing it to continue.
> [Incorrect use of the plural verb form "were"; "news" is defined in English dictionaries as a plural noun but is almost invariably treated as a singular noun.]
> The news about the drug trial was an obstacle to allowing it to continue.
> ["Was" is the correct form of verb for the singular term "news".]

Other terms may appear to be singular but can be properly used as a plural term.

The NIH were allotted their expected budgetary allowances.
["NIH" represents "National Institutes of Health" but appears to be singu
lar. The example sentence means that each institute in the NIH group
was allotted its budgetary allowance.]

English usage in British literature tends to be more careful than American
usage in distinguishing between the singular and plural meanings of some
nouns.

The task force agree on the priorities for research in this field.
[Individual members of the task force agree with each other on the prior-
ities.]
The task force recommends ten priorities for the research.
[After discussion and a vote, the task force was able, as a body (singular),
to present specific recommendations.]

COLLECTIVE NOUNS

Terms like "committee", "family", "personnel" are called collective nouns.
They represent a group of individuals considered as a single unit. The section immediately above illustrates a careful distinction between a task force
acting among themselves as differing individuals and a task force taking a
united step. A similar distinction can be drawn between "family" as representing persons sharing a relationship but acting as individuals and "family"
representing a group of persons functioning as a unit.

We know that the family disagree on what to do about the senile parents.
We have been told that the family agrees with our judgment about care of the
senile parents.

"FALSE COUSINS"

Some words spelled alike or closely similar in two languages can have quite
different meanings. A frequently quoted example is the pair "actuel,
actuelle" (French) and "actual" (English). In French "actuel" and "actuelle"
can mean "of current interest", "of present concern". In English "actual"
usually means simply "existing", "a matter of fact". Such confusions are usually readily corrected by journals' manuscript editors.

WORDS READILY CONFUSED

Many pairs or groups of words in English may be readily confused with regard to correct spelling or slight differences in meaning. Others are misused
through lack of knowledge of correct usage. This type of error is certainly

not restricted to nonanglophone authors and can be seen even in high-quality newspapers like *The New York Times*.

Similar Sound, Different Meaning

Some pairs of words sound similar when spoken but have different meanings. Such words are readily misspelled.

> principle [a noun: a rule governing conduct; a basic truth or law]
> "An important principle for medical care is "do no harm".
> principal [an adjective (modifier): leading or main]
> "A principal cause of death in elderly persons is stroke."

Some pairs sound closely, though not identically, similar.

> proceed [going on to carry out a new action]
> precede [an event happens before another]
>
> affect [as a noun in psychiatry and psychology, the external appearance of a mood or emotional state; as a verb, brings about a change, an effect]
> effect [as a noun, the result of having been affected (changed); as a verb, to bring about a change (rather formal usage)]

Spelling checkers in word-processing programs are of limited usefulness here. They will identify the correct spelling of either word but cannot recognize its misuse. Editorial offices usually correct errors of this kind easily.

Some words are readily misspelled because they belong to a category of words with very different meanings but similar word structures. Good examples are adjectives ending in -ible or -able and noun forms ending in -ibility or -ability.

> diffusible [not "diffusable"]   capable [not "capible"]
> responsibility [not "responsability"]   capability [not "capibility"]

There are rules that govern the spellings (see Chapter 3 in reference 4) but they are difficult to remember and apply. These errors are readily identified by spelling checkers in word-processing programs; this is a good reason to use these checkers.

Different Sound, Different Meanings (Misused Terms)

Some pairs or groups of words can be used erroneously through lack of attention to their proper uses. A classic example in medicine is the "case" and "patient" pair.

> case [in medicine, an instance, example, or episode of disease or injury]
> patient [a person with a disease or injury seen by a physician or other health-care professional]

Misuse of words in this category occurs as readily with anglophone authors as with nonanglophone authors. "Misuse" here often means "jargon" use. Fortunately journal editors will usually call attention to such misuses or even correct them.

Unfortunately, medical dictionaries do not, in general, draw desirable distinctions such as those properly drawn between "case" and "patient", or "morphology" and "structure", or "pathology" and "lesion" or "abnormality". An author tends to learn such distinctions through changes suggested by more experienced authors or made by editors.

There are many sources for guidance on how to avoid misspellings or misuses of confusable words. A good source for words used throughout English literature, nonscientific or scientific, is volume 4, *Confusable Words* (11), of the *Collins COBUILD English Guides* series. Two good sources for words used especially in sciences and clinical medicine are Chapter 3, "English Words That Are Often Confused", of the Perttunen book (4) mentioned above and Chapter 6, "Prose Style and Word Choice", of the Council of Biology Editors style manual (7).

DIFFERENCES IN AMERICAN AND BRITISH VOCABULARIES, SPELLING, AND PUNCTUATION

Differences in the English language as it is used by American medical journals and journals in British and Commonwealth countries can readily be seen in many aspects of usage.

- Different terms may be used for the same object or concept.

  For the place where surgery is carried out: operating room [American]; surgical theatre [British]
  For the place where patients are seen and treated by a physician or surgeon: clinic, office [American]; surgery [British]

- Different spellings may be used for the same words.

  meter [American]   metre [British]   edema [American]   œdema [British]

- Different styles may be applied to abbreviations and punctuation.

  His research grant came from the *NIH*. [American; no periods after the letters representing the abbreviation of a multiword term, here "National Institutes of Health"]   His research grant came from the *M.R.C.* [British; periods in the abbreviation for "Medical Research Council"]
  The best source for nomenclatural style in the animal sciences and medicine is Chapter 24, "Human and Animal Life." [American; period inside a closing quotation mark]
  The best source for nomenclatural style in the animal sciences and medicine

is Chapter 24, "Human and Animal Life". [British; period outside the closing quotation mark]

Descriptions of these differences can be found in many sources. For medicine the best source is the Council of Biology Editors style manual (7). In general, authors preparing papers for submission to British or Commonwealth journals should use British spellings and styles and for American journals American spellings and styles. Details in spelling and usage are readily changed by editorial offices to suit their preferences, and authors should not concern themselves with possibly having made errors in style.

OTHER ASPECTS OF SCIENTIFIC STYLE IN ENGLISH

This chapter covers only some of the more common errors made in English by nonanglophone authors (and some anglophone authors). Many other kinds of weaknesses in scientific prose style turn up in writing by both anglophone and nonanglophone authors—excessive use of abstract nouns, stacking of nouns as adjectives, and other kinds of weaknesses that careful authors will try to avoid. The preceding chapter (Chapter 17) considers many such weaknesses with examples showing how they can be corrected.

CONCLUSION

Authors for whom English is not the native language may have enough of a command of English to be able to write papers in English. But their knowledge of English may cover only the main elements of grammar, and they can readily err in many details of English style and usage. Errors in spelling are usually readily detected through use of a spelling checker in a word-processing program. Errors in word usage can sometimes be avoided by asking an anglophone colleague to read the paper before its final draft is prepared. Many errors are not serious problems for authors because they are detected and corrected in the editorial office of the journal accepting and publishing the paper. Some sources for guidance in proper usage have been cited and are listed below.

REFERENCES

1. Collins Cobuild English Dictionary. London (UK): HarperCollins; 1995.
2. Cambridge International Dictionary of English. Cambridge (UK): Cambridge University Press; 1995.
3. Berry R. Collins Cobuild English guides 3: Articles. London (UK): HarperCollins; 1993.
4. Perttunen JM. The words between: a handbook for scientists needing English, with examples mainly from biology and medicine. Helsinki (Finland): Kustannus oy Duodecim; 1990.
5. Brown L, editor. The new shorter Oxford English dictionary on historical principles. Oxford (UK): Clarendon Press; 1993:1980–1.
6. Robert P. Dictionnaire alphabétique & analogique de la langue Française. Paris (FR): S. N. L. Dictionnaire Le Robert; 1972:403.

7. Council of Biology Editors, Style Manual Committee. Scientific style and format: the CBE manual for authors, editors, and publishers. 6th ed. New York (NY): Cambridge University Press; 1994.
8. Campbell E. ESL resource book for engineers and scientists. New York (NY): John Wiley & Sons; 1995.
9. Collins Cobuild dictionary of phrasal verbs. London (UK): HarperCollins; 1989.
10. Publication manual of the American Psychological Association. 4th ed. Washington (DC): American Psychological Association; 1994.
11. Carpenter E. Collins Cobuild English guides 4: Confusable words. London: HarperCollins; 1993.

CHAPTER 19

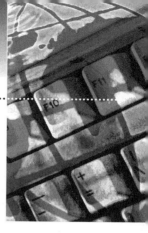

Scientific Style and References

All who write for formal publication—novelists, poets, compilers of catalogs, scientists—are expected to spell words in standard forms established by dictionaries. All who write in medicine are also expected to use accepted styles for units of measure, drug names, names of microorganisms, and other kinds of scientific terms. The journal for which you are preparing your paper may specify in its information-for-authors pages the details of scientific style it prefers. Be sure that you apply these in your text, tables, and illustrations.

This chapter describes briefly the main conventions of scientific style in clinical journals. You can find much more detailed guidance on scientific style in *Scientific Style and Format* (1) and other style manuals also described in Appendix E.

The other aspect of style in medical writing that calls for close attention is the formatting of references and how they are cited. Many clinical journals use the reference formats and citation system established by the International Committee of Medical Journal Editors (ICMJE) (2). Note, however, that many journals do not use the ICMJE formats and citation system and prefer other kinds of formats and citations. For this reason, you must pay close attention to the references and citation forms specified in the information-for-authors pages of the journal to which you plan to submit your paper. If that page does not specify the citation and reference system used by the journal, you can identify the system simply by looking through recent issues. A closing section of this chapter presents the ICMJE formats because a journal may specify these formats and not give examples of them.

ABBREVIATIONS AND SYMBOLS

Guides to scientific writing do not always make clear the difference between *abbreviation* and *symbol*. The two terms do not have the same meaning. Some symbols are not abbreviations, and most abbreviations are not used as symbols.

An abbreviation represents a word or a phrase in a short form derived from one or more of its letters: g is a short form of, and hence an abbreviation for, *gram;* Cl is an abbreviation of *chlorine;* HIV is an abbreviation for *human immunodeficiency virus.* DHHS is an abbreviation for *Department of Health and Human Services.*

A symbol represents a quantity, a unit, an element, a unit structure, an operation, or a relation. A symbol may be an abbreviation (Cl for *chlorine*) or may not be an abbreviation (pH for *negative logarithm of hydrogen ion concentration*).

The important difference between abbreviations and symbols is in their uses. Symbols are frequently joined to other symbols to form a representation with new meaning; for example, H for *hydrogen* and Cl for *chlorine* are joined as HCl to represent *hydrochloric acid.* Symbols may be used in equations that indicate the relations among the quantities they represent; for example, F for *force,* m for *mass,* and a for *acceleration* are combined in Newton's Second Law of Motion, $F = ma$, to indicate how the terms of the equation relate to each other. Authors must know this distinction between *abbreviation* and *symbol* because of what it implies for correct usage.

The uses of symbols in scientific publication are, in general, firmly established by a formal agreement within a professional society or among experts, or by long use. Authors must use established symbols lest what they write be misunderstood. To be sure that any symbols in your paper are standard symbols, check them against a standard source such as a scientific style manual (1) or the information-for-authors pages of the journal for which you are writing. If you must use nonstandard symbols, you must explain their meaning in your text.

Abbreviations in Text

Journals differ greatly in what abbreviations they will allow. Authors can often decide on acceptable usage by consulting the journal's information-for-authors pages and scanning recent issues. The more specialized the content of a journal, the more likely it will accept abbreviations widely used in its field even if they are informal ones unfamiliar to readers in other fields. If you can not find out whether an abbreviation is acceptable to a journal, write out the term. Editors rarely ask that terms be converted to abbreviations, but their requirements for revision are likely to stipulate that you not use certain abbreviations. Any abbreviations in your paper that are not standard for the journal must be explained at its first mention in the text by giving the full term followed by the abbreviation within parenthesis marks: "the acquired immunodeficiency syndrome (AIDS)". You may then use only the abbreviation in the rest of the text; if it appears in a table or figure, it must be explained there. Some abbreviations regarded by some journals as non-standard are acceptable in others.

Some authors use abbreviations freely (and coin new abbreviations) because they are too lazy to write out full terms or to pause to decide whether an abbreviation is truly needed in a particular sentence. Consider the example "SLE", widely used for *systemic lupus erythematosus*. In a paper solely about patients with systemic lupus erythematosus, a sentence about prognosis in its Discussion section might read "SLE patients without proteinuria at the first visit to a physician are likely to live longer than those with proteinuria." If only patients with systemic lupus erythematosus are considered in the paper, why not simply write, "Patients without proteinuria at the first visit . . ."?

The author who wants to hold down the use of abbreviations in a paper should read a near-final draft and pause at each abbreviation to ask two questions.

- If the abbreviation is used alone as the equivalent of a noun or a noun phrase, can it be dropped completely? Can "the prognosis with SLE" be replaced with "the prognosis" without loss of meaning in the context?
- If the abbreviation cannot be dropped without leading to confusion, can it be replaced with a short substitute noun? In a paragraph that refers to two transaminases, "The serum levels of ALT and AST were within the normal range" can be replaced with "The serum transaminase levels were . . ." without loss of meaning because no other transaminases are discussed in that paragraph.

Neither of these examples would be clear without the abbreviation if the sentence had to stand alone, but the altered form is likely to be clear in its place within a paragraph or longer section of the paper.

A third test to apply in eliminating abbreviations is the number of times each abbreviation is used after its first mention. The abbreviation SIADH for the *syndrome of inappropriate secretion of antidiuretic hormone* may conveniently substitute for the full term in a long review article about the syndrome written for nephrologists. But what if the abbreviation occurs only twice in a review of recently described paraneoplastic endocrine syndromes written for physicians in primary-care medicine? Is it asking too much of the author that he or she write out the full term at each of the two points?

Symbols generally should not be used alone in text. A case description can correctly note that a patient "was 1.82 m tall and weighed 68.2 kg" but a description of hospital-admission procedure should say "Patients' heights are measured in meters and their weights in kilograms", not ". . . measured in m and weights in kg". But well-established symbols representing long phrases are usually acceptable: "Measurement of pH is not useful in the differential diagnosis of pleural effusion", rather than "Measurement of fluid acidity expressed as the negative logarithm of hydrogen ion concentration is not useful . . ." or even the shorter equivalent, "Measurement of the fluid's hydrogen ion concentration . . .".

Abbreviations in Titles

Avoid using abbreviations in titles. It may be necessary, however, to use abbreviations for very long terms. Consider an oncologic paper with a title that begins, "A Modified-MOPP Regimen for Treatment of . . .". "MOPP" stands for *nitrogen mustard, oncovin, procarbazine, and prednisone.* A version of the title with MOPP written out would probably be rejected by the editor. The symbol pH would also be acceptable in a title ("Measurement of Pleural Fluid pH") because of the length of its full equivalent and the widely known meaning of *pH,* but the title, "The Influence of Gravity on the Heart", on a paper for a journal in cardiology probably would not be acceptable as "The Influence of *g* on the Heart".

Objections to abbreviations in titles may be increasingly relaxed with more searching of bibliographic databases online or in CD-ROM formats. Some searchers may expect to find papers about AIDS or HIV through searching for titles carrying those abbreviations. For this reason editors may become willing to let such abbreviations accompany their full terms in titles: "Central Nervous System Infections with the Human Immunodeficiency Virus (HIV)".

Abbreviations in Abstracts

Abstracts accompanying the published version of papers often are published separately as well, in another section of the journal or in a publication that reproduces abstracts from many journals. No matter where an abstract is to appear, it should be governed by the same rules for abbreviations and symbols that govern the rest of the paper. An abstract should be readable by itself, as an entity separate from the paper. Within its short format, terms are seldom used many times, and as noted above, it is not necessary to use abbreviations for terms occurring only once or twice within text. If an abbreviation is needed for a term frequently used in an abstract, that abbreviation must also be explained in the abstract when it first appears as well as when first used in the body of the paper.

Abbreviations in Tables and Illustrations

Just as in the text, widely accepted symbols for units of measure and statistical terms (such as *P* for *probability*) can be used in tables and figures without explanation. Nonstandard symbols and abbreviations must be explained in footnotes or in the legend; a reader should be able to understand the content of a table or illustration without having to refer to the text for explanations of abbreviations. Because of the space limits in tables and illustrations, editors may allow use of abbreviations in them that they would not accept in the text if the abbreviations are explained in a footnote or the legend.

NUMBERS

Rules for numbers, numerals, and numeric terms differ among journals and are too complex for a complete summary here. Some rules are widely accepted.

1. Use numerals with standard units of measure: "The diameter of the cyst was 15 mm".

2. Numbers accompanied by a unit in the text of scientific papers should be in numerals: "The patient had been bitten by 1 of her 10 cats".

3. Numbers 10 and smaller in a nonscientific paper or a nonscientific context in a scientific paper can be written as numeric terms: "Social upheavals of this kind developed in ten countries immediately after the end of the war".

4. Do not begin sentences with numerals; substitute numeric terms: "Thirty-five of the 120 patients were given the drug." If the number accompanies a unit, the name of the unit should be written out as well: "Ten grams per day was the usual dose." Such sentences can be rewritten to avoid using numeric terms rather than numbers: "The drug was given to 35 of the 120 patients." and "The usual dose was 10 g per day."

5. Because the comma is used as the decimal point in some countries, do not use the comma to separate 3-numeral groups in large numbers; space the groups. But when 4-digit numbers appear only with numbers of the same, or a smaller, class, do not separate the numerals.

Not	37,546,321	*But*	37 546 321
	6,732		6732

If 4-digit numbers appear with 5-digit, or larger, numbers, use the spaced style for all numbers.

. . . in 15 678 men and 4 632 women . . .

Note that European journals may apply the European convention of a comma for the decimal point.

. . . recorded a weight of 156,4 grams for the largest . . .

6. Very large numbers not representing precise values can be represented in the numeral-numeric term format.

. . . voted a budget of 56 million dollars for the immunization program.

7. Use a zero before the decimal point for all numbers smaller than 1.0.

> . . . with a birth length of 0.75 m . . .
> . . . and $P = 0.67$ with the resulting conclusion that . . .

A detailed discussion of the use of numbers in scientific writing can be found in Chapter 11 of the CBE style manual (1). Other sources are the additional style manuals described in Appendix E.

UNITS OF MEASUREMENT: METRIC USAGE

Virtually all journals publishing instructions for authors indicate their requirements for units of measurement. Most clinical journals now use metric units almost exclusively, with some allowing exceptions for body measurements like weight in pounds, height in feet and inches, and temperatures in degrees Fahrenheit rather than in kilograms, meters, and degrees Celsius.

Metric usage is not as simple for authors today as it was 20 or 30 years ago. Many journals have shifted to the international system of metric units, SI (from *Système International d'Unités*). The SI units include many of the older metric units, but emphasis is shifting to reporting in newer compound units in such fields as respiratory physiology and clinical chemistry (for example, millimoles per liter for concentrations rather than grams per 100 milliliters). Some journals in the United States now require SI units for clinical chemistry and hematology. Some journals are accepting manuscripts with non-SI metric units but are requiring authors to convert when the paper is accepted. Note that only SI metric units are used in most countries other than the United States, so authors planning to submit a paper to a non-US journal should check its information-for-authors pages for its requirements for units of measurement. Likewise, non-US authors planning to submit a paper to a US journal should check on its requirements for units.

Another difference between US and non-US journals is in the spelling and symbolization of some units. The terms *litre* and *metre* (and their use in derivatives like *centimetre*) are generally spelled *liter* and *meter,* forms that better represent English phonetics rather than French-language origins. The preferred US symbol for liter is L rather than the lowercase letter "ell", l, a preference based on eliminating possible ambiguities between the letter "ell" and the numeral "one".

Although hecto-, deka-, deci-, and centi- are SI prefixes, they should generally not be used except for the SI unit-multiples for area and volume and for the nontechnical use of centimeter. For measurements of length (and height) in the medical sciences, the meter and the millimeter should be used in preference to the centimeter. The diameter of a cyst, for example, should be given as 37 mm rather than as 3.7 cm; a patient's height should be given as 1.54 m rather than as 154 cm. The style rules for metric units and symbols are well-established. Incorrect usage in your manuscript will be corrected by the copy editor for the journal if your paper is published. Nevertheless, use of proper style in your manuscript will be evidence to the editor and peer reviewers that you know what you are doing.

The rules for metric style are worth knowing.

1. Names for metric units are capitalized only at the beginning of sentences and in other locations, such as titles, where capitalization is the rule for main words. Symbols for units named after persons are capitalized, but not the names of the units: the unit for pressure is the pascal; its symbol is Pa.

2. Upright letters are used for unit symbols, such as m for meter; quantity symbols, such as m for mass, are italicized (underlined in manuscript, m̲).

3. Periods (full stops) are not used after symbols except at the end of a sentence: "He was 1.71 m tall." and "His height was 1.71 m.".

4. If unit names are used, plural names are used for units with numeric values greater than 1, less than -1, or equal to 0: 1.1 meters, 0 degrees Celsius, -1.2 degrees Celsius; 0.95 meter, -1 degree Celsius.

5. Symbols for units are singular whether the units would be read as singular or plural: 1 m ("one meter"); 100 m ("100 meters").

6. No space should be left between the degree symbol (°) and the Celsius symbol: 37.1 °C, not 37.1° C; the paired symbols ° and C are combined unspaced as a single symbol for degree Celsius.

7. Squared or cubed units are designated by superscript powers, not words: 1.7 m^2 body surface area; not 1.7 square m body surface area.

8. In a symbol for a compound unit that is a product, use the product dot (raised period, centered dot) between the individual symbols: N · m.

9. Compound units with a denominator are written with "per" for the term but with a slant line ("slash") for the symbol: moles per liter; mol/L.

10. Compound units incorporating more than one unit in the denominator should not be written with more than one slant line. For example, 1.4 $mmol/cm^2/s$ should be written in one of these styles, in decreasing order of preference.

    1.4 $mmol \cdot cm^{-2} \cdot s^{-1}$
    1.4 $mmol/cm^2 \cdot s$
    1.4 $mmol/(cm^2 \cdot s)$

A helpful summary of the metric system, including the SI units, can be found in the CBE style manual (1) referred to above. A recently published source, *SI Units for Clinical Measurement* (3), includes a detailed description of SI units, their style requirements, and extensive detailed tables giving non-SI and SI units for many fields, including cardiovascular and pulmonary medicine, clinical chemistry, and hematology, with conversion factors and specifications for "significant digits".

STATISTICS

Quantitative evidence, for example, differences in group means in clinical trials, should be supported by appropriate statistical description and assessment, presumably available as the result of appropriate statistical tests described in the Methods section. Such statistical statements should appear wherever in the paper quantitative evidence is reported: abstracts, text, tables, and illustrations (or their legends). Statements of statistical assessment carried out by standard methods should be accompanied by a brief statement of the method by which they were derived, for example, "Fisher exact test".

Statistical statements of the form nn.n $\pm$ n.n must specify whether the $\pm$ n.n part represents a standard deviation or a standard error; a preferable form is nn, SD nn or nn, SE nn.

> *Not* 12.0 $\pm$ 0.4 *but* 12.0, SE 0.4

Statements of confidence intervals must specify the percentage span of the interval, as in "95%CI, -1.2 to 5.2". The two components that define the limits of the interval (in the example just given, -1.2 and 5.2) must be separated by the preposition *to;* a dash can be misread as a minus sign. Note that some journals may prefer the term "confidence limits" but "confidence interval" is to be preferred where possible because of its clearer implication of a span of values.

The symbols for the most frequently reported statistical variables are preferably italicized, in accordance with the recommendations of the International Standards Organization. Here are some examples.

sample size	n
standard deviation of a sample	s
probability	P
t statistic	t

Additional detail on statistical reporting can be found in Chapter 11 of the CBE manual cited above (1). A thorough, detailed, and highly specific discussion of statistical presentations is available in *How to Report Statistics in Medicine: Annotated Guidelines for Authors, Editors, and Reviewers* (4); in addition to including style rules for statistical statements, this source also presents many specific recommendations for statistical reporting in particular kinds of papers.

NOMENCLATURE
Chemistry and Biochemistry

Chemical compounds mentioned in clinical papers can be identified by either a formal chemical name or a shorter "trivial" (from the chemist's point of view) name. An example is one of adrenocortical hormones.

11B,17,21-trihydroxypregn-4-ene-3,20-dione   [formal chemical name]
hydrocortisone   [trivial name]

Formal chemical names are rarely used outside of the chemical, biochemical, and endocrinologic literature. Papers written for clinical journals should usually use the "trivial", or common, name for an organic compound. An organic compound not widely known by a standard common name should be identified, however, by its formal chemical name, at least at its first mention in a paper (after which it may be conveniently identified by the common name or, in some cases, by an abbreviation). Inorganic compounds should be identified by their standard common names rather than by older nonstandard names: *hydrochloric acid* rather than *muriatic acid*. An authoritative source for verification of full chemical names and common names is *The Merck Index* (5).

Drug Names

A drug should be identified by its generic (nonproprietary) name. If the drug's chemical structure is important for some aspect of the paper, such as discussion of its metabolites, its formal chemical name also may have to be given. If you need to identify the particular brand of drug (such as for acknowledgment of supply of the drug by a pharmaceutical firm, comparisons of several brands of the same generic drug, a report of an adverse effect that may be attributable to a particular brand), use the brand name of the drug at least in the Methods section (along with the generic name) to make clear the specific product. Brand names of drugs should, like other trademark names, have their initial letter capitalized; generic names of drugs start with a lowercase letter except where capitalization is needed for another style convention, as in a title.

Generic drug names can be verified in the most recent edition of *USAN and the USP Dictionary of Drug Names* (6); this source carries additional useful information, including formal chemical names of drugs, trade names, previously used generic names, and code numbers for investigational drugs.

Disease Names and Eponyms

If a disease is known by several names, use the name most familiar among your probable readers. If one of the synonyms for a disease is an eponym (name derived from a proper name, like *Addison disease*), use the noneponymic name unless the eponym is more widely known. Your decision may have to be arbitrary. For example, *Crohn disease* and *regional enteritis* are probably equally well-known; regional enteritis should be preferred because it concisely characterizes the disease as localized inflammation of the bowel. Osteitis deformans is probably more widely known by *Paget disease of bone;* hence the eponym may be preferred for a clinical audience, the descriptive, noneponymic *osteitis deformans* for an audience of pathologists. If you choose the eponym, be sure that it refers to no more than one disease or is the complete eponymic name. *Paget disease*, for example, is used in *Paget disease of bone, Paget disease of the breast,* and *Paget disease of the vulva;* if you are writing about one of these diseases, you should use the full eponym, not simply "Paget disease". This last point also applies to compound terms. To avoid any ambiguity with *lupus vulgaris, lupus erythematosus* should not be amputated to the jargon form "lupus".

Increasingly the preferred form for eponyms is the nonpossessive form: *Crohn disease,* not *Crohn's* disease; *the Cushing syndrome,* not *Cushing's syndrome.* Some journals still use some possessive forms; for these journals, two rules can be easily applied to most eponyms: if the eponym is derived from the name of a single describer, use the possessive form: *Parkinson's disease, Hodgkin's disease;* if the eponym is derived from the names of 2 or more describers or from the name of a patient, family, or place, use the nonpossessive form: *Creutzfeldt-Jakob disease, Hippel-Lindau disease; Christmas disease, Byler disease; Minamata disease.*

Note that eponymic terms ending with *syndrome* should open with the article *the: the acquired immunodeficiency syndrome, the CREST syndrome.*

Eponyms are capitalized but not adjectives or nouns derived from them. Thus, *addisonian* in *addisonian crisis* (from *Thomas Addison*) is not capitalized, nor is *parkinsonism* from *Parkinson disease.*

Disease names derived from capitalized names of microorganisms are not capitalized: *brucellosis* from *Brucella; salmonellosis* from *Salmonella.*

Names in Microbiology, Zoology, and Botany

Binomial taxonomic names for organisms (genus and species) should be italicized (indicated in manuscript by underlining): <u>Staphylococcus aureus</u> in manuscript, *Staphylococcus aureus* in published form. Formal names at a higher level (order, family, and tribe) are capitalized but generally not italicized, thus *Pseudomonas* for the genus but Pseudomonadaceae for the family.

A genus name may be abbreviated after its first mention only if it is followed by a specific epithet: *Staphylococcus aureus,* subsequently *S. aureus.* If you are referring to species in several genera whose names begin with the same letter, use several letters for the abbreviation of the generic name:

Staph. for *Staphylococcus, Sh.* for *Shigella.* The best way to avoid confusion of similar abbreviations, however, is to write out the full generic name.

Common names for bacterial species, like *the gonococcus* for *Neisseria gonorrhoeae,* are acceptable in many contexts, but these should not be used as an equivalent to the formal taxonomic name. Because the common names for the same organism may differ in some countries, the first use of a common name in a paper should be followed by the formal name within parenthesis marks.

Adjectival forms like "streptococcal" and "staphylococcal" are well known and acceptable. If a genus name has to be used adjectivally because a specifically adjectival form (7) is not well established, italic type and initial capitalization are not used: pseudomonas meningitis, not "*Pseudomonas* meningitis".

Taxonomic names in zoology and botany call for similar styles: *Drosophila melanogaster* for the fruit fly; *Rhus toxicodendron* for the poison oak.

CITATIONS AND REFERENCES

Two systems for references and their citations in text are in wide use among clinical and medical-science journals: the citation-sequence system (also known as the "Vancouver system") and the name–year system (also known as the "Harvard system"). The name "Vancouver system" represents the origin of the citation-sequence system in the form recommended by the International Committee of Medical Journal Editors (2) at a conference in Vancouver, British Columbia, in 1978. The origin of the term "Harvard system" was explained in a 1988 paper in the *British Medical Journal* (8).

The Citation-Sequence ("Vancouver") System of Citations and References

More than 500 journals around the world use the citation-sequence system in the form specified by the International Committee of Medical Journal Editors (2).

References are listed and numbered at the end of a paper in the sequence in which they are first cited in the text. Any references not cited in the text but only in a table or a figure legend are sequenced in accordance with the location of the table's or figure's identification in the text.

Citations

Citations in the text (or tables or figures) are Arabic numerals within parenthesis marks that are the references' numbers in the references list.

> Citation: We know little about exactly how women decide when to start requesting mammography (1) despite the wide attention in the press to . . .

Reference: 1. Jones C, Booth K. A survey of decision-processes among women seeking periodic examinations. J Women's Med 1999;78:105–9.

Note that many journals style citations as superscript numbers.

We know little about exactly how women decide when to start requesting mammography[1] despite the wide attention in the press to . . .

A journal's preference can be identified by examining recent issues or consulting its information-for-authors pages.

References

The formats for references recommended by the International Committee of Medical Journal Editors (ICMJE) (2) are based on formats developed by the National Library of Medicine for use in its MEDLINE system and in *Index Medicus*. The ICMJE formats are not all identical with the Library's formats.

The ICMJE formats are presented here in the form of examples given beneath the type of document to be referenced. These formats are, as mentioned above, used in hundreds of medical journals, but authors must be sure to check the information-for-authors pages in the journal for which they are preparing a paper on whether the journal specifically accepts the ICMJE formats and citation system. If it does not, it probably specifies the formats and citation system it prefers.

Note in the ICMJE examples below that article and book titles are not capitalized as in their original form; only the initial word is capitalized. Proper names (personal names, organization names, names of geographical entities, for example) are, however, capitalized in accordance with their normal form. Exceptions to this rule are government documents and "classical" literature titles such as Shakespeare's plays.

The abbreviations for journal titles are those used in MEDLINE and the *Index Medicus*.

Page numbers represent first and last pages of an article. The closing page is represented by the minimal number of digits needed for identification.

980–3 [pages 980 to and including 983]   980–95 [pages 980 to and including 995]

• Standard Journal Article with Six Authors or Fewer

Vega KJ, Pina I, Krevsky B. Heart transplantation is associated with an increased risk for pancreato-biliary disease. Ann Intern Med 1996 Jun 1;124(11):980–3.

Note that if the journal uses continuous pagination throughout a volume, the month and issue number can be omitted, a standard practice in many journals.

Vega KJ, Pina I, Krevsky B. Heart transplantation is associated with an increased risk for pancreato-biliary disease. Ann Intern Med 1996;124:980–3.

- Standard Journal Article with More Than Six Authors

  Parkin DM, Clayton D, Black RJ, Masuyer E, Friedl HP, Ivanov E, et al. Childhood leukaemia in Europe after Chernobyl: 5 year follow-up. Br J Cancer 1996;73:1006–12.

Note that references in the National Library of Medicine's MEDLINE and *Index Medicus* list all authors up to 25 authors.

- Article with an Organization as Author

  The Cardiac Society of Australia and New Zealand. Clinical exercise stress testing: safety and performance guidelines. Med J Aust 1996;164:282–4.

- Article with No Author Given

  Cancer in South Africa [editorial]. S Afr Med J 1994;84:15.

- Article Not in English

  Ryder TE, Haukeland EA, Solhaug JH. Bilateral infrapatellar seneruptur hos tidligere frisk kvinne. Tidsskr Nor Laegeforen 1996;116:41–2.

Note that an alternative form could be an English translation of the title placed within square brackets as in *Index Medicus*.

- Article in a Volume Supplement

  Shen HM, Zhang, QF. Risk assessment of nickel carcinogenicity and occupational lung cancer. Environ Health Perspect 1994;102 Suppl 1:275–82.

- Article in an Issue Supplement

  Payne DK, Sullivan MD, Massie MJ. Women's psychological reactions to breast cancer. Semin Oncol 1996;23(1 Suppl 2):89–97.

- Article in a Part of a Volume

  Ozben T, Nacitarhan S, Tuncer N. Plasma and urine sialic acid in non-insulin dependent diabetes mellitus. Ann Clin Biochem 1995;32(Pt 3):303–6.

- Article in a Part of an Issue

  Poole GH, Mills SM. One hundred consecutive cases of flap lacerations of the leg in ageing patients. N Z Med J 1994;107(986 Pt 1):377–8.

- Article in an Issue and No Volume Designation

  Turan I, Wredmark T, Fellander-Tsai L. Arthroscopic ankle arthrodesis in rheumatoid arthritis. Clin Orthop 1995;(320):110–4.

- Article in a Journal or Other Type of Serial without Issues or Volumes

   Browell DA, Lennard TW. Immunologic status of the cancer patient and the effects of blood transfusion on antitumor responses. Curr Opin Gen Surg 1993:325–33.

- Article with Pagination in Roman Numerals

   Fisher GA, Sikic BI. Drug resistance in clinical oncology and hematology. Introduction. Hematol Oncol North Am 1995 Apr;9(2):xi–xii.

- Type of Article Identified

   Enzensberger W, Fischer PA. Metronome in Parkinson's disease [letter]. Lancet 1996;347:1337.
   Clement J, De Bock R. Hematological complications of hantavirus nephropathy (HVN) [abstract]. Kidney Int 1992;42:1285.

- Article Containing a Retraction

   Garey CE, Schwarzman AL, Rise ML, Seyfried TN. Ceruloplasmin gene defect associated with epilepsy in EL mice [retraction of Garey CE, Schwarzman AL, Rise ML, Seyfried TN. In: Nat Genet 1994;6:426–31]. Nat Genet 1995; 11: 104.

- Retraction of Article

   Liou GI, Wang M, Matragoon S. Precocious IRBP gene expression during mouse development [retracted in Invest Ophthalmol Vis Sci 1994;35:3127]. Invest Ophthalmol Vis Sci 1994;35:1083–8.

- Article with Published Erratum

   Hamlin JA, Kahn AM. Herniography in symptomatic patients following inguinal hernia repair [published erratum appears in West J Med 1995;162:278]. West J Med 1995;162:28–31.

- Book or Other Kind of Monograph with Personal Author(s)

   Ringsven MK, Bond D. Gerontology and leadership skills for nurses. 2nd ed. Albany (NY): Delmar Publishers; 1996.

- Book or Other Kind of Monograph with Editor(s) or Compiler(s) as Author

   Norman IJ, Redfern SJ, editors. Mental health care for elderly people. New York: Churchill Livingstone; 1996.

- Book or Other Kind of Monograph with Organization as Author and Publisher

Institute of Medicine (US). Looking at the future of the Medicaid program. Washington: The Institute; 1992.

- Chapter in a Book

Phillips SJ, Whisnant JP. Hypertension and stroke. In: Laragh JH, Brenner BM, editors. Hypertension: pathophysiology, diagnosis, and management. 2nd ed. New York: Raven Press; 1995. p. 465–78.

- Conference Proceedings

Kimura J, Shibasaki H, editors. Recent advances in clinical neurophysiology. Proceedings of the 10th International Congress of EMG and Clinical Neurophysiology; 1995 Oct 15–19; Kyoto, Japan. Amsterdam: Elsevier; 1996.

- Conference Paper

Bengtsson S, Solheim BG. Enforcement of data protection, privacy and security in medical informatics. In: Lun KC, Degoulet P, Piemme TE, Rienhoff O, editors. MEDINFO 92. Proceedings of the 7th World Congress on Medical Informatics; 1992 Sep 6–10; Geneva, Switzerland. Amsterdam: North-Holland; 1992. p. 1561–5.

- Scientific or Technical Report Issued by a Funding or Sponsoring Agency

Smith P, Golladay K. Payment for durable medical equipment billed during skilled nursing facility stays. Final report. Dallas (TX): Dept of Health and Human Services (US), Office of Evaluation and Inspections; 1994 Oct. Report Nr: HHSI-GOEI69200860.

- Scientific or Technical Report Issued by Performing Agency

Field MJ, Tranquada RE, Feasley JC, editors. Health services research: work force and educational issues. Washington: National Academy Press; 1995. Contract Nr: AHCPR282942008. Sponsored by the Agency for Health Care Policy and Research.

- Doctoral Dissertation

Kaplan SJ. Post-hospital home health care: the elderly's access and utilization [dissertation]. St. Louis (MO): Washington Univ.; 1995.

- Patent

Larsen CE, Trip R, Johnson CR, inventors; Novoste Corporation, assignee. Methods for procedures related to the electrophysiology of the heart. US patent 5,529,067. 1995 Jun 25.

- Newspaper Article

Lee G. Hospitalizations tied to ozone pollution: study estimates 50,000 admissions annually. The Washington Post 1996 Jun 21;Sect. A:3 (col. 5).

- Audiovisual Medium

  HIV+/AIDS: the facts and the future [videocassette]. St. Louis (MO): Mosby-Year Book; 1995.

- Government Document: Public Law

  Preventive Health Amendments of 1993, Pub. L. No. 103–183, 107 Stat. 2226 (Dec. 14, 1993).

- Government Document: Unenacted Bill

  Medical Records Confidentiality Act of 1995, S. 1360, 104th Cong., 1st Session. (1995).

- Government Document: Code of Federal Regulations

  Informed Consent, 42 C.F.R. Sect. 441.257 (1995).

- Government Document: Hearing

  Increased Drug Abuse: the Impact on the Nation's Emergency Rooms: Hearings Before the Subcomm. on Human Resources and Intergovernmental Relations of the House Comm. on Government Operations, 103rd Cong., 1st Sess. (May 26, 1993).

- Map

  North Carolina. Tuberculosis rates per 100,000 population, 1990 [demographic map]. Raleigh: North Carolina Dept. of Environment, Health, and Natural Resources, Div. of Epidemiology; 1991.

- Biblical Reference

  The Holy Bible. King James Version. Grand Rapids (MI): Zondervan Publishing House; 1995. Ruth 3:1–18.

- Dictionary and Other Reference Works

  Stedman's medical dictionary. 26th edition. Baltimore: Williams & Wilkins; 1995. Apraxia; p. 119–20.

- Classical Literature

  The Winter's Tale: act 5, scene 1, lines 13–16. The complete works of William Shakespeare. London: Rex; 1973.

- Forthcoming publication ("In press")

Leshner AI. Molecular mechanisms of cocaine addiction. N Engl J Med. In press 1996.

• Electronic Medium: Journal Article

Morse SS. Factors in the emergence of infectious diseases. Emerg Infect Dis [serial online] 1995 Jan–Mar [accessed 1996 Jun 5];1(1):24 screens. Available from: URL: http://www.cdc.gov/ncidod/EID/eid.htm

• Electronic Medium: CD-ROM Monograph

CDI, clinical dermatology illustrated [monograph on CD-ROM]. Reeves JRT, Maibach H. CMEA Multimedia Group, producers. 2nd ed. Version 2.0 San Diego: CMEA; 1995.

• Electronic Medium: Computer File

Hemodynamics III: the ups and downs of hemodynamics [computer program]. Version 2.2. Orlando (FL): Computerized Educational Systems; 1993.

Some journals apply their own typeface styles to references, for example, italicizing titles. In general, authors need not try to style their references in imitation of the journal's style; such characteristics are applied by the journal's manuscript editor.

Further details on, and additional examples of, reference types can be found in Chapter 30 of the Council of Biology Editors style manual (1) and other style manuals described in Appendix E.

The Name–Year ("Harvard") System of Citations and References

The name–year system of citations and references exists in many variant forms but they adhere to a similar pattern.

References are listed at the end of an article or chapter in an alphabetic sequence determined by the surname of the first author and following elements. If two references have identical author names, they are listed by year of publication. More detailed rules can be found in Section 30.15, Chapter 30, of the Council of Biology Editors style manual (1). The year of publication is generally given following the author name or names.

Brown K, Braun TM, Jones CP. 1998. Biliary disease related to surgery in other systems. Surg Proc 79:114–6.

Vega KJ, Pina I, Krevsky B. 1996. Heart transplantation is associated with an increased risk for pancreato-biliary disease. Ann Intern Med 124:980–3.

The text citations include the author name(s) and the year of publication.

In reviewing the literature (Vega et al 1996; Brown et al 1998), we found that . . .

The journals of the American Psychological Association (APA) use the name–year system, and the Association's style manual (9) is a helpful source of examples of reference formats for this system. Note, however, that the APA style places the year datum in references within parenthesis marks and includes punctuation and other devices not used in the ICMJE's citation-sequence references.

> Vega, K. J., Pina, I., & Krevsky, B. (1996). Heart transplantation is associated with an increased risk for pancreato-biliary disease. Ann Intern Med 124:980–3.

Because of the many variations of reference formats in the name–year system, authors writing papers for a journal using this kind of system must consult its information-for-authors pages for guidance and examine some recent issues for examples of citation-reference style if that page gives inadequate help.

Some journals use a variant of the name–year system in which references are listed in the alphabetic sequence. The citations in text are not by name and year but by the sequential numbers assigned to the references in the alphabetically arranged References section.

CONCLUSION

This chapter has only touched on some of the main principles and rules that guide scientific style in clinical fields. Many fields of medical science such as biochemistry, genetics, immunology, microbiology, pulmonary physiology, and radiology have their own well-developed and detailed conventions for nomenclature and symbolization; many of these are summarized in Chapters 16 through 24 of the Council of Biology Editors style manual (1). They may also be specified in the information-for-authors pages of journals in these fields. The journal for which you are writing your paper is likely to specify the conventions most likely to be needed by its authors. If it does not, it may nevertheless have its own internal rules that will be applied when the manuscript of your paper is marked for the printer.

Be sure you know the citation and reference system of the journal for which you are writing. It should be specified in the journal's information-for-authors pages; if it is not, you will have to examine recent issues for guidance on how to cite your references and on their correct formats.

REFERENCES

1. Style Manual Committee, Council of Biology Editors. Scientific style and format: the CBE manual for authors, editors, and publishers. 6th ed. New York (NY): Cambridge University Press; 1994.
2. International Committee of Medical Journal Editors. Uniform requirements for manuscripts submitted to biomedical journals. Ann Intern Med 1997; 126:36–47. Note that this document is available at the American College of

Physicians' Web site (http://www.acponline.org/journals/resource/info 4aut.htm).

3. Young DS, Huth EJ. SI units for clinical measurement. Philadelphia (PA): American College of Physicians; 1998.

4. Lang TA, Secic M. How to report statistics in medicine: annotated guidelines for authors, editors, and reviewers. Philadelphia (PA): American College of Physicians; 1997.

5. Budavari S, editor. The Merck index: an encyclopedia of chemicals, drugs, and biologicals. 12th ed. Whitehouse Station (NJ): Merck; 1996.

6. USAN and the USP dictionary of drug names. Rockville (MD): United States Pharmacopeial Convention. Published annually.

7. [Huth EJ.] Style notes: taxonomic names in microbiology and their adjectival derivatives. Ann Intern Med 1989;110:419–20.

8. Chernin E. The "Harvard system": a mystery dispelled. Br Med J 1988; 297: 1062–3.

9. Publication manual of the American Psychological Association. 4th ed. Washington (DC): American Psychological Association; 1994.

CHAPTER 20

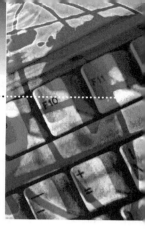

Preparing the Final Manuscript

You have revised your paper thoroughly and carefully. You are now ready to prepare the manuscript to be sent to the journal. Prepare the final manuscript in three steps.

Step 1. Review the manuscript requirements of the journal stated in its information-for-authors pages. Does the journal expect to receive an electronic version of the manuscript (diskette or e-mail transmission) in addition to the paper manuscript?

Step 2. Review the final version of your paper to be sure that it contains all the needed elements (title page, abstract, text pages, references, and so on) and that these meet the journal's requirements.

Step 3. Get the manuscript keyboarded ("typed") in accordance with the journal's requirements.

If you read a copy of the journal's information-for-authors pages before you began to write the paper and followed the instructions while you worked on the first and later drafts, these three steps may not take much time. But even if you proceeded that way, do not shortcut these steps; details in content and format should not be neglected if a final manuscript is to fit the journal's requirements.

Note that *manuscript* should refer only to the physical vehicle for the paper, specifically the sheets of paper, the typing on them, and any photographs and drawings serving as illustrations. The *paper* is the intellectual content carried in the manuscript; the term *paper* is properly applied whether it is published or exists only in manuscript form. A paper is submitted to a journal as a manuscript, but the editor judges and comes to a decision on a paper, not a manuscript.

REVIEW OF THE JOURNAL'S MANUSCRIPT REQUIREMENTS

Journals differ greatly in how much detail they provide in their information-for-authors pages. Some do little more than specify the number of copies to be submitted and give the address of the editor. Some provide authors with detailed checklists. If the journal for which you have written your paper does not provide a detailed list, you may find helpful the list below abstracted from "Uniform Requirements for Manuscripts Submitted to Biomedical Journals" (1) with a few details added. This list covers only requirements for content and format; those for keyboarding ("typing") are given near the end of this chapter.

Manuscripts: Content and Format

1. Title page

- Title. If you wish to use a subtitle, you may place it following the title closed with a colon (:) but a less ambiguous arrangement would be starting it below the title proper, indicating, perhaps at the left-hand margin of the page, which is which by parenthetic notes such as "(title)" and "(subtitle)". You should scan issues of the journal to see whether it allows subtitles.
- Author names: First name, middle initial(s), and last (surname, family name) name of each author, with highest academic degree(s). If your name carries the surname (family) name first as in Chinese, you should explain this arrangement in your letter of submission that will accompany the manuscript (see Chapter 21).
- Department(s) and institution(s) to which the paper should be attributed.
- Disclaimers, if any.
- Author responsible for correspondence about the paper: Name, postal address, telephone number, and any other addresses such as those for a telex, for facsimile transmission ("fax"), or for electronic-mail (e-mail).
- Author responsible for receiving reprint requests: name and address or statement that reprints will not be available.
- Grant support or other type of support, such as provision of study materials, financial assistance.
- Running head or footline of no more than 40 characters and spaces (also known as short title), labeled as such.

Note that some journals will expect to receive some of these details on sheets separate from the manuscript itself or in the letter of submission.

2. Abstract page

- Abstract with a length not exceeding that allowed by the journal. Many journals have allowed lengths up to only 150 words but now that the National Library of Medicine (Bethesda, Maryland, USA) will accommodate abstracts running up to 250 words, some journals have changed their policy to allow this length. The greater length may be needed to accommodate the structured abstracts requested by *Annals of Internal Medicine, British Medical Journal,* and other journals using this innovation.
- Key or indexing terms: 3 to 10 words or short phrases, preferably drawn from the Medical Subject Headings (MeSH) list (2) of *Index Medicus* and the MEDLINE system. These suggested key terms will not be used by many journals; inspect recent issues of the journal to which you will send your paper to identify whether it uses such terms with abstracts.

3. Text

- Headings appropriate to the type and sequence of the paper (such as Introduction, Methods, Results, and Discussion for research papers)
- Subheadings (within headed sections) in long papers. If subheadings are used, they must be clearly distinguished from headings by choice of typeface. For example, text headings could be in all-capital letters and subheadings (first level below headings) in capitals and lowercase letters. Journal papers rarely carry more than two levels of headings (headings and subheadings). Your preferences may be changed by the journal.
- Citations in the text of references. The journal's information-for-authors pages will almost certainly specify whether these should be arabic numerals (as in the citation-sequence ["Vancouver"] system; within parenthesis signs or superscripted) assigned in the order of citation in the text or the parenthetic name and year type of citation, such as "(Smith 1999)".

4. Acknowledgments

- Names of persons (with their institutional affiliations) who have contributed substantially to the content of the paper but do not qualify as authors or who have given technical or financial assistance. You should have written permission from them to list their names.

5. References

- Listed in order of their first citation in the text if the journal specifies the citation-sequence ("Vancouver") system. For the name–year ("Harvard") system, list them in the alphabetic sequence determined by the first-author name; see Chapter 19 for more details.
- Verified against the referenced documents.

- Content and format based on styles specified in "Uniform Requirements for Manuscripts Submitted to Biomedical Journals" (1) for journals using the citation-sequence ("Vancouver") system or the style specified by journals using the name–year ("Harvard") system. See Chapter 19.
- Journal titles abbreviated as in MEDLINE and the *Index Medicus*.
- Unpublished observations and personal communications should not, in general, be used as references; some journals will allow in-text parenthetic citations of such materials. Papers accepted for publication but not yet published can be given as references but should be identified at the end of the reference as "In press" or a similar term. Some journals may allow research papers submitted to a journal but not yet accepted to be treated as "unpublished observations".

6. Tables

- Each table on a separate page.
- Tables numbered (arabic numerals) consecutively in accordance with their order of citation in the text.
- Title for each table.
- Explanatory text in footnotes, not in title.
- Nonstandard abbreviations explained in footnotes.

7. Illustrations

- Photographic copies, not original art work or films
- Number of sets of illustrations corresponding to number of manuscript copies
- Photographic prints not larger than 20.3 by 25.4 cm (8 by 10 inches)
- Figures numbered consecutively in accordance with their order of citation in the text
- Each figure identified on its back by applied label with figure number, names of authors, and identification of top of figure
- Prints not marred by impressions of writing on their backs or by paper clip marks
- Photomicrographs with an internal scale

8. Legends for illustrations

- Legends on manuscript page(s), not on backs of figures

Note that although more than 500 journals around the world that subscribe to the *Uniform Requirements* document already cited (1) have agreed to receive manuscripts prepared in accord with most of the details specified above, some of these requirements may not be appropriate for some journals in medicine and related fields. If you use this list, check its details against the information-for-authors pages of the journal for which you have written the paper. The section below points out some departures from these uniform requirements. Note that a few journals in the "Uniform Requirements . . ." agreement change some style details (notably in references) for publication. But journals in the agreement should not ask authors to make such changes.

REVIEW OF THE FINAL VERSION OF THE PAPER

After you have worked on your paper through two or more revisions to this final stage, its content and prose style should be beyond need of further reworking. But you may need to correct a few remaining details before you have the final manuscript typed.

Title Page

Title, Running Head, or Footline

Be sure the title describes the content of the paper as specifically as possible. If you drafted the title when you wrote the first version, the title may no longer be fully accurate. Omission of some text when you worked on the first or second revisions may have made the present title inaccurate. Remove such empty phrases as "A Study of . . ." and "Observations on . . .". Shorten an excessively long title by moving some of its content into a subtitle (if the journal allows subtitles; check some recent issues). Titles with more than 100 characters (letters and spaces) usually are too long.

Some journals place highly abbreviated titles representing the content of the paper at the top or foot of each page after the title page to assist readers in orienting themselves. These "running heads" or "footlines" must be much shorter than titles, usually not exceeding 40 characters and spaces. Their terms should be drawn from the paper's title.

Authors

All persons listed as authors must have read and approved this final version. Exceptions might be made if an author has waived this right in advance, but many journals expect to receive signatures of all authors on a form that affirms that all authors have approved the version of the paper submitted. Signatures could be legitimately thus supplied by authors who will see the final manuscript just before it is mailed to the journal or will see the paper at the proof stage.

Disclaimers and Acknowledgment of Support

If you have written your paper as part of your duties in a governmental agency or with an industrial employer, you may be required to make a statement on the title page of the paper that separates your employer from any responsibility for its content. If you are not sure of how to word the required statement, ask the appropriate person in your organization.

Be sure that the paper carries acknowledgments of support from all sources in the form and location specified by the journal; see "Acknowledgments" below.

Abstract Page

Abstract

Be sure that the length of the abstract does not exceed that allowed by the journal. Check to see that numeric data in the abstract agree with these data as they appear in text and tables. For a more detailed discussion of abstract content and structure, see Chapter 12.

Key or Indexing Terms

Journals differ in how they select terms under which their papers are listed in the journal's index. Some use only terms appearing in the titles of papers. Some have an indexer who searches each paper for additional topics under which the paper should be indexed. Some journals use only the Medical Subject Headings (MeSH) terms developed by the US National Library of Medicine for the subject index of *Index Medicus*. This practice prevents the often-confusing use of several synonyms as entry terms in the index for different papers on the same subject. The MeSH terms are recommended in the *Uniform Requirements* . . . document (1) for key words, or indexing terms, to be placed on the abstract page of the manuscript. Authors can find copies of the MeSH compilation (2) in hospital and medical-center libraries. MeSH terms can also be found in the Library's Grateful Med program and at its Web site.

Text Pages

Text Heading and Subheadings

Unless your paper is short (for example, an editorial or a book review), you have probably divided its text with headings for the main divisions. If it is a paper on experimental findings in laboratory research, for example, the headings probably include Introduction, Methods, Results, and Discussion. The text of a review paper about a disease might carry headings such as Definition, Etiology, Pathogenesis, Pathology, Epidemiology, Diagnosis, Differential Diagnosis, Treatment, and Prognosis. Before the final manuscript is prepared, make sure that these headings are at the right divisions in the text. If you have written a very long paper, you have probably divided the text additionally with subheadings appropriate to kinds of headings described above. The section of a review article headed with Diagnosis might carry subheadings such as History, Physical Examination, Laboratory Tests, and Imaging Studies. The main headings are often called *first-order headings;* subheadings at the next level down are *second-order headings* and two levels down, *third-order headings.*

In addition to checking all text headings for location and appropriateness, you should, at this point, identify headings as to their levels (first-order, second-order, and so on) so that the keyboarder will use the type conventions corresponding to those in the journal. If the journal prints first-order headings like Results and Discussion in all capital, or "upper case", letters (RESULTS, DISCUSSION), you should write in pencil on the left-hand margin of your manuscript adjacent to each heading the instructions, "first-order heading: all capitals". If second-order headings (the subheadings or next level of headings) are printed in the journal with initial capitals, the pencilled instructions in the margin should be "second-order heading: capitals and lower case". Such instructions can be abbreviated as "1st, all caps" and "2nd, caps and lc". Italicized headings should be typed with an italic typeface (easy to do in many word-processing programs) or underlined in accordance with the manuscript convention for indicating italicization.

Citation of References

Be sure that each reference is cited at the right point in the text. As you read through the text and come to a citation, look back at the references to be sure that the citation is appropriate to the immediately preceding text. Also make sure that every reference is cited at least once in the text, a table, or a legend to a figure.

This is also the time to be sure that the system of citations corresponds to that used in the journal. If you have carried citations through successive drafts of the paper as name-and-year designations such as "(Gurwith and Jones, 1978)", as suggested in Chapter 12, and the journal uses citation by numbers (the citation-sequence system), now is the time to assign numbers to the references and place these numbers at the right points in the text, substituting them for the temporary name-and-date citations. A large fraction of clinical journals, especially those in the "Uniform Requirements . . ." agreement (1), specify that references be arranged in the order in which they are first cited in the paper. For this citation-sequence system (the "Vancouver style"), check the order in which each reference is first cited and be sure that the references are arranged and numbered in the same order. Then replace the name-and-date citations in the text, if you have carried the citations in this form through the successive drafts, with the reference numbers. If a reference is cited only in a table or legend to a figure, and not in the text, treat the first mention of that table or figure as the first mention of the reference.

Some journals in medicine and related fields do not use the citation-sequence system ("Vancouver style") but require that references be listed in the alphabetic order determined by the family name (surname) of the first author. For these journals you must be sure that your references are in this order. Authors find it easy to arrange most names of European origin in the right alphabetic order, but uncertainties may arise with names carrying definite articles or particles (such as *van* in *Ludwig van Beethoven*) in the family name, with compound family names (such as in Spanish names), or with Oriental names. A thorough guide to alphabetizing author names can be found in Section 30.15, Chapter 30, of the Council of Biology Editors style manual (3); a shorter guide can be found in Chapter 6 of the American Chemical Society style manual (4). In journals that publish references in alphabetical order by the family name of the first author, the text citations for references are likely to be parenthetic statements of the name of the author (or authors) and the year of the referred-to document's publication, such as "(Huth 1982)" for the book you are reading. This system, known as the name–year system (see Chapter 19), is widely used among disciplines outside of science and some journals in science. If you have carried name–year citations in your text from the first draft and the journal does use the name–year system, you now need only check those citations to be sure that each is in its right place, that each refers to the reference you intend it to, and that the name–year designations correspond to those in each cited reference.

Some journals, notably European journals, publish references in alphabetical order (arranged by first-author family name) but use citation numbers in the text. If your paper is going to such a journal, you now need to check that your references are in correct alphabetical order (see comments above on alphabetization), to number the references, and to replace the name–year citations with the newly assigned reference numbers.

Acknowledgments

Many journals allow authors to append an Acknowledgments statement at the end of the text to credit assistance that does not justify authorship. Such assistance should be credited only to persons willing to have it thus acknowledged. Giving the names of persons who may have had some connection with the study or with preparing the paper but who have not consented to mention of their names could be a breach of scientific ethics. A colleague who read your paper in draft and disagreed with some of its content may not wish to be associated with its publication. To acknowledge his or her reading of the paper in draft can imply approval of its content even if your Acknowledgment does not state such approval. For this reason, you should have in hand the written consent of all persons mentioned in an Acknowledgments note before the paper is submitted.

Some journals designate the Acknowledgments section as the place for authors to identify grant support, donors of equipment or supplies, other kinds of assistance, or potential conflicts of interest (such as equity holdings).

References

Order

The section above, "Citation of References", discusses the two sequences for references: arrangement by order of first citation in the text and its accompanying tables or figure legends, and alphabetical order based on the family names of first authors. Some other basis for order of references, such as year of publication, is unlikely in medical journals.

Content and Format

Two errors in preparing references for the final manuscript may lead to a required further revision if the paper is accepted: failure to include the data elements expected in references by the journal; failure to place the elements in the specified format. At this point be sure to check the journal's requirements on references. If the journal does not include requirements or formats for references in its information-for-authors pages, examine the references in papers in recent issues for guides to the kinds of data required, the arrangement, and the punctuation.

If some of your references are to documents of kinds not frequently cited in clinical journals, such as government reports, newspapers, legal papers, and dissertations, you may be unable to find appropriate example references in recent issues of the journal. Chapter 19 illustrates reference formats for some such documents, as well as the more frequently cited journal articles and books. Additional examples can be found in Chapter 30 of the Council of Biology Editors style manual (3) and in some of the style manuals described in Appendix E. Note that all references should designate an author or authors. The "author" for some kinds of documents may be a committee or government agency. If no organization can be identified as "author" (specifically known as a *corporate author* or *collective author*) and the document is likely to have been written by an unnamed person or unnamed persons (but not a corporate group), the author can be designated as "[Anonymous]".

Abbreviations of Journal Titles

The journal for which you are preparing your paper may use the full titles of journals in references, but the odds are that if it uses abbreviated titles those titles are abbreviated in accordance with the rules used by MEDLINE and the *Index Medicus*. Abbreviated titles for most journals likely to be cited in medical papers can be found in each January issue of the *Index Medicus*.

Submitted but Unpublished Papers

Because references should refer only to widely available documents or those that can be consulted in libraries by scholarly authors (such as manuscripts), many journals will not allow references to papers that have been submitted to journals but not yet accepted for publication. In some journals such papers may be cited in the text within parenthesis marks by the author's name and designated as "unpublished".

Most journals will allow references to papers accepted but not yet published because an acceptance can be independently verified with the editorial office of the journal that has issued it. These references should be used in the usual format, with the year given but "[In press]" replacing year, volume number, and page numbers.

Abstracts, Personal Communications, and Unpublished Observations

The acceptability as references of informal documents and of mentions of unpublished observations differs widely among journals. Most journals will not allow references to such sources; among such journals some will allow citation of them in the text, usually within parenthesis marks. Abstracts are sometimes treated as informal documents (because their content has not passed through formal peer review), and formal reference to them is not allowed; some journals will accept references to them if they are designated as abstracts. As with mention of persons in an Acknowledgments section, personal communications should not be cited in the text (if the journal allows such citations) without written permission from the cited person or persons; the journal may ask for copies of permissions.

Verification of References

The completeness and accuracy of all data elements in all references must be checked against the documents given as the references. You should be able to verify all of your references because you should not cite any documents you have not seen; such citation would be intellectual dishonesty. Your check should include author names, the title of the document and the title of a publication within which it appears (journal title, book title, and so on), and relevant further identification (such as volume and page number, year of publication). Not all of the available identifying data will necessarily have to be carried in your references; some journal articles, for example, have subtitles as well as main titles, and subtitles are rarely included in references. The example references in Chapter 19 illustrate the kinds of data you have to check.

If you find errors in the identifying data in the original document (such as misspelled names of authors), do not correct the errors for your references. The published form of the data element, even if in error, will have to be used by a reader looking for the document; if the search goes through an automated system, the corrected form could obstruct the search. Errors you have identified can be signaled as such by the Latin word *sic* (meaning *thus*) within square brackets after the error. For example, if you know that "Seabright" in a title with the term, "Seabright bantam syndrome", should be spelled *Sebright,* that error can be indicated as "Seabright [sic] bantam syndrome".

Tables

If in revising your paper through successive drafts you have deleted unneeded text but have not dropped tables or illustrations, the total number of tables and illustrations may be excessive in relation to the length of the text. Too many tables and illustrations can produce difficulties in page layout for the journal. If limits on the number of tables and illustrations are not specified in the journal's information-for-authors pages, examine some recent issues to see how many are usually carried in articles with various lengths of text. A useful guideline to most journals' limits is no more than 1 table or illustration per 1000 words of text (roughly 4 pages of text typed double-spaced).

The title of a table should be sufficiently detailed to enable the reader to understand the purpose and content of the table without going to the text for an explanation. Footnotes can explain details that could not be described in the title without making it too long. Be sure that nonstandard abbreviations in the table are explained in footnotes.

Illustrations

Check on whether you have enough photographic copies of all illustrations to match the number of copies of the final manuscript you must submit.

KEYBOARDING THE FINAL MANUSCRIPT

After you have checked all elements of the paper with attention to the points made above, the final manuscript can be keyboarded. Again, check the journal's information-for-authors pages for instructions. If it does not provide guidelines for whoever is going to keyboard the manuscript, the points made below may be helpful.

Close attention to a journal's manuscript requirements is most critical for papers going to journals printed from camera-ready copy or manuscripts prepared as digital records for direct typesetting.

Manuscripts that are to serve as camera-ready copy (pages to be printed as photographic reproductions of the typed manuscript) must be prepared exactly as specified by the journal. These requirements may include the kind of paper and other technical details. The journal will probably provide sheets of paper with outlines delineating the area within which typed text must be confined.

Some journals are beginning to use for typesetting by their printer the digital records of manuscripts on disks ("floppy disks") generated by word-processing programs. In these systems, the author may be asked to introduce code symbols or words into the text; these codes instruct the computer typesetter on choices of typefaces and other details in the page format of the journal. The manuscript will probably be reviewed by the editor and manuscript consultants in the present conventional procedure, with the codes to be inserted into the manuscript only after the journal has accepted the paper and is ready to prepare it for the printer.

Typewriter or Computer-linked Printer

The preceding versions of the paper (drafts) have probably been prepared with a word-processing program, and the final version can be readily printed out with a laser or ink-jet printer. If a dot-matrix printer is used, it should be able to produce letter-quality or near letter-quality characters; one should not be used to print manuscripts with draft-quality characters (in which individual dots forming the characters are readily visible). If the final version is to be typed, the typist should use a typewriter ribbon producing a strong black impression. The typist should not use a typewriter with an unusual typeface, such as one having only capital letters or one imitating handwriting.

Paper

A good-quality white bond paper in a standard size should be used: the US standard size of 8.5 by 11 inches (roughly 22 by 28 cm) or, for journals in countries using metric sizes, 212 by 297 mm (ISO A4 size). US journals prefer to receive manuscripts prepared with the 8.5 by 11 inch dimensions.

If the manuscript is typed, the typist should not use one of the patented bond papers advertised as making erasures easy; type impressions on such papers usually smear readily with handling. Do not use carbon paper for the original manuscript or for copies; copies are preferably prepared on a xerographic machine.

Continuous-form papers for computer printers should be of the micro-perforated type so that the manuscript pages do not carry little tufts of paper on their edges.

Spacing

Double-space all lines throughout the manuscript, including not only text pages but also title page, abstract, references, tables, and legends for illustrations. Double-spacing of references means double-spacing between lines of individual references, as well as between adjacent references. Double-spacing is likely to be needed by the journal's manuscript editor for room for instructions to the printer. Do not single-space any part of the manuscript. Avoid the temptation to fool an editor into thinking a paper is shorter than one might guess from the number of pages by typing with 1½ spaces between lines rather than double-spacing or by making the margins excessively narrow. An experienced editor readily catches such ruses and dislikes them.

Numbering Pages

Use arabic numerals and place the page number in a righthand corner (top or bottom) of each page; the righthand bottom corner is preferred. Some journals may prefer page numbers centered in the bottom margin. Number pages consecutively, beginning with the title page.

Sequence and Division Sections

Begin each of the sections on a separate page and in this sequence: title page, abstract (with keywords, if requested by the journal), text, acknowledgments, references, tables (no more than one to a page), and legends for illustrations.

Format on Each Page

Type on only 1 side of each sheet of paper. Leave margins of 2.5 to 4 cm (1 to 1.5 inches) at the top, bottom, and sides of each page. Avoid dividing words at the ends of lines. Indent the beginning line of each paragraph.

If the manuscript is prepared with a word-processing program, do not "right-justify" the text at the right margin (vertical alignment of terminal characters of all lines). In many programs, right-justification often produces excessively long spaces between words in each line, which impedes reading.

CHECKING AND CORRECTING THE FINAL MANUSCRIPT

Whoever keyboards the final manuscript (author or typist) should read the completed manuscript first for keyboarding errors. If the manuscript has been prepared with a word-processing program, most errors can be caught with the program's spelling checker.

The manuscript should then be read twice after typographical errors have been corrected, at least once with someone else reading the corrected version from which the final manuscript was prepared. In one of these two readings, close attention should be given to accurate placement of citations in text, accuracy of quotations, and correctness of spelling of names and technical terms. If the manuscript has been prepared with a word-processing program, corrections can readily be inserted. If the manuscript has been typed, minor corrections can be noted in the space above the line and the insertion points in the line marked with an inverted "vee-mark", also known as a caret. If long corrections are needed, the entire page (and following pages if necessary) should be keyboarded again.

COPIES

Journals expect to receive either original copies of the manuscript or xerographic copies. If the manuscript has been prepared with a word-processing program, the additional copies requested by most journals can readily be provided as multiple copies with a laser or inkjet printer as cheaply as xerographic copies.

Be sure to retain at least one complete copy of the final manuscript, including illustrations, in your own files (as well as the digital record of the manuscript if it was prepared with a word-processor). Coauthors should also have complete copies for their files.

If the journal also expects to receive a copy of the manuscript as a word-processing file on a diskette or transmitted by e-mail, its information-for-authors pages will specify which form and the relevant technical details.

CONCLUSION

Before the final version of your paper is computer-keyboarded or typed, review the manuscript requirements of the journal and be sure that your paper contains all the needed elements and that these are in accordance with the journal's requirements. Many details will have to be checked on the title page, the abstract page, in the text (especially the citation of references), the references (for data elements and format), and the tables and illustrations. Be sure the final manuscript is prepared as expected by the journal and that the requisite number of copies will be available.

REFERENCES

1. International Committee of Medical Journal Editors. Uniform requirements for manuscripts submitted to biomedical journals. Ann Intern Med 1997;126:36–47. Note that this document is available at the American College of Physicians' Web site (http://www.acponline.org/journals/resource/info 4aut.htm).
2. National Library of Medicine. Medical subject headings. Bethesda (MD): National Library of Medicine. Published annually as Part 2 of the January issue of *Index Medicus*. The MeSH terms compilation is also published as a separate publication and can be consulted at the Library's Web site; see Chapter 3.
3. Style Manual Committee, Council of Biology Editors. Scientific style and format: The CBE manual for authors, editors, and publishers. 6th ed. New York (NY): Cambridge University Press; 1994.
4. Dodd JS. The ACS style guide: a manual for authors and editors. 2nd ed. Washington (DC): American Chemical Society; 1997.

PART 4

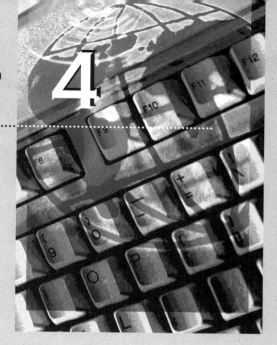

You and the Journal

CHAPTER 21

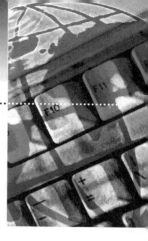

Submitting the Paper to the Journal

The final version of your paper is ready to be sent to the journal for which you have prepared it. You have in hand the numbers of manuscript copies and illustrations the journal asks for in its information-for-authors pages and additional copies for your file and your coauthors. Six steps remain.

- Preparing the submission letter to accompany the manuscript.
- Getting the signatures of all authors on forms required by the journal with submissions.
- Assembling all other items that also have to be sent with the manuscript.
- Packing the letter, manuscript, illustrations, and other documents.
- Checking again in the journal's information-for-authors pages on whether it expects submission of papers as a word-processing file on a "floppy" disk or via e-mail.
- Mailing the manuscript package.

THE SUBMISSION LETTER

The editor of the journal to which you are submitting the paper will need some information about you and your paper. You may wish to send additional information that could help the editor in processing the manuscript for review and coming to a decision. All of this information should be in the submission letter, also sometimes called "the covering letter". What should the letter say? What additional information might be included? The journal's information-for-authors pages may define what information it expects to find in a submission letter.

Identification of the Paper

The paper should be identified by its full title and the full names of all authors. The editor will probably assume that all of the listed authors have read the final version and agreed to its content; some journals expect an explicit signed statement on such agreement. The institutional affiliations of the authors and the name of the institution in which the paper has its origin need not be given in the letter; this information should be carried on the title page (for some journals on the following page); see "Title Page" in Chapter 20.

Description of the Paper

If the title of the paper may not adequately summarize the content of the paper, perhaps because of complexity of its content, you may wish to describe the content more fully.

If the journal publishes various types and formats of papers (such as research reports, brief communications, reviews, editorials), the right category will probably be clear to the editor when he scans the manuscript for a first impression of the paper. You may wish, however, to indicate the category you believe to be appropriate. Presumably you selected the category from the journal's information-for-authors pages or a scan of the journal's content before you began to write the paper. The editor may disagree with your choice but if the paper is accepted you should be happy to accept his or her decision!

Selection of the Journal

That the content of the paper is relevant to the journal's scope and audience may be clear to the editor from the paper's title, abstract, or quickly scanned text. But if the paper might be appropriate for more than one kind of journal, you may wish to explain briefly why you selected the editor's journal. A paper on more efficient procedures for nurses in pediatricians' offices might be submitted to a journal in nursing or one in pediatrics. If the described study finds that the savings in time and costs may benefit the pediatrician more than the nurse, you may decide to prepare the paper for, and send it to, a pediatrics journal. Perhaps you should briefly make this point in your letter lest the editor of the pediatrics journal conclude as soon as he or she looks at the manuscript that it should have been sent to a nursing journal.

Repetitive Publication and Duplicate Submission

Professional journals are expensive to publish, and editors make the best use of their pages by publishing as much as possible only new information. Editors feel ethically obliged to do what they can to prevent clogging bibliographic indexes like MEDLINE with references to papers describing the same findings from a single study. For these reasons you should indicate in your letter that the content of your paper, in its entirety or in part, has not been published already and is not in any paper already, or about to be, submitted to another journal. A statement this specific is needed because to the editor *repetitive publication* refers not only to exact duplication of a paper (exactly the same title, abstract, text, references, tables, and illustrations) but also to repeated publication of essentially the same information whether or not it is presented in precisely the same way.

If any part of the submitted paper's content has been, or shortly will be, published but you believe that its publication again should not thereby be precluded, you should tell the editor why you believe publication of your submitted paper in his or her journal is justified and specify the extent of the duplication. The editor may be aided by your including with the manuscript (see below) a copy of any possibly related paper.

A paper should be sent to only one journal and not to another until it has been rejected by the first. Editors resent having to spend time and effort in processing papers also submitted to other journals that are subsequently withdrawn because of an acceptance elsewhere. What you might gain through saving time in getting an acceptance more quickly, you may lose in reputation. Your letter should include a statement that the paper is being submitted only to that journal and has not been, or will not shortly be, submitted to another journal.

Conflicts of Interest

Some journals may expect a statement in the submission letter identifying any real or potential conflict of interest among the authors between objective reporting of properly designed research and financial or contractual interests with organizations that might bias what data are reported and how they are interpreted. This kind of information may be expected in a separate form. The journal's information-for-authors pages should be checked again for such requirements.

Conditions on Publication

State in the submission letter any conditions you feel you must place on publication of the paper by the journal if it is accepted. You may wish, for example, to read a version of the paper at a professional society meeting in May and to do so must respect the policy of the society that only papers not already published may be read at its meeting. Hence, you will have to ask of the editor that if the paper is accepted it not be published earlier than June. Or you may wish to have the paper also published in a proceedings of a scientific meeting to be issued at a date far enough in the future so that it will appear after its publication in the journal; you want to be sure that the journal will grant you permission for the republication in the proceedings. This situation should be described to the editor so that he or she can decide whether the time needed for review of the manuscript, the journal's backlog (if any), and the press schedule are such that your request could be met. Another example is that of color illustrations; you may wish to have the editor agree to publish the paper, if accepted, only with the color, rather than black-and-white, illustrations.

Whatever condition you may wish to place on publication, be sure that you do need it. The rejection rate is necessarily high in a major journal popular with authors; its editor may not wish to have to deal with conditions that may limit the scope of editorial decisions and the flexibility of schedules. The editor may prefer to reject the paper immediately to avoid possibly being burdened later with the condition asked for.

Copyright

Most professional journals expect to have the copyright on an article to be transferred to the journal by the author when the paper is submitted or when it is accepted. An author will not be free to transfer copyright in two circumstances: if he or she has written the paper as a Federal employee, or if the copyright became the property of a private organization at the time of the paper's creation because of the author's acceptance of that arrangement as an employee of the organization. If the author cannot transfer copyright to the journal for one of these two reasons or any other reason, that constraint should be stated in the submission letter. Some journals will not accept a paper for which copyright cannot be transferred (except papers from Federal employees).

Content for Optional Publication

What if your paper is very long, in part because of an unusually large number of large tables, but you feel that all of its content should be available to at least some readers? You could point out in your letter that you would be willing to have those portions of the paper not critically needed for most readers filed in an archival repository from which interested readers would be able to get copies of the part deleted from the version of the paper published. A journal may be willing to let authors state that they will supply readers with copies of large tables (or other material) that could not be included in the published version of the paper. Such materials might also be posted at an institutional Web site.

Alternatives in Format

A Methods section might be very long because, for example, it includes a detailed description of a statistical method rarely used in medical research. The author might suggest to the editor that the description could be placed at the end of the paper in an appendix, where it would not distract readers interested in the paper but unable to understand the principles and application of the statistical method.

Suggestions on Reviewers

Most editors maintain files with the names of potential manuscript reviewers who are expert in the fields covered by their journals, but these files may not be adequate for some highly specialized topics. If you believe that the topic of your paper is one not frequently covered by the journal, you may wish to suggest experts on the topic who could pass critical judgment on your paper. If you do so, you might assure the editor that the suggested reviewers have not participated in any way in preparing the paper, have not read the paper before its submission, and are not friends who might be uncritically biased toward the paper.

If your research is in a highly competitive field, you may not wish to have your paper reviewed by rivals; you may feel that they might be tempted to hinder or try to block its publication. You can properly ask the editor not to use as reviewers the persons you specify. You should not, however, give the editor such a long list of reviewers to be avoided that he or she will suspect you of eliminating all persons expert enough in the field to find any weaknesses in the paper.

The Responsible Author

The letter must make clear who will be responsible for receiving correspondence and phone calls from the editor or other members of the journal's staff and who will be responsible for revising the paper. Usually, but not always, the two will be the same person, probably you. The letter should include the name(s), postal address(es), and phone number(s). Other useful addresses may include those for an electronic-mail system ("e-mail") or a facsimile ("fax") or telex terminal. If the previously agreed-upon responsible author may be away in the near future for a long vacation, a business trip abroad, or a sabbatical leave, an alternative responsible author should be designated, also with address and telephone information.

If your paper is being submitted by an editor in your institution (an "author's editor"), the letter should indicate whether the journal editor is free to correspond with, or telephone, the responsible author for revisions and meeting other requests or should direct all inquiries and requests to the author's editor.

Payment for Manuscript Handling

Some journals charge a fee to cover the costs of processing and reviewing manuscripts; those that do will indicate so in their information-for-authors pages. If the journal to which you are sending the paper expects to receive payment with the manuscript, indicate in the letter that payment is enclosed and identify the document of payment (check, bank draft, or money order).

Cost of Color Illustrations

Some journals will take on the cost of publishing color illustrations, which is far higher than for black-and-white illustrations, but many journals expect the author to meet that cost. Indicate in the letter whether you will be willing to pay for this cost if your paper includes color illustrations.

What Not to Include in the Letter

Probably all editors feel that they, their editorial associates, their editorial boards, and their manuscript reviewers are collectively competent enough to judge the importance and validity of papers in the fields their journals cover. You may have doubts about a particular journal, but presumably that is not the journal to which you are sending your paper. Do not risk slurring the editor's competence by including in the letter what the advertising industry calls a "hard sell"; do not claim that the paper reports the greatest breakthrough in medical science since Pasteur demolished the theory of spontaneous generation of life or reports the greatest advance in therapeutics since Fleming stumbled onto penicillin. If your paper is so important, it will be recognized as such. If it is not so recognized, your effusions will probably not change anyone's judgment; the manuscript reviewers will probably not see your letter anyway.

REQUIRED SUBMISSION FORMS

As already indicated in this chapter, some journals expect to receive some of the information relevant to the submitted paper on specific forms. Such forms may include a transfer-of-copyright form, an affirmation-of-authorship form, a form for reporting real or potential conflicts-of-interest. Requirements for inclusion of such forms in the submission package will be stated in a journal's information-for-authors pages and the forms may even be published in some issues of the journal adjacent to the information pages. You may have noted such requirements weeks or months ago when you consulted the journal's information pages before beginning to write the paper (as suggested in Chapters 2 and 4), but if you did not, be sure to check for them now.

THE NEXT STEP

After you have prepared your submission letter (see Figure 21.1 for an example), you should be ready to prepare the manuscript and accompanying materials for mailing.

Rosena Happenstance, DM
Editor, Journal of Therapeutic Science
999 Rocky Lane
Butterbush DN 10001-4323

Dear Dr Happenstance: 31 December 1987

Enclosed are three copies of "Aspirin for Treatment of Headaches: A
Double-blind Comparison with a Placebo", by TX Stone, RM Rock, and J
Doe. The paper is submitted to be considered for publication as a
research report in your journal. Neither the entire paper nor any part of
its content has been published or has been accepted by another journal.
The paper is not being submitted in its entirety or in part to any other
journal.

We believe the paper may be of particular interest to your readers
because the study reports a new and more precise method of
estimating subjective relief of pain.

Correspondence and phone calls about the paper should be directed to
me at the following address and phone number:

Jan Doe, BSN, PhD
Institute for Analgesic Research
4321 Main Road
Asberdelphia, UZ 12345-999
(234) 567-8912

Thank you for your attention to our paper.
Sincerely yours,

Jan Doe, BSN, PhD

FIGURE 21.1. A typical, but fictional, submission letter.

The Manuscript Package

Contents

It is clear to you already that more than the manuscript must be mailed to
the editor. Here is a checklist that includes items which must be sent and
items needed only in some circumstances. This checklist may not be complete for some journals. Check the journal's information-for-authors pages
for what it expects to receive in the submission package; it may expect, for
example, to receive, as indicated above, a "floppy" disk version of the paper
in the form of a word-processing file.

- Submission letter.
- Manuscript copies: the number requested by the journal; illustrations in
  separate envelopes for each set.

- Transfer-of-copyright form (unless the submission letter indicates transfer of copyright).
- Copies of related manuscripts or papers (see above, "Repetitive Publication and Duplicate Submission")
- Reply postal card or letter with self-addressed and stamped envelope for acknowledgment of receipt of the manuscript (not wanted by some journals)
- Copies of permissions to publish pictures of patients, to cite unpublished communications, to acknowledge help with the paper
- Stiffening cardboard

The items to be sent should be mailed in a sturdy envelope large enough to accommodate them without difficulty but small enough to protect its contents against shifting about. Photographs can be protected against creasing by including cardboard inserts fitting snugly into the envelope.

Addressing the Envelope

Be sure that you have the correct address to which the manuscript package should be mailed; check the journal's information-for-authors pages if you are not sure. Occasionally authors erroneously mail manuscripts to the journal's advertising office or its publisher's office, which may not be at the same location as the editorial office.

Mailing

Unless you must meet a very close deadline, the manuscript package can usually be sent to the editorial office within the country by first-class mail; when you consider the time likely to be required for peer reviewing of the paper (see Chapter 22) the small gain in time from sending it by one of the express-mail services is rarely worth their greater cost. If you are mailing it to another country or to another continent, use air mail.

Before you mail the package be sure that you, and perhaps your coauthors, have retained copies of all that you are about to mail. Mail service is not flawless anywhere; some manuscripts do get lost.

CONCLUSION

Submitting a paper to a journal calls for preparing a submission letter that will give the editor the information he or she will need about you and the paper, assembling any items that will have to be sent along with the manuscript, packing the manuscript and other items in a suitable envelope, and mailing the package.

CHAPTER 22

Peer Reviewing and the Editor's Decision

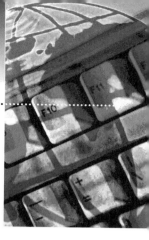

You wrote and revised your paper with great care. The manuscript of the final version was typed and assembled with close attention to the journal's requirements. You mailed the manuscript to the editor and received notice of its arrival at the journal's office. What happens next?

WHAT DETERMINES EDITORIAL DECISIONS?

Journals differ greatly in how their editors decide what to accept and what to reject. The chief editors of some journals, notably those in the basic medical services, divide the reading of submitted papers and responsibility for decisions on them, with or without peer reviews, among associate editors and members of a large editorial board. Editors of journals in clinical medicine and closely related fields may be aided in assessing papers by one or more associate editors but are highly likely to also ask peer reviewers (manuscript reviewers) to read papers critically, suggest possible decisions, and recommend revisions the editor may request before acceptance of papers.

Factors Bearing on Decisions

Exactly what procedure is followed by an editor in coming to decisions is less important for authors than the factors the editor may have to take into account in each decision. Most journals receive far more papers than they can carry in the pages allotted by the publisher. For this reason, rejection rates necessarily run at some arbitrary level, which for the more prominent clinical journals is between, roughly, 50% and 90%. Thus editors must decide on criteria to sort out which papers will be accepted and which will not.

At least five criteria are likely to be applied at some time by most editors.

- Relevance of the paper to the journal's scope and audience.
- Importance of the paper's message to most of the journal's audience.
- Newness of the paper's message.
- Scientific validity of the evidence supporting the paper's conclusions.
- Usefulness of the paper to the journal in its maintaining a desirable range of topics.

Even if a paper is acceptable when judged by these five criteria, the editor may have to apply two more.

- Effect of acceptance on the journal's backlog of already accepted papers.
- Quality and pertinence of the presentation in the manuscript and the extent of revision that would be needed for an acceptance.

Editors do not wish to have their journals known as slow to get papers into print, so they have to hold down the backlog of papers accepted but not yet published. The backlog does have to be large enough to ensure an adequate supply of papers for publication in the face of fluctuations from week to week in the numbers of papers submitted. But the backlog also must be kept small enough not to lead to a delay in publishing accepted papers. A paper rejected when the backlog is large might have been accepted if the backlog had been small. The quality of presentation may be a decisive factor. Two papers with equal merit in content may compete with each other for acceptance; if one has an equal potential importance but has been poorly written and its manuscript carelessly prepared, it is likely to be the one rejected.

Even though an editor may apply most of these criteria in coming to a decision on your paper, you may never know exactly how your paper was judged. Editors are unlikely to assign exact quantitative judgments to all papers for each criterion. If they did, they would probably not have the time to dictate decision letters that would explain in detail all the criteria applied to each paper and how it ranked for each criterion. The decision letter you receive will almost certainly not explain why your paper was accepted if that is the good news. If the letter brings the bad news of rejection, it is likely to carry at least one reason for rejection, but it is not likely to describe all the factors that were assessed by the editor for the decision. Some of them may be apparent in comments by peer reviewers prepared for the author.

PEER REVIEWING

Virtually no editors of either clinical or basic-science journals are expert enough in enough topics within their fields to be able, by themselves, to come to critical judgments on what to publish and what not to publish. They may have associate editors with expertise in topics beyond what they know well but even then they must rely heavily on getting critical judgments from external reviewers ("peer reviewers"; in some fields called "referees") on most of the papers they even consider possibly publishing.

Policies and Procedures

Policies of journals on what papers to send out for external critical readings differ widely. Some of the major clinical journals may send out only 40 or 50% of submitted papers and reject the other 50 or 60% without peer reviewing. These rejections will be based on one or more of the criteria laid out above.

- The paper's topic is outside the journal's scope.
- The paper's message is "stale"; the paper is not sufficiently "new".
- The paper has obvious and irremediable flaws in scientific validity.

And so on. Such a policy is quite understandable. Peer reviewing is expensive in clerical and mailing costs. Good peer reviewers must not be overburdened with requests for reviews lest they become unavailable. Many authors do feel that all papers submitted to a journal should have external readings. Certainly they could benefit from criticisms returned by reviewers even if the journal does not wish to publish the paper. Indeed, some journals do send all papers out for critical readings, perhaps through the editorial-board members or a large group of external associate editors. How can you find out the policy of a journal on peer reviewing?

Many journals now publish detailed statements on their policies and procedures on peer reviewing, generally in their information-for-authors pages. Procedures in peer reviewing are changing and such statements may not cover all possible points. In general, reviewers are still kept anonymous. Some journals attempt to "blind" their reviewers by trying to conceal the authorship of papers. With the development of rapid electronic communication and Web sites, some journals may move to a much more open kind of peer reviewing. If you cannot find a published statement by a journal on its policy and procedure, some of your colleagues who have dealt with that journal may be able to give you a sense of how it proceeds.

What Do Editors Ask of Peer Reviewers?

Some authors misunderstand the function of peer reviewers and think that they are asked by editors, in effect, to "vote" on whether a paper should be accepted, to give the editor the decision. A few journals may work this way but most do not. Most editors regard peer reviewers simply as advisors, persons who give their own expert opinions on a paper. What questions may be posed to elicit those opinions?

- What would be the potential importance of a paper if it is published? Would it represent truly new information? Would it represent only confirmation of recently published new information? Would it strengthen the evidence for an apparently important newly developed concept or diagnostic procedure or treatment? What kind of priority should the paper be given if the editor must choose among many papers with equal merit? What would be its audience?
- What is the strength of evidence for the paper's conclusions? Was the research design adequate? Was the research properly executed? Were the data properly analyzed? Are there probably remediable defects that could be mended in a revised version?
- Is the paper clear enough? Properly structured and sequenced?
- What criticisms and recommendations would you wish to pass on to the authors for revision of the paper?
- Do you suggest acceptance? Possible acceptance after revision? Rejection? Note, as commented above, that editors do not take such recommendations as "votes" on what the editor should do but, rather, as summary statements on the worth of the paper, as the reviewer sees it, for the journal.

Editors generally seek such opinions from reviewers by supplying them with forms that indicate the kinds of judgments sought and provide space for the reviewers to write out in detail the basis for their judgments. In general, reviewers are asked to not state their judgments on the publishability (for the particular journal) of a paper in comments they prepare for authors.

How Many Reviewers Are Asked to Review a Paper?

How many reviewers are asked to read a paper can depend on the journal's general policy on reviewing and on the paper itself. In general, most journals that ask for peer reviews seek to get reviews from at least two reviewers. The two may be selected so as to try to ensure a balance of judgments, one reviewer expected to probably have some bias toward the paper's content and the other likely to have some anti-bias. If the paper has complex content and a wider range of expertise is needed, more than two reviewers will be sought. If two reviewers were sought and one returned an unsatisfactory, cursory review, a third may be sought.

What Do Editors Do with Peer Reviews?

As pointed out above, editors treat reviewers' critiques and judgments as advisory. An externally reviewed paper will probably be discussed at one of the periodic meetings of the journal's editorial board or the journal's group of editors. If both of the opinions of the peer reviewers are clearly adverse, the editor may come to his or her decision alone. Even if the paper is brought to a board or editorial group meeting, a decision may be postponed until further critical judgments on the paper are available, for example, a close reading by an expert in epidemiologic methods or a statistician.

Even if a journal decides to reject a paper after peer reviewing, it will probably send the author copies of the reviewers' comments prepared specifically for the author or authors. Occasionally reviewers, despite instructions to keep their comments impersonal, will indulge in *ad hominem* comments or will allow opinions on publishability of the paper to get into the comments. Careful editors remove such content. Even if the journal's policy calls for reviewer anonymity, some reviewers ask that they be identified and the journal may allow that.

TIME NEEDED FOR A DECISION

How soon can you expect to receive a decision? If the editor reads your paper, decides not to send it to peer reviewers, and rejects it, you may receive that decision promptly. But even if the editor decides on rejection as soon as he reads the paper, the typing and mailing of a decision letter take time. So no less than two or three weeks are likely to pass before you hear from the editor.

If the paper is sent to external reviewers for reading, more time will pass before a decision. Reviewers are asked to review papers promptly, often within a specified period such as ten days or two weeks, but even those who agree to a time limit may exceed it because of illness or unanticipated demands on their time. The many differences in editorial-office procedures and consultant response make it hard to predict the time needed for a decision on a peer-reviewed paper. A fair range of time is four to eight weeks. If you have not received a decision within this period, the editor may have had difficulties in getting adequate consultant critiques or the office staff may have been burdened with an unusually heavy load of work. Sending an inquiry by letter to the editor on the status of your paper after eight weeks have passed and you have not received a decision is a reasonable step to take.

DECISIONS AND RESPONSES

Acceptances: Immediate and Provisional

Few authors, particularly those whose papers have not been invited, receive immediate and unconditional acceptances. Even authors fortunate enough to have their papers accepted immediately for important and valid content are likely to be asked to revise the paper to improve its presentation: shortening text, restructuring tables, eliminating informal abbreviations, improving illustrations, or other changes. If you do receive an immediate acceptance with such requests for revision, be pleased with your good fortune and carry out the requests. The revisions are, from the editor's point of view, needed for good reasons, such as space available, format limits on number of tables, and other technical problems. If the requests seem unclear, unreasonable, impossible to carry out, or likely to cripple the paper's capacity to carry its message, do not simply refuse to carry out the revisions and return the paper unrevised. Reply by letter to the editor about the difficulties you see in revising the paper along the lines requested and why. The editor may insist on the revisions or, if your objections seem justified, may compromise on the first requests.

Acceptances are often provisional, with final acceptance depending on how well the author can revise the paper to meet criticisms of its content, the requests for revision of its presentation, or both. As with immediate acceptances calling only for technical revisions of the manuscript, do your best to revise the paper without delay along the lines recommended by the reviewers and requested by the editor. If recommendations from the reviewers are contradictory, you may have to ask the editor for guidance on how to proceed if his letter has not mediated between the conflicting comments. Not all recommendations from reviewers may have to be accepted, but you will have to justify to the editor (see below) why you have not made those changes. Before you conclude that revision is not needed because the consultant apparently did not read your paper closely, be sure that the paper does not suffer from faulty presentation, such as unclear writing, conflicting data, or some other defect. If you disagree with most, if not all, of the reviewers' recommendations and the editor's requests, you can appeal to the editor for exemptions. Do not simply ignore the reviewers' comments and the editor's decision letter and return the paper unchanged. You may prefer withdrawing the paper from further consideration by the journal, but if you take this step, inform the editor so that the journal's records of your paper can be kept up-to-date.

Returning a Revised Paper

Review of your revised paper will be easier for the editor, the journal staff, and reviewers who read the new version if you send with it a letter not only identifying it as a new version but also specifying exactly what changes were made, their locations, and their relation to the reviewers' recommendations and the editor's requests. Changes asked for and not made should be pointed out, and you should justify having not made them. If each consultant was not identified in some way so that you can link your changes to specific recommendations, you may wish to make copies of the reviewers' sheets and mark them for ready reference in your letter, such as "recommendations A1, A3 and recommendations B2, B6, and B7" (from Consultant A and Consultant B).

Rejections

What if the paper is rejected? Do not get angry and take a rash step. The rejection may be fully justified from the editor's point of view. Keep in mind how authors are competing for limited space in journals, especially the most widely read journals. Consider carefully the comments from the reviewers, if the paper was sent out to reviewers. They may point out sound reasons that figured in the editor's decision. If the reviewers seem to have misread the paper, the fault may lie in unclear writing, misplaced emphasis, or some other defect in the paper's structure or style. If the editor's letter simply tells you that the paper could not be given a high enough priority, or that space cannot be made for the paper (another way of stating priorities), you are likely getting the truth. This is a shorthand way to tell you that the paper's information is not new enough or important enough for the journal at this time. That kind of rejection is not necessarily a slur on the soundness of the paper's content or on how well it presents its message.

Should you appeal the decision? If you think you can meet major objections to the paper by revising it, the editor may be willing to reconsider a new version but do not send in a new version without getting the editor's consent. If you seek that consent, do it by correspondence. The editor may have reasons not given in the rejection letter as to why the paper was rejected, and you may be able to save yourself time by getting those reasons.

Should you send the paper to another journal? This response is usually the better step, unless you decide not to go on with seeking to get it published. The paper may be readily accepted by a journal of lesser reputation or a more specialized journal. Before you send the paper to a new journal, however, do what you can to improve the odds that it will be accepted. Consider carefully the comments from reviewers and from the editor. These may enable you to improve the paper greatly. Do not overlook the possibility that the reviewers who will read the paper for the second journal may include one or more of the reviewers who read it for the first journal; if so, a failure to revise the paper in response to fair criticism could bias a reviewer against the paper in this second submission. Be sure that the manuscript you send is a clean manuscript, bearing no marks from its submission to the first journal, no restapling holes, no other indications to the second journal's editor that he is not the first editor to see it! Be sure, too, that the new manuscript meets all the technical requirements of the second journal. In brief, be sure that the manuscript looks as if it had been prepared specifically for the second journal.

CONCLUSION

Journals differ in the procedures used for review of submitted papers and decisions on which to accept. Most use some variation of the peer review system in which experts are asked to give the editor judgments on papers' validity and importance. The editor is likely to apply additional criteria in coming to decisions. If your paper is ac-
continued

Conclusion continued.

cepted, some revision is still likely to be needed to meet reviewer and editorial re-quests. If your paper is rejected, consider carefully, not angrily, whether the rejection was justified and whether the paper should be carefully revised again, even if you de-cide to submit it to another journal rather than give up efforts to get it published.

CHAPTER 23

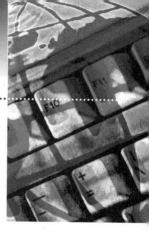

Correcting Edited Manuscript or Proof

The editor has accepted your paper. The acceptance letter may also tell you when you can expect to receive proof of the paper to read and correct and in what issue the paper will be published.

When journals were printed from lead type, authors could expect to receive eventually a proof of their papers for correction. A proof was a version of your paper set in type and printed out on paper. The proof would show you what changes were made in the paper by one of the journal's editors when the manuscript was prepared for the printer. Proof was usually sent to the author in the form of galley proof, long single-columns of the text of the paper as it was set in type. Authors got from the proof some impression of how the paper was going to look in print, but the main reason for sending authors proof was to enable them to catch errors in typesetting the paper and to correct them. The proof might carry questions from the manuscript editor about some details in the paper on which he or she needed some explanation. After galley proof was corrected by you and by the manuscript editor, the columns of type were assembled into pages. Proof of the pages would be checked by the journal for adequacy of corrections, but, generally, authors would not be sent page proofs for review.

With the development of computer-based equipment and procedures for publishing, journals have changed radically in what they provide authors between acceptance of a paper and its appearance in the published journal.

PRESENT-DAY PREPUBLICATION PROCEDURES

Journals now differ widely in what they send to authors as the main step in actually publishing a paper.

265

Return of an Edited Manuscript; No Proof

Most journals have a manuscript editor ("subeditor" in British usage) prepare the finally accepted version of a paper so that when it appears in the journal it will conform in details of style and format to the standards of the journal. Such changes typically deal with matters like the style of references and the structure of tables. In this procedure the journal will send you the edited version of the manuscript for approval and any needed corrections. The manuscript may show what text has been deleted, if any, and what text has been added by the manuscript editor, if any. The manuscript may carry queries in the margin from the manuscript editor or the manuscript may be accompanied by a letter with queries. These have to do with clarifying some details in your manuscript. They must be answered. The manuscript editor may or may not have rewritten any of the text. Any rewriting has probably been done solely to produce a clearer prose style. Nevertheless, there is some risk that the meaning of the text has been altered. If the journal publishing your paper follows this procedure, you must be sure to read the edited manuscript carefully.

Any rewriting done by the manuscript editor probably has improved the clarity of the text. You should avoid a knee-jerk reaction to such changes; some authors consider each and every word of their text to be virtually sacred and resent any changes. If errors have resulted, they must, of course, be corrected. Text to be inserted must be carefully printed above the line where it is to be inserted or in an adjacent margin; a caret ($\wedge$) should be placed just below the line of text at the point of the needed insertion. If the text to be inserted is too long, this addition may have to be typed or printed on a slip of paper that can be attached to the edge of the page at the level of the line to which you are adding it. Resist any temptation to rewrite the text except for obviously needed correction. Changes other than corrections are likely to be taken by the manuscript editor to the journal's editor for a judgment on its acceptability. Text that should be deleted can be crossed out with a horizontal line. The manuscript editor may be helped if you make marginal notes such as "Add" or "Delete", but such notes should be circled to indicate unequivocally that they are directions and not text itself.

Queries from the manuscript editor must be, as indicated above, answered. They may be answered by your making additions or deletions on the manuscript, but they may call for explanations or additional text. The journal probably expects you to answer such queries in a letter you return with the manuscript. Such answers should not only reply to the query but indicate, if necessary, where you have, in response, made changes in the manuscript. If you cannot answer a query, state that too.

If the editing of your manuscript is grossly unacceptable, you will probably have to get in touch with the journal's editor and explain your position and what you expect in response. You should, however, be careful about taking such a step; it might result in the editor's postponing publication of the paper.

The letter from the journal accompanying the edited manuscript may indicate the publication date, but not necessarily so. Some journals have a manuscript editor prepare a paper as soon as it is accepted so that with your acceptance or correction of the edited version, it can be scheduled immediately or held for a later issue. Editors' decisions on scheduling particular papers can be determined by many factors, such as priorities they have for getting some papers out quickly, the balance of topics in an issue, and similar matters.

Journals proceeding this way may or may not subsequently provide proof, so you must take great care with making corrections and answering queries. The edited manuscript may be the last time you see your paper until it appears in an issue of the journal.

Proof in Page Form

With modern computer-based composition of journal pages, proof of a paper is sent by the composing house or printer to the journal in a page format. It may resemble the appearance of pages of the paper as it will finally be seen in the journal. Some journals send to authors both the edited manuscript and the same proof for reading and approval with or without corrections. The suggestions above on how to handle an edited manuscript also apply to review and correction of proof. Again, any queries from the manuscript editor must be answered.

The journal may or may not send, with the manuscript and the proof, a sheet showing marks that can be used on proof to indicate succinctly needed changes. If such a sheet is provided, do your best to apply marks where changes are needed. If one is not, your instructions will have to be encircled marginal notes on needed changes and markings like those suggested above for marking manuscripts.

The "page proof" you are sent is probably not the final, true page proof that the journal alone will receive so that it can check on how satisfactorily the compositor or printer has responded to requested changes. But the journal is usually solely responsible for that check.

WHAT TO DO IN READING EDITED MANUSCRIPT OR PROOF

Read proof to be sure that it says what the edited manuscript says. If you are reading an edited manuscript and deletions by the manuscript editor are not indicated, you should first have your original manuscript read for you by a coauthor as you follow the edited manuscript so that you do not miss deletions or additions by the manuscript editor. If you have reviewed the edited manuscript yourself and you are now reading the proof, your colleague should read for you the edited manuscript as you follow in the proof.

Read proof to be sure that all content of the paper agrees with itself, that the same numbers for the same findings or observations appear in the abstract, the text, the tables, and the illustrations.

Read proof to be sure that nothing needed in the paper has been left out by the manuscript editor or the compositor or printer in preparing the proof.

Some Details Meriting Your Close Attention

Spelling

Even if you are only slightly uncertain about the correct spelling of a word, verify its spelling in a dictionary. Be careful about misuse of such sound-alike words as "principal" and "principle". Be especially careful about scientific terms not familiar to you and about personal names. Personal names cited in the text from your references should be checked against those names as they appear in the references; a disagreement should lead to a check against the original document.

Word Division

Some words will have been broken at the end of lines to "justify" the right margin of the text (to keep the right-hand ends of lines of the text aligned). Such divisions usually follow one of two practices. British practice divides words by etymologic units; American practice divides words by pronunciation units. The newer computer typesetters, in general, divide words according to American practice. Most dictionaries indicate word divisions and can be used to check on the correctness of a break in a word at the end of a line.

Other Details

Focus attention on details readily missed in the first (two readers) reading, such as correct use of italics for scientific names and proper alignments within equations.

Cross-Checking

Verifying authors' names cited in the text against the references has been mentioned above. Other cross-checks should also be carried out. Do the citation numbers in the text match the right references? Are the same numeric values given for the same data at all points where they are mentioned: abstract, results, text, tables, figures?

Checking Tables

Tables should be checked for correctness of title, row and column headings, and numeric values for the data in the field. Any arithmetic operations represented by data, such as addition for column totals or percentage calculation, should be verified. These checks may have been carried out before the final version of the paper was typed, but a check again at this time is a wise precaution. The correctness of alignment of data under column headings and beside row headings should be checked. Be sure that all footnote symbols in the table have corresponding footnotes and that the footnote symbols are in the proper order: They should read left to right, top to bottom.

Checking Illustrations

Proofs of line illustrations such as graphs and diagrams must be checked closely to be sure that data have not been lost, that lines have not been broken where they should not be, and that no other errors have occurred in reproduction. Continuous-tone illustrations such as roentgenograms and photomicrographs should be checked for defects that might be interpreted by readers as part of the original. Orientation should be checked to be sure that "top" is where the top should be; note, however, that the "top" you designated in a photomicrograph might have become "side" if the editor decided that a change in orientation was needed.

WHAT NOT TO DO WITH EDITED MANUSCRIPT OR PROOF

An edited manuscript or proof is sent for correction, not for rewriting the paper. When the paper was accepted, the editor was accepting that paper and not a new version rewritten at the proof stage. If you or any coauthors have changed your mind about content in the paper, you may have to get either permission from the editor to withdraw it from publication or permission for an addendum at the end of the text with the new material.

Resist a temptation to polish your prose at this last minute. Changes at this stage are expensive; the editor will probably disregard changes that have nothing to do with correctness of content.

Do not treat proof lightly, reading it quickly and casually as if it were sent to you only to have you confirm that yes, this is your paper.

RESPONSIBILITY FOR RESPONSES

What if the editor or publisher has not told you when you can expect to receive the edited manuscript or proof? What if you might be away on a business trip or vacation in the months ahead? You should ask when the manuscript or proof is likely to arrive, so that, if necessary, you can change the time of your absence or arrange to have a coauthor or another responsible colleague read and correct the manuscript or proof for you. The responsibility should not be shirked. If none of the authors takes it, the journal will probably proceed to publish the paper just as its manuscript editor prepared it. Any errors will be your fault. Journals cannot tolerate a delay in return of corrected manuscript or proof from the author. The schedule for an issue must be held to.

CONCLUSION

A journal-edited manuscript or proof (the paper as composed with a typeface) is sent to authors not for rewriting of the paper but for correction of errors made by the manuscript editor or in composition of the paper by a compositor or printer. Careful, systematic reading of the edited manuscript or proof will sharply reduce the chances that any errors will go uncorrected. Readings should look not only for errors committed after the paper was accepted but also for errors that might have escaped attention when the final manuscript was read before being sent to the journal, such as disagreement between data in the abstract and in the main body of the paper.

Chapter 24

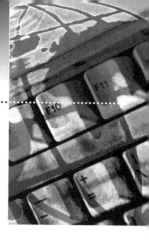

Between Proof and Publication

After you have received edited manuscript or proof, corrected it, and returned it to the journal, you can be reasonably sure that the paper will appear in the journal in the issue indicated to you. If you have not been told the issue of publication, the paper will probably appear in a few weeks to a few months. Between the date on which you returned the manuscript or proof and the publication date, some questions may come up that merit comment here.

REPRINTS AND PREPRINTS

Forms for ordering reprint are usually sent with proof. If an order form has not been sent and you wish to purchase reprints, request the form from the publisher. Reprints may be more expensive if ordered after publication of the issue with your paper.

Some authors may wish to provide colleagues elsewhere with copies of a paper in advance of publication by mailing them copies of the manuscript or of the proof rather than sending reprints. They should remember that after a paper is accepted and its copyright transferred to the journal by the author, the journal acquires by that copyright the legal right to decide how the paper is handled up to and after its publication. The journal may not wish to have copies of the paper circulated before the issue for which it is scheduled appears. If the journal wishes, for example, to have no mention of the content of the paper appear in another journal or in a newspaper before its own publication date, that wish may have been stated in the acceptance letter as a condition of acceptance. If no such condition of acceptance was stated, the journal may wish, nevertheless, that the paper not circulate before it appears in print. The prudent author who wants to send out preprint copies will consult the journal's editor before doing so; the journal may be willing to let you send out preprints.

With the ease of "publishing" papers in a Web site for Internet access, an author may be tempted to post a version of a just-accepted paper in a Web site to which he or she has access. Such a posting might be considered by the journal that just accepted the paper as the equivalent of sending out preprints. Before providing such Internet access, the author should ask the journal's permission to do so.

PREPUBLICATION DISCLOSURES

If your paper is reporting new scientific information likely to be of interest to a much wider audience than that of the journal, your institution or the journal itself may wish to send out press releases about it in advance of its publication. If you do not wish to have a press release go out and the journal has not queried you on this point, you should notify the editor of your wish when you return the edited manuscript or proof. Presumably, your institution would not prepare and mail press releases without your consent.

If you read your paper (or a shorter version of it) at a scientific meeting, you may face the risk that a reporter will inquire about its acceptance and publication date to prepare a news story about your findings. Such inquiries should be directed to the journal's editor. Many journals have "embargoes" on papers they have accepted. These "embargoes" are agreements with news organs that, in exchange for the journal's providing enough advance information on a paper to enable a reporter to prepare an accurate news account, the reporter's news medium will not publish or broadcast the story until the day of publication of the journal's issue carrying the paper.

You or the journal editor may be approached by other parties for information about the content of the paper. Stock market analysts may get wind of a drug trial and wish to know the details of the findings; a favorable outcome could lead to a big price rise in the stock of the firm marketing the drug. A pharmaceutical firm may hear of a new serious adverse effect of one of its drugs and wish to get details about your findings before the paper reporting the effect is published. In circumstances like these you may be visited or telephoned by someone seeking information about your paper but not known to you as a professional colleague. Do not forget that as soon as your paper was accepted and your copyright passed to the journal, the paper and any of its content became the property of the journal, with the right to decide whether any preprint disclosure of content should be allowed. Hence, any inquiries to you of this kind about the paper should be referred to the editor or the publisher. If the editor is approached for similar prepublication release of information and believes such release is acceptable from the journal's point of view, you are likely to be contacted by the editor for permission for the release despite the journal's holding the copyright.

CITING ACCEPTED PAPERS

Chapter 20 points out that in deciding which references can be used in the formal list of references at the end of the paper, cited papers can be identified as "in press" after they have been accepted (finally, not only provisionally) by a journal. If you have written or are writing another paper that cites the paper you have "in press", references to your paper "in press" can now be changed to give more precise identification. At least you should be able to add the journal's volume number, or publication date, or both in place of "in press". After you have returned the edited manuscript or proof, the editorial office may be able to give you the details you need for a clear identification of the paper.

PUBLICATION

In a few weeks or months your paper will appear in print, probably touching off in you a well-justified pride. But do not be surprised if on reading the paper in the journal you are hit by a wave of nausea or some other unpleasant sensation. You may suddenly see a defect you did not catch in the last revision. You may see how you could have said something better. Hold on; do not flog yourself. You will do better in your next paper!

Keep in mind that a serious error undetected before publication can be corrected in many journals by your sending the journal a letter-to-the-editor for publication describing the error and its specific location in the paper and giving the correction.

RETRACTIONS

A rare but nevertheless distressing trauma that we all hope will never hit us as an author is discovering that we have unwittingly written a paper with fraudulent or otherwise unreliable data and with erroneous conclusions derived therefrom. In circumstances like these, we are obliged by generally accepted ethical standards for scientific publication to call attention to the invalidity of a paper with flawed data. Such information must be conveyed to the editor of the involved journal. If the paper has not been accepted, it can be withdrawn from further editorial process. If the paper has been accepted but not yet scheduled for an issue, the editor will probably be willing to let you withdraw it from publication. If the paper has been, or is about to be, published, you should prepare a letter indicating that you wish to "retract" the paper and the reasons for this request. Coauthors who agree with your position should be cosigners of the letter. The journal will probably eventually publish your notice of retraction, which will be identified by the National Library of Medicine and an entry for it in the MEDLINE database linked to the entry for the retracted paper.

A similarly troubling discovery is that one or more of our coauthors have already published some, or even all, of what we are to report in a paper just accepted or already published. If the paper does not unequivocally identify such prior publication, there is the ethical obligation to notify the involved journal of the repetitive publication. Its editor will probably wish to identify the repetitive publication in the journal. As with retracted papers, the National Library of Medicine will link a notice of repetitive publication to the entry for the offending paper.

CONCLUSION

Between acceptance of a paper and its publication, authors may have to pay attention to matters that will require continuing communication with the journal. You may wish to order reprints or ask for permission to distribute preprints. You may be approached by persons with commercial interests who could profit from advance knowledge of what you are publishing; the journal would have to be alerted to such approaches. If you are beset by such mishaps as involvement with a defective paper (fraud or serious errors) or with unidentified repetitive publication, you will have to decide how to deal with such breaches of publication ethics.

PART 5

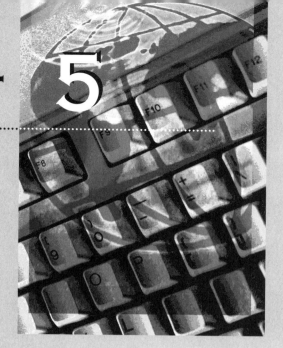

Books

CHAPTER 25

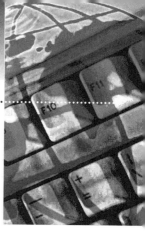

Writing or Editing a Book

Writing a book, yourself or with coauthors, or preparing a contributor text as its editor is a task far more complex and time-consuming than writing papers for journals. Getting guidance on how to proceed is likely to be more difficult than getting help from colleagues with writing papers. Many more of your colleagues will have published extensively in journals than have written or edited books. This chapter cannot cover every detail in book publishing but it does try to orient authors who have had no experience in book authoring and publishing on how they may proceed and what will be expected of them by a publisher.

The task in writing a book yourself, or with a few coauthors, differs from that in serving as the editor of a contributor text.

The differences between authored books and contributor texts cannot be defined sharply. Authored books, in general, are those written entirely by a solo author or a small number of coauthors. The author (or authors) takes full responsibility for all of the content of a book. Contributor texts, in general, are those assembled from individual chapters, each of which is written by a single author or coauthors. Contributions are indicated by an author byline at the heads of chapters. The editor (or editors) of the contributor text is named on the book's title page; the names and affiliations of the contributors are usually listed in a "Contributors" section in the opening pages ("front matter"). The editor takes responsibility for the text's overall content and works closely with contributors to ensure relevancy and accuracy of content and adherence to the text's format.

ESTABLISHING THE NEED FOR A BOOK

A decision to write or edit a book is likely to come about through one of two routes. The first is your seeing a need for a book not satisfied by currently published books. In the second route, you are approached by a publisher who sees a need for a book and wishes to convince you to write it or, for a contributor text, serve as its editor.

Personally Seeing a Need for a Book

If you are an expert in your field, you are probably teaching or training medical students, or residents, or doctoral candidates, or postdoctoral fellows. You know what books already represent your field and are available for teaching and training or for consultation by more experienced clinicians or investigators. You may feel that existing books are out-of-date or present their information inadequately. If you are in a newly developed field or one with rapid recent advances, there may be no books at all in your field. Another possibility is your seeing a need for a book on a medical topic for the general reading public.

Inquiry or Invitation from a Publisher

You are prominent in your field through publishing many papers in leading journals or attention by news media to your research or clinical achievements. A publisher may approach you about writing a book based on your experience or putting one together as its editor. Publishers constantly monitor market needs and possibilities for books that will sell well. These are likely to be books on newly developed or rapidly advancing fields or on topics not already adequately represented by books in print. The publisher (usually represented by an acquisitions editor) may have decided to approach you on his or her own initiative. Or the publisher may have consulted other professionals for suggestions for possible authors on the field or topic. This approach may be simply an inquiry as to your possible interest in writing or editing the proposed book. If your position in your field is widely known and respected, the approach may bring an outright invitation.

DECIDING TO WRITE OR EDIT A BOOK

Whether you have seen a need for a book yourself or have been approached by a publisher, you will have to decide on whether you wish to proceed.

If you were approached by a publisher, you will have to decide on whether to respond with "yes, I will write the proposed book" or "yes, I will serve as the editor". There are many questions you should ask yourself.

- Do I have a clear and convinced view of the need for the book? Do I agree with the publisher's assessment of a need?
- Do I have a clear sense of what its content should be? Can I write out a preliminary table of contents?
- Would I write it myself, or with one or two coauthors? Or would I put the book together from contributions by other authors? If so, will I be able to solicit qualified authors for the various chapters?

- If I would need coauthors, could I find coauthors with whom I could work conveniently, efficiently, and effectively?
- Can I spare the time to write or assemble a book? For most medical professionals, writing a book will probably have to be squeezed into early morning hours, evenings, weekends. The task will run on through months or even years.
- Can the materials needed for the book's contents—such as bibliographic references, photographs, and other similar materials—be readily assembled?
- If you are going to respond with a detailed proposal for a contributor text, can you get at least preliminary indications of interest and possible commitment from persons you believe would be competent authors? You would owe them detailed enough descriptions of topics to be covered, probable length of contributions, and an at least tentative schedule for writing and submitting their pieces. A publisher will probably wish to have preliminary commitments of this kind in considering your proposal.
- For a contributor text: Do I have the resources needed for a large project—an administrative assistant, a writing assistant, adequate secretarial help?
- Will I be able to suggest to the publisher the possible markets for the book?
- Am I likely to be satisfied with rewards for the work that would be involved? The rewards might simply be the satisfactions that can come from organizing your thinking for an audience, or from the prestige, if not dollars, that might follow. Most medical books do not earn enough in royalties to make them attractive income-producers. Some do if they come to be standard textbooks adopted for courses or training programs and hence widely used by medical students or residents.
- What do I think of the publisher myself?
- After looking at books currently published by the publisher, what do I think of the quality of their content, of the attractiveness of their design and layout?
- What is the reputation of the publisher among my colleagues? Have any of them published books with this publisher? What are the opinions of medical librarians in my institution?

If you are approached by a publisher with a proposal for a contributor text for which you would serve as editor, you should find out in detail what help you would be given by the publisher in contacting potential authors, in giving them instructions on how to proceed if they accept the invitation to take part in the project, in monitoring authors' progress, and in holding authors to the schedule.

A publisher might have approached you to serve as the editor of a contributor text to be based on the proceedings of a symposium or conference. Organizing and assembling such a text is a still more complex task because it is likely to involve not only the publisher but also the organization responsible for the program.

- Would all papers invited for the program be provided for publication?
- Would you be free to have all papers peer reviewed and revised to meet criticisms?
- Would you be free to reject any papers?
- Would you, as editor, have any say in who is invited to speak and what topics are to be covered?

A proposal for this kind of text may have been already developed collaboratively with the organization responsible for the program. The organization may have recommended you as a desirable editor.

If you were not approached by a publisher but saw a need for a book yourself, many of the questions posed above would be just as relevant for deciding on whether to proceed and look for a possible publisher.

TYPES OF PUBLISHERS

If you decided on your own that the book you have in mind should be published, you will have to find a possible publisher and submit your proposal. There are several routes to finding a possible publisher. Some of your colleagues who have had books published may recommend some publishers. Medical librarians are usually familiar with a range of publishers and can suggest standard reference catalogues of books in print. These catalogues have listings of books by their subject. A review of books listed under topics akin to the topic you have in mind will show you what books, if any, on that topic have been published and are in print.

Before you decide on approaching a publisher with a proposal, you should know the types of publishers, their characteristics, and, hence, their possible suitability as publisher of the book you have in mind.

Commercial Scholarly Publishers

The biggest publishers of books for the professions and scholarly disciplines are the commercial firms that publish for profit and know how to market books in the audiences they aim to sell to. These firms specialize in publishing books for various disciplines, for example, the physical sciences, the legal profession, or some other definable field. Most books in medicine and the closely allied fields are published by firms that specialize in these fields. Sometimes such specialized publishing is carried out by a division within a larger company that also publishes what are called "trade books" (see the section below, "Trade Publishers"). The names of most of the publishers widely known as "medical publishers" will be familiar names throughout medicine. There are, however, some smaller commercial medical publishers that are less well known. They will almost certainly be known to medical librarians, who will probably have a good grasp on the quality of what they publish.

Most potential authors of medical books would probably opt to have one of such commercial publishers publish their book. These firms advertise and market widely, both to the profession and to medical librarians. They also exhibit their books at national medical meetings. The visibility of their books in the profession is, in general, high.

Organization Presses

Some professional organizations have developed book-publishing units ("presses") and can effectively market books dealing with topics in their fields to their members. Some examples are the American Psychiatric Press (American Psychiatric Association), the American Hospital Association Press (books on medical economics, quality control, personnel management), the Publishing Division of the American College of Physicians, and the BMJ Publishing Group (British Medical Association). Such units may be willing to publish books that are thought by a commercial house to have too small a market. Their marketing capacities may be assisted by arrangements with another organization to also list their books in its catalog.

University Presses

Much of the scholarly publishing outside of large professional fields like medicine, law, and the physical sciences is done by presses operating as part of a university. University presses, in general, tend to publish in the humanities or on topics of regional importance, but some have published books on medical topics, especially books likely to have relatively wide audiences. They maintain high standards in what they publish, but their capacity for marketing to medical audiences is likely to be limited.

Trade Publishers

Large commercial publishers of books aimed at the large markets of readers of fiction and nonfiction of wide appeal are known as "trade publishers" and the books they publish as "trade books". In general they are not interested in publishing books aimed specifically at professional fields like law and medicine, but, as mentioned above, they may have a division devoted specifically to medicine and the allied health fields.

If the book you have in mind is one you think might have a wide appeal in the general reading public, a trade publisher would probably be the best choice. Keep in mind, however, that competition for getting a book published for the general market is intense. Some university presses have become quite successful in publishing books of this kind.

Vanity Publishers

Vanity publishers are commercial firms that specialize in publishing books whose authors are willing to pay to have them published. They may publish books on any topic if the author will meet the cost of publishing. Their marketing is usually sharply limited, and they will be seen by most medical authors as not being an option.

Self-Publishers

With the methods of "desktop publishing" with personal computers, it is possible for authors to produce and sell their own books. But this is a risky route to take. You would be likely to need technical assistance in preparing the materials a printer would need for printing the book. You would have to negotiate with a printer to print the book and bind it. You would have to figure out how to advertise the book to its market. You would have to arrange for "fulfillment", the receiving of orders and payment and the mailing out of ordered books. You would have to bear the cost of production and marketing. You would, however, be able to pocket all of the profit. Few medical professionals are likely to be able to take on such chores in addition to writing the book.

SUBMITTING A PROPOSAL TO A PUBLISHER

Whether you decided on your own to write a book or assemble a contributor text and to try to find a publisher for it or you have been approached by a publisher, you will be expected to submit a formal proposal. Most publishers have detailed guidelines on what they expect to receive in a proposal. Following these guidelines closely and submitting all of the expected materials will improve the odds that you will get a favorable response from the publisher. Some materials are highly likely to be asked for.

- Justifications for the book:
  - What is the need?
  - What is the potential competition from other books?
  - What are the features of potentially competing books?
  - How would your book be better?
  - What do you see as the market for the book?

If you were approached by a publisher, he or she may have already answered these questions but they may still wish to have your judgments.

- A physical picture of the book: How big a book might it be, in pages? Many illustrations? What kind? Only black-and-white line drawings or roentgenographs? Color illustrations?
- A detailed table of contents. You may be asked to submit a sample chapter as well.
- What schedule might you be able to hold to?

If you are approaching the publisher yourself, a curriculum vitae and a personal bibliography may be asked for so that your qualifications for writing or editing the book are clear.

Keep in mind that you should not submit a proposal to more than one publisher at a time. You might be tempted to save some time in approaching another publisher, or several, if the first one turns down your proposal. You might get to an acceptance faster but you would run the risk of blackening your professional name with a publisher who offers you a contract only to find that another publisher has already closed an agreement with you.

WRITING A BOOK AND THEN LOOKING FOR A PUBLISHER

If you decided at some point to write a book you thought was needed and went ahead and wrote it, you have the task of finding a publisher interested in publishing it. Your approach should be much the same as suggested in the preceding section, "Submitting a Proposal to a Publisher". The difference is that you can ship the manuscript of your completed book along with the materials the publisher has indicated in guidelines are needed for a proposal.

This is a highly risky approach. You may not be able to find any publisher interested in publishing the book despite your having labored in preparing a complete manuscript. Your view of a need for the book may be faulty. The market may be saturated. The potential market is seen by the publisher as too small. The cost of producing the proposed book is too high. The publisher may already have such a book in development. Even if a publisher shows some interest in the proposed book, there may be seen a need for a radically different scope or presentation, which could require a major revision of your manuscript.

If you proceed this way nevertheless, there are some precautions you should take before sending off the manuscript. Review your manuscript again. Is the content complete and up-to-date? Is the organization logical and effective? A section within "The Author's Responsibilities" below outlines the conventional format usually used for books. You may have to consider delaying submitting the manuscript until you revise it into the format a publisher will expect to find. The second precaution is producing at least one additional paper copy or electronic file of the manuscript; you should never send out a sole copy of a manuscript, even via certified mail.

BETWEEN SUBMITTING A PROPOSAL
AND SIGNING A CONTRACT

On receiving the proposal, the acquisitions editor of the publisher will almost certainly have to discuss the proposal with others in the firm but will probably also seek external opinions about the desirability of publishing the book. This can take some weeks. If you have not received a decision after two or three months, you are justified in asking about the state of your proposal. If as much as six months goes by without a decision, you may wish to inform the publisher that you are withdrawing your proposal. If you had submitted a manuscript, you should ask for its return.

If the publisher decides immediately to publish the proposed book, you may be offered a contract right away. This outcome is unlikely. Even if the publisher does wish to proceed with publishing the book, the odds are high that some revision of your proposal will be expected before you are offered a contract.

A contract is a legal document that specifies the responsibilities of the author and of the publisher. Contracts can cover many details. Some of the usual points dealt with are the nature of the proposed book, a schedule for delivery of the manuscript, the length of the manuscript, the basis for royalty payments, the rights of the publisher on such matters as translations into other languages, possible use of the book in other media, and copyright. Details in a contract are typically negotiable. Before you sign a contract you may wish to consult colleagues who have published books for their opinions on the proposed contract. You can consult published sources of further information, for example, the section "The Contract" in Chapter 4, "Working with Your Publisher" in Luey's *Handbook for Academic Authors* (1). You can get legal counsel from a lawyer specializing in publication law. If you have been presented a contract by a widely respected medical publisher, you are likely to be offered an entirely reasonable contract. Royalty rates are similar among major publishers; some of your colleagues may be willing to discuss what royalty arrangements were in their contracts.

One of the most frequent questions about a contract is about transfer of copyright. An author who writes a book owns the copyright as of the creation of the work. Nevertheless, publishers expect, in general, to get a transfer of that copyright to them as part of the contract. An author may feel that such a transfer is undesirable, a kind of loss of his or her property. But it must be kept in mind that in exchange for the transfer a publisher will provide many services an author would probably not be able to deal with, such as negotiating with another publisher on a foreign-language edition. Most medical authors are familiar with transfer of copyright on their journal papers to journals in exchange for their services. These considerations are discussed in more detail in "Transfer of Copyright", a section in Chapter 5, "Working with Your Publisher" in Luey's book (1).

If you are going to serve as the editor of a contributor text, you may wish to try to get a written commitment from the publisher before you sign the contract for help in contacting potential authors, in setting out schedules, and monitoring the authors' progress.

THE AUTHOR'S AND THE EDITOR'S RESPONSIBILITIES

You have signed a contract. Who is now responsible for doing what? The author, or editor of a contributor text, has responsibilities.

Manuscript Preparation

Publishers differ in what instructions they supply to book authors; if you do not receive specific instructions on what they expect to receive after you sign a contract, you should ask for instructions. Some book publishers have quite detailed guidelines for submission of manuscripts, as well as style manuals, and will supply authors with copies. For example, the publisher of this book, Williams & Wilkins, has a style manual assembled mainly for its own editors but one likely to be useful to its authors as well. Its coverage includes such matters as proper treatment of abbreviations and acronyms, proper spelling and hyphenation of frequently mishandled words, gender issues, proper phrases and terms, undesirable jargon, instructions on permissions, references citations and formats, and MEDLINE abbreviations of journal titles.

Many points are likely to be covered in a publisher's instructions.

- Overall format of the book. Formats are widely standardized; Table 25.1 indicates the usual kind of format widely used among English-language publishers. Publishers in other countries may have somewhat different formats; for example, many French publishers place the contents pages at the end of the book, rather than in the "front matter".
- Manuscript-page formats, including such details as margins, spacing of text and sentences, codes for text headings, and so on.
- Text citations of references (citation-sequence numbers or name–year citations), styles for references. Style for unpublished references.
- Tables: placement in the manuscript, numbering system, type of footnote signs.
- Illustrations: numbering system, numbers of illustrations to be supplied, legends for figures.
- Abbreviations: where and how acceptable; punctuation.
- Scientific style: system of units (for example, only SI units or any consistent system); handling of numbers (numerals, number-words); drug names (generic, trade); nonpossessive eponyms or older styles.
- Number of copies of the manuscript (printed "hard-copy"); electronic

TABLE 25.1. Typical book formats among English-language publishers[a]

Section	Content
Front matter	Title page: book title, authors' names. Additional details may include academic degrees, affiliations. Pages that may precede the title page include a right-hand "half-title" page carrying a short version of the book's title and a left-hand page listing other books by the publisher or another kind of explanatory material. The half-title page and "other titles" page are usually prepared by the publisher.
	Copyright page ("verso" of title page): such information as the copyright notice, cataloguing designation, International Standard Book Number (ISBN), edition, and publication-date details. The copyright page is usually prepared by the publisher.
	Dedication.
	List of contributors.
	Contents page or pages ("table of contents").
	Illustrations list.
	Tables list.
	Abbreviations list.
	Foreword (not "forward"!): a statement by someone not an author on the need, importance, utility of the book; often requested by the publisher to serve as a quotable text helpful in promotion of sales.
	Preface: a statement by the author(s) on such matters as his or her intent in writing the book, on its probable utility and for whom, or other points.
	Acknowledgments and credits.
	Introduction: Not always present; may be an explanation of how to use the book, of why it has been structured as it is.
Text	Chapters (which may be grouped in topically logical parts).
	Illustrations and tables accompanying the chapter texts.
Back matter	Addendum: text material that had to be added late in the publishing process.
	Appendix(es): detailed text that supplements the main text and is placed here so that it does not interrupt the flow of the main text.
	Glossary: definitions of terms used in the main text.
	Notes: Arranged by relevant chapter.
	Bibliographies.
	Index. Note that an index cannot be compiled until the text of the book has been completed; in general, publishers prefer to index a book themselves or have the index prepared by a professional indexer.

[a]Not all of these format elements are present in all books. A publisher can supply instructions on which ones are needed or acceptable.

version of the manuscript (including acceptable word-processing formats, graphic formats).

• Responsibilities for transfer of copyright.
• Responsibilities for permissions to reproduce illustrations or tables or to quote long passages.

If potential details about an acceptable manuscript or its electronic equivalent occur to you and are not covered in the publisher's explicit instructions, you should raise questions about them before you begin work on the book.

The Editor's Tasks with Contributor Texts

Serving as the editor for a book assembled with contributions from many different authors is a much more complex task than writing a book as the sole author or with a few coauthors.

You (and any coeditors) will have a number of responsibilities. You will have to define the expected content and length of chapters and get firm commitments from competent authors to write them. You will have to set schedules for submission of manuscripts and see that they are adhered to. You will have to make sure that the contributions cover the proposed topics adequately and that they have a consistency in point of view and an adequate similarity in style. You may have to consider getting peer reviews of contributors' chapters as a means of ensuring their adequacy and quality. You will also have to be prepared to get contributors to respond to feedback from the publisher and the publisher's reviewers.

Adherence to Schedules

The publisher's schedule for getting a book produced and marketed involves a complex sequence of events: editorial, production, manufacturing, marketing. Any failures of authors to hold to agreed-upon schedules can interrupt that sequence. Hence authors of complete books and editors of contributor texts must strive to hold to those schedules. Slippage from schedules can affect the marketability of a book: a competing text comes out first, the information in a book on a rapidly developing field can become stale. You will be expected to hold to the schedule stipulated in the contract. Publishers are aware that that can be difficult for busy professionals and may be willing to tolerate some delay. But if you do see a delay ahead, you should inform the publisher of it.

Responsibility for Artwork

Authors tend to think of writing a book as just writing text. Many medical texts carry illustrations. Plans to assemble needed illustrations or getting them produced should have as high a priority as planning for writing the book's text. If line drawings are needed—as in a book describing and illustrating surgical techniques—an artist will have to be engaged and instructed on what will be needed. If photographs of patients are to be used, permissions to use them will have to be secured.

Help with Marketing

Publishers are skilled in marketing, but they may ask for an author's help. They may wish to know whether because of your attendance at national meetings you might be available to spend some time at the publisher's exhibit of books, including your book. They may wish to know if you have a sense of how the book might be advertised in other countries or in particular markets. They may wish to know if potentially competing books have come out just before yours.

Before the book goes into production, you may be asked to supply biographical information about yourself, and perhaps a photograph, that the publisher can use in preparing content for the book's "dust jacket" (paper cover, with description of the book and a note on who you are). You should respond as well as you can, and quickly, to such requests; your help is clearly in your interests.

THE PUBLISHER'S RESPONSIBILITIES

A publisher's responsibilities with an author cover three main areas: editorial management, production, and marketing. These are divided among persons with differing responsibilities. Not all publishers have exactly the same types of staff persons with the same responsibilities and titles, but a general pattern of staff persons who sequentially see a book through from the signing of the contract to its marketing is common to all publishers. Your contacts with the publisher will be contacts with these staff persons.

Editorial Management

By the time you get to signing the contract and preparing to write the book, you have already had dealings with one or more of the publisher's representatives, at least with someone who has raised the question of your writing a book or responded to your proposal. This person is usually known as an "acquisitions editor". He or she will probably be the person who discussed with you what the book should be and presented the contract.

Once the contract has been signed, responsibility for seeing work on the book progress will probably move to a managing editor. This is the person likely to be the one who will follow your progress in working on the book and answer questions about how you should proceed in developing the manuscript. This person may also manage steps toward getting the book into production, such as checking for adequacy of your manuscript, illustrations, and so on. Some of these functions may be carried out by a developmental editor.

Production

The production staff of the publisher manages such details as design of the book, copyediting the manuscript, getting the manuscript (paper, or electronic, or both) to the printer, supplying you with proof, and other practical matters. You are likely to have contact with these staff on various details about the book. You may be asked to review designs for the book and give back your opinions. You will certainly be expected to respond to queries from the copy editor, who will be responsible for correcting errors in style and other details in the manuscript. When there are differences in judgment on, for example, style details, you may be able to negotiate changes to what you regard as preferable style. Keep in mind, however, that some details of style may be standard for the publisher and hence nonnegotiable.

Marketing

You probably took some part in the marketing operations of the publisher when, before you signed the contract, you supplied detailed information about the projected content of the book and your view of its probable audiences (markets). As noted above under "Help with Marketing" you have the responsibility of cooperating with the publisher in marketing efforts. During the production process you may be contacted again for any revised views you may have about the book's potential markets (medical fields, professional levels, countries).

WORKING ON THE BOOK

Many aspects of writing and revising successive drafts of text have been covered in preceding chapters. They are as relevant to writing or editing a book as they are to writing papers for journal publication. There are two points that need emphasis here: the author's or editor's need for full knowledge of the publisher's expectations and the need for a firm schedule for work on the book and adherence to it.

The preceding section, "The Author's and the Editor's Responsibilities", indicates the many details you need to know before you start to write and need to pay attention to as you write. These include, for example, format, style, and manuscript characteristics (paper and electronic). If you do not have this information before you start, you could have substantial additional amounts of work to undertake before you can present the publisher with a final, acceptable manuscript. Get this information before you start and raise any questions that do not seem to be covered by the publisher's instructions.

For help in dealing with format and style matters as you write, you can consult your contact at the publisher's office. You may find helpful working out a collaboration with someone closer at hand. Such technical help can be gotten from an "author's editor", someone familiar with publication methods, procedures, and standards. Your own institution or department may have an editorial unit able to serve as an "author's editor" and prepared to offer such help. If it does not, you can be directed to qualified author's editors by one of the organizations that includes them among its members. Note that for correct e-mail and Web-site addresses given below you should omit the semicolons and periods that follow them in this listing as conventional needed punctuation (for example, amwa@amwa.org and not amwa@amwa.org;).

- American Medical Writers Association, 9650 Rockville Pike, Bethesda, MD 20814-3998, USA. Telephone (301) 493-0003; fax (301) 493-6384; e-mail, amwa@amwa.org; Web site, http://www.amwa.org/amwa.
- Board of Editors in the Life Sciences, c/o Miriam Bloom, SciWrite, 4433 Wedgwood Street, Jackson, MS 39211, USA. Telephone (601) 982-1800; fax (601) 982-1933; e-mail, sciwrite@umsmed.edu.
- Council of Biology Editors, Drohan Management Group, 11250 Roger Bacon Drive, Reston, VA 20190. Telephone (703 437-4377); fax (703 435-4390); e-mail, cbehdqts@aol.com.
- European Association of Science Editors. EASE Secretariat, Attention Mrs Jenny Gretton, PO Box 426, Guildford, GU4 7ZH, United Kingdom. Telephone and fax +44 1483 211056; e-mail secretary@ease.org.uk; Web site, http://www.ease.org.uk.

Alternatively, your publisher could probably recommend an author's editor who has worked with some of their authors and hence knows the publisher's requirements. The help of an author's editor may be especially valuable for authors for whom English is not the native language.

Your second important need is having a schedule you can hold to. Writing for publication is not easy except for some highly experienced authors; writing a book is an especially demanding task and there is no simple formula that could make it easy. Each author has his or her own best way of working. Probably a majority of authors write most readily in the morning; if you are a busy professional you may have to plan to start your day with some writing each morning before the main work of your day. This was the way the Canadian pathologist, William Boyd, wrote his many highly successful, widely used textbooks of pathology. You may prefer some other scheme: a regular hour each evening, a half-day on Saturdays and Sundays, some other program. But try to settle on one and stick to it, no matter what it is.

AFTER SUBMITTING THE MANUSCRIPT

Your responsibilities for the book do not end with your submitting the manuscript. Many publishers will send it out to external reviewers for critical readings, much as journal editors send submitted papers out to peer reviewers. The publisher may ask you for the names of suitable critical readers. You should welcome critical readings of this kind; a "second pair of eyes" on your own work may see errors, gaps in needed content, or redundant content you did not catch. The publisher's editor may recommend revisions. The improvements resulting from revisions recommended by external readers and the editor will probably only help to ensure the value of your book and how it will be seen by potential buyers.

As with journal papers, you can expect to see an edited version of your manuscript or proof of your text and tables, which will almost certainly be proof in page form. The proof should be read carefully as recommended in Chapter 23 and without delay. Avoid temptations to try to rewrite any of the text at this point; your markings on the proof should be confined to answering any questions and correcting definite errors in format or content. If any changes have been made by the copy editor that seem to you to be incorrect, you should discuss the apparent problem directly with the copy editor.

ADDITIONAL GUIDANCE

This chapter cannot cover every possible detail relevant to conceiving of, proposing, and writing a book. Some other sources offer sound advice. The *Handbook for Academic Authors* (1) has already been mentioned in connection with contracts. It additionally offers help on finding a publisher, working with the publisher, proposing and assembling a contributor book, and the preparation of electronic manuscripts, along with other topics. A good source on conference proceedings that is also relevant to organizing a contributor text is "B4. Editing Conference Proceedings", a chapter in the handbook of the European Association of Science Editors (2). Chapter 29, "Books, Technical Reports, and Monographs", of the Council of Biology Editors style manual (3) covers book formats in detail. Similar coverage is available in Chapter 1, "The Parts of a Book", of *The Chicago Manual of Style* (4).

CONCLUSION

Writing or editing a book is usually a much more complex task than writing a journal article and should not be undertaken lightly even if you have been approached by a publisher. The proposed scope and content of the book and its probable place in the market for medical books need to be carefully considered whether you were approached or you made the proposal. Once agreement on your writing or assembling the book has been reached with the publisher and a contract signed, you will need a detailed set of instructions from the publisher on your responsibilities for the book's format, style conventions, and the schedule.

REFERENCES

1. Luey B. Handbook for academic authors. 3rd ed. New York (NY): Cambridge University Press; 1995.
2. Science editors' handbook. Guildford, Surrey, United Kingdom: European As-

sociation of Science Editors; [issued in parts at various dates]. See the section "Working on the Book" in this chapter for the publisher's address.

3. Style Manual Committee, Council of Biology Editors. Scientific style and format: the CBE manual for authors, editors, and publishers. 6th ed. New York (NY): Cambridge University Press; 1994.

4. The Chicago manual of style. 14th ed. Chicago (IL): University of Chicago Press; 1993.

APPENDIX A

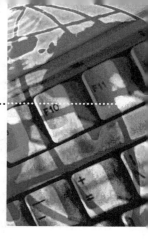

Guidelines on Authorship

[This appendix is an excerpt from "Guidelines on Authorship of Medical Papers" (Huth EJ. Ann Intern Med. 1986;104:269–74),which draws on principles developed by the International Committee of Medical Journal Editors and represented in its statements on authorship in successive editions of the Committee's *Uniform Requirements* document; the 1997 edition was published in *Annals of Internal Medicine* 1997 Jan 1;126(1):36–47. Note that this document is also available at the American College of Physicians' Web site (http://www.acponline.org/journals/resource/resortoc.htm). This Web site also lists all the journals that subscribe to the *Uniform Requirements* standards. Note that some journals state their own guidelines on authorship in their information-for-author pages; some medical schools and research institutions have their own guidelines on authorship.]

PRINCIPLES FOR AUTHORSHIP

Principle 1. Each author should have participated sufficiently in the work represented by the article to take public responsibility for the content.

Investigators in the sciences and others who use scientific information must have confidence in its accuracy and validity. Such confidence rests in part on knowing that at least one person has taken public responsibility for the information, and for published information the responsible persons are authors .... "Public responsibility" means that an author can defend the content of the article, including the data and other evidence and the conclusions based on them. Such ability can come only from having participated closely in the work represented by the article and in preparing the article for publication .... This responsibility also requires that the author be willing to concede publicly errors of fact or interpretation discovered after publication of the article and to state reasons for error.

In the case of fraud or other kinds of deception attributable to one or more of the authors, the other authors must be willing to state publicly the nature and extent of deception and to account as far as possible for its occurrence.

293

Principle 2. Participation must include three steps: (1) conception or design of the work represented by the article, or analysis and interpretation of the data, or both; (2) drafting the article or revising it for critically important content; and (3) final approval of the version to be published.

The work represented by a scientific article includes forming the hypothesis tested by the research it reports or forming the question it answers, developing the means of gathering the reported data or other evidence, collecting the data or other evidence, critically analyzing the evidence and any counter-evidence, and writing the article so that it accurately reports all of these steps and their products in the structure of critical argument . . . . Authors could not publicly defend the intellectual content of an article unless they understand thoroughly the basis for its origin (conception) and can testify to the validity of its argument (critical analysis of evidence). Authors must also have sufficient involvement in writing the [article], either in drafting the initial version or revising subsequent versions to insure validity of the argument and conclusions, to be able to defend the article as an accurate report . . . of the work that led to it.

Principle 3. Participation solely in the collection of data (or other evidence) does not justify authorship.

Data and other evidence bearing on the conclusions and validity of a scientific article may be gathered by persons who know little or nothing of the steps critical to its main intellectual substance: the genesis, design of the work, and the critical analysis of evidence. Such persons could not take public responsibility for the main elements of an article and could testify only to the validity of elements of evidence and not to how they support the argument and its conclusion. Contributions of data by persons for whom authorship is not justified can be acknowledged by other means (see Principle 5).

Principle 4. Each part of the content of an article critical to its main conclusions and each step in the work that led to its publication (steps 1, 2, and 3 in Principle 2) must be attributable to at least one author.

. . . Each element of a scientific article vital to its conclusions . . . must be publicly defensible or its validity is open to question. Therefore, the authorship of [an article] must include one or more persons able to defend any of its critically vital elements . . . .

Principle 5. Persons who have contributed intellectually to the article but whose contributions do not justify authorship may be named and their contribution described— for example, "advice", "critical review of study proposal", "data collection", "participation in clinical trial". Such persons must have given their permission to be named. Technical help must be acknowledged in a separate paragraph.

Contemporary research can involve persons whose contributions are not vital to the argument and conclusions of the article but that have been supportive for authors. Lest authors misrepresent themselves as being solely responsible for all that the article represents, they should indicate who provided intellectual assistance and its nature. Purely technical assistance includes building equipment, collecting data (specimen gathering and laboratory measurements), locating and abstracting literature, and work in preparing a manuscript that is not intellectual work on its scientific content.

GUIDELINES FOR SPECIFIC KINDS OF ARTICLES

Principle 2 defines participation in three steps as a requirement for authorship.

Step 1.   Conception of the work represented by the article, design of the work, analysis and interpretation of data or other evidence presented in the article, or all of these.

Step 2.   Drafting the article or revising it for critically important content.

Step 3.   Approving the final version of the article for publication.

Steps 2 and 3 necessarily apply to all types of articles. Specific contributions in Step 1 may differ for the various types of articles written for a clinical journal.

Step 1 for Articles Reporting Clinical, Epidemiologic, or Laboratory Research

Conception: Framing a specific hypothesis to be tested or specific question to be answered.

Design of the work: Drafting and deciding on the structure and methods for the research.

Analysis and interpretation of the data: This function includes assessing the precision, accuracy, and relevance of data, and statistical analysis. It also includes reviewing the literature for supportive evidence and counter-evidence.

Participation solely in study design or in data analysis or in both may represent adequate participation in Step 1 to justify authorship. Providing technical help, simple referral of patients, or collecting data do not by themselves represent adequate participation in Step 1. In epidemiologic studies the referral of a problem for study does not by itself represent adequate participation in Step 1, but recognizing in the problem an hypothesis to be tested or a specific question to be answered may be adequate.

Step 1 for Articles Reporting a Case-Series Analysis

Conception: Framing the specific question or questions the analysis is expected to answer.

Design of the work: Defining the characteristics of the cases to be analyzed and the scope of the literature to be considered for supportive evidence and counter-evidence.

Analysis and interpretation of the case data and literature evidence: Critical assessment; structuring and presentation; statistical analysis.

Locating and abstracting case data or literature do not by themselves represent adequate participation in Step 1 for this kind of article. Providing case data ("routine examination and tests") that would have been obtained even if the case-series analysis was not to be carried out is not participation justifying authorship (see Principle 3).

Step 1 for Individual Case Reports

Conception: Recognizing and defining the case characteristics that appear to justify further study of the case and eventually the report.

Design of the work: Deciding on and securing additional case data and relevant literature evidence that support the importance identified in "Conception".

Analysis and interpretation of the case data and literature evidence: Critical assessment and selection of case data and literature evidence.

Providing case data (such as "routine tests", laboratory estimations, roentgenographic or other imaging studies, cardiac studies) does not by itself represent adequate participation in Step 1 to justify authorship. Just the referral of the patient (case) to the person or persons responsible for "Conception" does not justify authorship.

Step 1 for Review Articles, Editorials, and Similar Articles Based on Critical Assessment of the Literature

Conception: Framing the specific question or questions to be answered.

Design of the work: Defining the characteristics of the literature to be reviewed.

Analysis and interpretation of the evidence considered: Selection of evidence through critical assessment.

Locating and abstracting the literature are not by themselves participation in Step 1. . . .

APPENDIX B

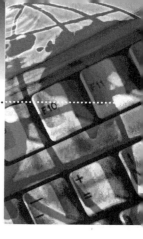

The "Uniform Requirements" Document: An Abridged Version

The editorial policies and technical requirements of many medical journals, especially those with preponderantly clinical content, are based at least in part on the document *Uniform Requirements for Manuscripts Submitted to Biomedical Journals* (1). It is intended to, and can serve, as a guide to authors on many aspects of writing and submitting articles. It is published here to serve as a reference document for many points made in the main text of this book. For the convenience of users of this book, the examples of formats for references have been omitted here and placed in the section "Citations and References" in Chapter 17, "Scientific Style and Format". This document is available in its full form at various Web sites, for example, that of the American College of Physicians, http://www.acponline.org (designated as ACP Online). The ACP Web site also includes a list of all journals that subscribe to the *Uniform Requirements* standards.

Authors must note that the manuscript and submission requirements of many journals may differ in at least some details even if the journal states that it subscribes to the principles and procedures set forth in this document. As stated at many points in this book, authors should read carefully the information-for-authors pages of any journal to which they plan to submit a paper.

UNIFORM REQUIREMENTS FOR MANUSCRIPTS SUBMITTED TO BIOMEDICAL JOURNALS

International Committee of Medical Journal Editors

A small group of editors of general medical journals met informally in Vancouver, British Columbia, in 1978 to establish guidelines for the format of manuscripts submitted to their journals. The group became known as the Vancouver Group. Its requirements for manuscripts, including formats for bibliographic references developed by the National Library of Medicine, were first published in 1979. The Vancouver Group expanded and evolved into the International Committee of Medical Journal Editors (ICMJE), which meets annually; gradually it has broadened its concerns.

The committee has produced five editions of the Uniform Requirements for Manuscripts Submitted to Biomedical Journals. Over the years, issues have arisen that go beyond manuscript preparation. Some of these issues are now covered in the Uniform Requirements; others are addressed in separate statements. Each statement has been published in a scientific journal.

The fifth edition (1997) is an effort to reorganize and reword the fourth edition to increase clarity and address concerns about rights, privacy, descriptions of methods, and other matters. The total content of Uniform Requirements for Manuscripts Submitted to Biomedical Journals may be reproduced for educational, not-for-profit purposes without regard for copyright; the committee encourages distribution of the material. Journals that agree to use the Uniform Requirements (over 500 do so) are asked to cite the 1997 document in their instructions to authors.

It is important to emphasize what these requirements do and do not imply.

First, the Uniform Requirements are instructions to authors on how to prepare manuscripts, not to editors on publication style. (But many journals have drawn on them for elements of their publication styles.)

Second, if authors prepare their manuscripts in the style specified in these requirements, editors of the participating journals will not return the manuscripts for changes in style before considering them for publication. In the publishing process, however, the journals may alter accepted manuscripts to conform with details of their publication style.

Third, authors sending manuscripts to a participating journal should not try to prepare them in accordance with the publication style of that journal but should follow the Uniform Requirements.

Authors must also follow the instructions to authors in the journal as to what topics are suitable for that journal and the types of papers that may be submitted—for example, original articles, reviews, or case reports. In addition, the journal's instructions are likely to contain other requirements unique to that journal, such as the number of copies of a manuscript that are required, acceptable languages, length of articles, and approved abbreviations.

Participating journals are expected to state in their instructions to authors that their requirements are in accordance with the Uniform Requirements for Manuscripts Submitted to Biomedical Journals and to cite a published version.

ISSUES TO CONSIDER BEFORE SUBMITTING A MANUSCRIPT

Redundant or Duplicate Publication

Redundant or duplicate publication is publication of a paper that overlaps substantially with one already published.

Readers of primary source periodicals deserve to be able to trust that what they are reading is original unless there is a clear statement that the article is being republished by the choice of the author and editor. The bases of this position are international copyright laws, ethical conduct, and cost-effective use of resources.

Most journals do not wish to receive papers on work that has already been reported in large part in a published article or is contained in another paper that has been submitted or accepted for publication elsewhere, in print or in electronic media. This policy does not preclude the journal considering a paper that has been rejected by another journal, or a complete report that follows publication of a preliminary report, such as an abstract or poster displayed for colleagues at a professional meeting. Nor does it prevent journals considering a paper that has been presented at a scientific meeting but not published in full or that is being considered for publication in a proceedings or similar format. Press reports of scheduled meetings will not usually be regarded as breaches of this rule, but such reports should not be amplified by additional data or copies of tables and illustrations.

When submitting a paper, the author should always make a full statement to the editor about all submissions and previous reports that might be regarded as redundant or duplicate publication of the same or very similar work. The author should alert the editor if the work includes subjects about which a previous report has been published. Any such work should be referred to and referenced in the new paper. Copies of such material should be included with the submitted paper to help the editor decide how to handle the matter.

If redundant or duplicate publication is attempted or occurs without such notification, authors should expect editorial action to be taken. At the least, prompt rejection of the submitted manuscript should be expected. If the editor was not aware of the violations and the article has already been published, then a notice of redundant or duplicate publication will probably be published with or without the author's explanation or approval.

Preliminary release, usually to public media, of scientific information described in a paper that has been accepted but not yet published violates the policies of many journals. In a few cases, and only by arrangement with the editor, preliminary release of data may be acceptable—for example, if there is a public health emergency.

Acceptable Secondary Publication

Secondary publication in the same or another language, especially in other countries, is justifiable, and can be beneficial, provided all of the following conditions are met.

1. The authors have received approval from the editors of both journals; the editor concerned with secondary publication must have a photocopy, reprint, or manuscript of the primary version.

2. The priority of the primary publication is respected by a publication interval of at least one week (unless specifically negotiated otherwise by both editors).

3. The paper for secondary publication is intended for a different group of readers; an abbreviated version could be sufficient.

4. The secondary version faithfully reflects the data and interpretations of the primary version.

5. The footnote on the title page of the secondary version informs readers, peers, and documenting agencies that the paper has been published in whole or in part and states the primary reference. A suitable footnote might read: "This article is based on a study first reported in the [title of journal, with full reference]." Permission for such secondary publication should be free of charge.

Protection of Patients' Rights to Privacy

Patients have a right to privacy that should not be infringed without informed consent. Identifying information should not be published in written descriptions, photographs, and pedigrees unless the information is essential for scientific purposes and the patient (or parent or guardian) gives written informed consent for publication. Informed consent for this purpose requires that the patient be shown the manuscript to be published.

Identifying details should be omitted if they are not essential, but patient data should never be altered or falsified in an attempt to attain anonymity. Complete anonymity is difficult to achieve, and informed consent should be obtained if there is any doubt. For example, masking the eye region in photographs of patients is inadequate protection of anonymity.

The requirement for informed consent should be included in the journal's instructions for authors. When informed consent has been obtained it should be indicated in the published article.

REQUIREMENTS FOR SUBMISSION OF MANUSCRIPTS

Summary of Technical Requirements

- Double space all parts of manuscripts.
- Begin each section or component on a new page.
- Review the sequence: title page, abstract and key words, text, acknowledgments, references, tables (each on separate page), legends.
- Illustrations, unmounted prints, should be no larger than 203 × 254 mm (8 × 10 inches).
- Include permission to reproduce previously published material or to use illustrations that may identify human subjects.

- Enclose transfer of copyright and other forms.
- Submit required number of paper copies.
- Keep copies of everything submitted.

Preparation of Manuscript

The text of observational and experimental articles is usually (but not necessarily) divided into sections with the headings Introduction, Methods, Results, and Discussion. Long articles may need subheadings within some sections (especially the Results and Discussion sections) to clarify their content. Other types of articles, such as case reports, reviews, and editorials, are likely to need other formats. Authors should consult individual journals for further guidance.

Type or print out the manuscript on white bond paper, 216 × 279 mm (8.5 × 11 inches), or ISO A4 (212 × 297 mm), with margins of at least 25 mm (1 inch). Type or print on only one side of the paper. Use double spacing throughout, including for the title page, abstract, text, acknowledgments, references, individual tables, and legends. Number pages consecutively, beginning with the title page. Put the page number in the upper or lower right-hand corner of each page.

Manuscripts on Disks

For papers that are close to final acceptance, some journals require authors to provide a copy in electronic form (on a disk); they may accept a variety of word-processing formats or text (ASCII) files.

When submitting disks, authors should:

1. be certain to include a print-out of the version of the article that is on the disk;

2. put only the latest version of the manuscript on the disk;

3. name the file clearly;

4. label the disk with the format of the file and the file name;

5. provide information on the hardware and software used.

Authors should consult the journal's instructions to authors for acceptable formats, conventions for naming files, number of copies to be submitted, and other details.

Title Page

The title page should carry 1) the title of the article, which should be concise but informative; 2) the name by which each author is known, with his or her highest academic degree(s) and institutional affiliation; 3) the name of the department(s) and institution(s) to which the work should be attributed; 4) disclaimers, if any; 5) the name and address of the author responsible for correspondence about the manuscript; 6) the name and address of the author to whom requests for reprints should be addressed or a statement that reprints will not be available from the authors; 7) source(s) of support in the form of grants, equipment, drugs, or all of these; and 8) a short running head or footline of no more than 40 characters (count letters and spaces) at the foot of the title page.

Authorship

All persons designated as authors should qualify for authorship. Each author should have participated sufficiently in the work to take public responsibility for the content.

Authorship credit should be based only on substantial contributions to 1) conception and design, or analysis and interpretation of data; and to 2) drafting the article or revising it critically for important intellectual content; and on 3) final approval of the version to be published. Conditions 1, 2, and 3 must all be met. Participation solely in the acquisition of funding or the collection of data does not justify authorship. General supervision of the research group is not sufficient for authorship. Any part of an article critical to its main conclusions must be the responsibility of at least one author.

Editors may ask authors to describe what each contributed; this information may be published. Increasingly, multicenter trials are attributed to a corporate author. All members of the group who are named as authors, either in the authorship position below the title or in a footnote, should fully meet the above criteria for authorship. Group members who do not meet these criteria should be listed, with their permission, in the Acknowledgments or in an appendix (see Acknowledgments).

The order of authorship should be a joint decision of the coauthors. Because the order is assigned in different ways, its meaning cannot be inferred accurately unless it is stated by the authors. Authors may wish to explain the order of authorship in a footnote. In deciding on the order, authors should be aware that many journals limit the number of authors listed in the table of contents and that the U.S. National Library of Medicine (NLM) lists in MEDLINE only the first 24 plus the last author when there are more than 25 authors.

Abstract and Key Words

The second page should carry an abstract (of no more than 150 words for unstructured abstracts or 250 words for structured abstracts). The abstract should state the purposes of the study or investigation, basic procedures (selection of study subjects or laboratory animals; observational and analytical methods), main findings (giving specific data and their statistical significance, if possible), and the principal conclusions. It should emphasize new and important aspects of the study or observations.

Below the abstract authors should provide, and identify as such, 3 to 10 key words or short phrases that will assist indexers in cross-indexing the article and may be published with the abstract. Terms from the Medical Subject Headings (MeSH) list of *Index Medicus* should be used; if suitable MeSH terms are not yet available for recently introduced terms, present terms may be used.

Introduction

State the purpose of the article and summarize the rationale for the study or observation. Give only strictly pertinent references and do not include data or conclusions from the work being reported.

Methods

Describe your selection of the observational or experimental subjects (patients or laboratory animals, including controls) clearly. Identify the age, sex, and other important characteristics of the subjects. The definition and relevance of race and ethnicity are ambiguous. Authors should be particularly careful about using these categories.

Identify the methods, apparatus (give the manufacturer's name and address in parentheses), and procedures in sufficient detail to allow other workers to reproduce the results. Give references to established methods, including statistical methods (*see* below); provide references and brief descriptions for methods that have been published but are not well known; describe new or substantially modified methods, give reasons for using them, and evaluate their limitations. Identify precisely all drugs and chemicals used, including generic name(s), dose(s), and route(s) of administration.

Reports of randomized clinical trials should present information on all major study elements, including the protocol (study population, interventions or exposures, outcomes, and the rationale for statistical analysis), assignment of interventions (methods of randomization, concealment of allocation to treatment groups), and the method of masking (blinding).

Authors submitting review manuscripts should include a section describing the methods used for locating, selecting, extracting, and synthesizing data. These methods should also be summarized in the abstract.

Ethics. When reporting experiments on human subjects, indicate whether the procedures followed were in accordance with the ethical standards of the responsible committee on human experimentation (institutional or regional) and with the Helsinki Declaration of 1975, as revised in 1983. Do not use patients' names, initials, or hospital numbers, especially in illustrative material. When reporting experiments on animals, indicate whether the institution's or a national research council's guide for, or any national law on, the care and use of laboratory animals was followed.

Statistics. Describe statistical methods with enough detail to enable a knowledgeable reader with access to the original data to verify the reported results. When possible, quantify findings and present them with appropriate indicators of measurement error or uncertainty (such as confidence intervals). Avoid relying solely on statistical hypothesis testing, such as the use of P values, which fails to convey important quantitative information. Discuss the eligibility of experimental subjects. Give details about randomization. Describe the methods for and success of any blinding of observations. Report complications of treatment. Give numbers of observations. Report losses to observation (such as dropouts from a clinical trial). References for the design of the study and statistical methods should be to standard works when possible (with pages stated) rather than to papers in which the designs or methods were originally reported. Specify any general-use computer programs used.

Put a general description of methods in the Methods section. When data are summarized in the Results section, specify the statistical methods used to analyze them. Restrict tables and figures to those needed to explain the argument of the paper and to assess its support. Use graphs as an alternative to tables with many entries; do not duplicate data in graphs and tables. Avoid nontechnical uses of technical terms in statistics, such as "random" (which implies a randomizing device), "normal", "significant," "correlations," and "sample." Define statistical terms, abbreviations, and most symbols.

Results

Present your results in logical sequence in the text, tables, and illustrations. Do not repeat in the text all the data in the tables or illustrations; emphasize or summarize only important observations.

Discussion

Emphasize the new and important aspects of the study and the conclusions that follow from them. Do not repeat in detail data or other material given in the Introduction or the Results section. Include in the Discussion section the implications of the findings and their limitations, including implications for future research. Relate the observations to other relevant studies.

Link the conclusions with the goals of the study but avoid unqualified statements and conclusions not completely supported by the data. In particular, authors should avoid making statements on economic benefits and costs unless their manuscript includes economic data and analyses. Avoid claiming priority and alluding to work that has not been completed. State new hypotheses when warranted, but clearly label them as such. Recommendations, when appropriate, may be included.

Acknowledgments

At an appropriate place in the article (the title page footnote or an appendix to the text; *see* the journal's requirements), one or more statements should specify 1) contributions that need acknowledging but do not justify authorship, such as general support by a departmental chair; 2) acknowledgments of technical help; 3) acknowledgments of financial and material support, which should specify the nature of the support; and 4) relationships that may pose a conflict of interest (*see* Conflict of Interest).

Persons who have contributed intellectually to the paper but whose contributions do not justify authorship may be named and their function or contribution described—for example, "scientific adviser," "critical review of study proposal," "data collection," or "participation in clinical trial." Such persons must have given their permission to be named. Authors are responsible for obtaining written permission from persons acknowledged by name, because readers may infer their endorsement of the data and conclusions.

Technical help should be acknowledged in a paragraph separate from that acknowledging other contributions.

References

References should be numbered consecutively in the order in which they are first mentioned in the text. Identify references in text, tables, and legends by Arabic numerals in parentheses. References cited only in tables or figure legends should be numbered in accordance with the sequence established by the first identification in the text of the particular table or figure.

[Use the style of the example references given in the section "Citations and References" in Chapter 19, "Scientific Style and References"] . . . , which are based on the formats used by the NLM in *Index Medicus.* The titles of journals should be abbreviated according to the style used in *Index Medicus.* Consult the *List of Journals Indexed in Index Medicus,* published annually as a separate publication by the library and as a list in the January issue of *Index Medicus.* The list can also be obtained through the library's web site (http://www.nlm.nih.gov). Avoid using abstracts as references. References to papers accepted but not yet published should be designated as "in press" or "forthcoming"; authors should obtain written permission to cite such papers as well as verification that they have been accepted for publication. Information from manuscripts submitted but not accepted should be cited in the text as "unpublished observations" with written permission from the source.

Avoid citing a "personal communication" unless it provides essential information not available from a public source, in which case the name of the person and date of communication should be cited in parentheses in the text. For scientific articles, authors should obtain written permission and confirmation of accuracy from the source of a personal communication. The references must be verified by the author(s) against the original documents. The Uniform Requirements style (the Vancouver style) is based largely on an ANSI standard style adapted by the NLM for its databases. . . .

Tables

Type or print out each table with double spacing on a separate sheet of paper. Do not submit tables as photographs. Number tables consecutively in the order of their first citation in the text and supply a brief title for each. Give each column a short or abbreviated heading. Place explanatory matter in footnotes, not in the heading. Explain in footnotes all nonstandard abbreviations that are used in each table. For footnotes use the following symbols, in this sequence: *, †, ‡, §, ‖, ¶, **, ††, ‡‡.

Identify statistical measures of variations, such as standard deviation and standard error of the mean.

Do not use internal horizontal and vertical rules.

Be sure that each table is cited in the text.

If you use data from another published or unpublished source, obtain permission and acknowledge them fully.

The use of too many tables in relation to the length of the text may produce difficulties in the layout of pages. Examine issues of the journal to which you plan to submit your paper to estimate how many tables can be used per 1000 words of text.

The editor, on accepting a paper, may recommend that additional tables containing important backup data too extensive to publish be deposited with an archival service, such as the National Auxiliary Publication Service in the United States, or made available by the authors. In that event an appropriate statement will be added to the text. Submit such tables for consideration with the paper.

Illustrations (Figures)

Submit the required number of complete sets of figures. Figures should be professionally drawn and photographed; freehand or typewritten lettering is unacceptable. Instead of original drawings, x-ray films, and other material, send sharp, glossy, black-and-white photographic prints, usually 127 × 173 mm (5 × 7 inches) but no larger than 203 × 254 mm (8 × 10 inches). Letters, numbers, and symbols should be clear and even throughout and of sufficient size that when reduced for publication each item will still be legible. Titles and detailed explanations belong in the legends for illustrations not on the illustrations themselves.

Each figure should have a label pasted on its back indicating the number of the figure, author's name, and top of the figure. Do not write on the back of figures or scratch or mar them by using paper clips. Do not bend figures or mount them on cardboard.

Photomicrographs should have internal scale markers. Symbols, arrows, or letters used in photomicrographs should contrast with the background.

If photographs of people are used, either the subjects must not be identifiable or their pictures must be accompanied by written permission to use the photograph (*see* Protection of Patients' Rights to Privacy).

Figures should be numbered consecutively according to the order in which they have been first cited in the text. If a figure has been published, acknowledge the original source and submit written permission from the copyright holder to reproduce the material. Permission is required irrespective of authorship or publisher except for documents in the public domain.

For illustrations in color, ascertain whether the journal requires color negatives, positive transparencies, or color prints. Accompanying drawings marked to indicate the region to be reproduced may be useful to the editor. Some journals publish illustrations in color only if the author pays for the extra cost.

Legends for Illustrations

Type or print out legends for illustrations using double spacing, starting on a separate page, with Arabic numerals corresponding to the illustrations. When symbols, arrows, numbers, or letters are used to identify parts of the illustrations, identify and explain each one clearly in the legend. Explain the internal scale and identify the method of staining in photomicrographs.

Units of Measurement

Measurements of length, height, weight, and volume should be reported in metric units (meter, kilogram, or liter) or their decimal multiples.

Temperatures should be given in degrees Celsius. Blood pressures should be given in millimeters of mercury. All hematologic and clinical chemistry measurements should be reported in the metric system in terms of the International System of Units (SI). Editors may request that alternative or non-SI units be added by the authors before publication.

Abbreviations and Symbols

Use only standard abbreviations. Avoid abbreviations in the title and abstract. The full term for which an abbreviation stands should precede its first use in the text unless it is a standard unit of measurement.

SENDING THE MANUSCRIPT TO THE JOURNAL

Send the required number of copies of the manuscript in a heavy-paper envelope, enclosing the copies and figures in cardboard, if necessary, to prevent the photographs from being bent. Place photographs and transparencies in a separate heavy-paper envelope.

Manuscripts must be accompanied by a covering letter signed by all coauthors. This must include 1) information on prior or duplicate publication or submission elsewhere of any part of the work as defined earlier in this document; 2) a statement of financial or other relationships that might lead to a conflict of interest (*see* below); 3) a statement that the manuscript has been read and approved by all the authors, that the requirements for authorship as stated earlier in this document have been met, and that each author believes that the manuscript represents honest work; and 4) the name, address, and telephone number of the corresponding author, who is responsible for communicating with the other authors about revisions and final approval of the proofs. The letter should give any additional information that may be helpful to the editor, such as the type of article in the particular journal that the manuscript represents and whether the author(s) would be willing to meet the cost of reproducing color illustrations.

The manuscript must be accompanied by copies of any permissions to reproduce published material, to use illustrations or report information about identifiable people, or to name people for their contributions.

SEPARATE STATEMENTS

Definition of a Peer-Reviewed Journal

A peer-reviewed journal is one that has submitted most of its published articles for review by experts who are not part of the editorial staff. The number and kind of manuscripts sent for review, the number of reviewers, the reviewing procedures, and the use made of the reviewers' opinions may vary, and therefore each journal should publicly disclose its policies in its instructions to authors for the benefit of readers and potential authors.

Editorial Freedom and Integrity

Owners and editors of medical journals have a common endeavor—the publication of a reliable and readable journal, produced with due respect for the stated aims of the journal and for costs. The functions of owners and editors, however, are different. Owners have the right to appoint and dismiss editors and to make important business decisions in which editors should be involved to the fullest extent possible. Editors must have full authority for determining the editorial content of the journal. This concept of editorial freedom should be resolutely defended by editors even to the extent of their placing their positions at stake. To secure this freedom in practice, the editor should have direct access to the highest level of ownership, not only to a delegated manager.

Editors of medical journals should have a contract that clearly states the editor's rights and duties in addition to the general terms of the appointment and that defines mechanisms for resolving conflict.

An independent editorial advisory board may be useful in helping the editor establish and maintain editorial policy.

All editors and editors' organizations have the obligation to support the concept of editorial freedom and to draw major transgressions of such freedom to the attention of the international medical community.

Conflict of Interest

Conflict of interest for a given manuscript exists when a participant in the peer review and publication process—author, reviewer, and editor—has ties to activities that could inappropriately influence his or her judgment, whether or not judgment is in fact affected. Financial relationships with industry (for example, through employment, consultancies, stock ownership, honoraria, expert testimony), either directly or through immediate family, are usually considered to be the most important conflicts of interest. However, conflicts can occur for other reasons, such as personal relationships, academic competition, and intellectual passion.

Public trust in the peer review process and the credibility of published articles depend in part on how well conflict of interest is handled during writing, peer review, and editorial decision making. Bias can often be identified and eliminated by careful attention to the scientific methods and conclusions of the work. Financial relationships and their effects are less easily detected than other conflicts of interest. Participants in peer review and publication should disclose their conflicting interests, and the information should be made available so that others can judge their effects for themselves. Because readers may be less able to detect bias in review articles and editorials than in reports of original research, some journals do not accept reviews and editorials from authors with a conflict of interest.

Authors. When they submit a manuscript, whether an article or a letter, authors are responsible for recognizing and disclosing financial and other conflicts of interest that might bias their work. They should acknowledge in the manuscript all financial support for the work and other financial or personal connections to the work.

Reviewers. External peer reviewers should disclose to editors any conflicts of interest that could bias their opinions of the manuscript, and they should disqualify themselves from reviewing specific manuscripts if they believe it to be appropriate. The editors must be made aware of reviewers' conflicts of interest to interpret the reviews and judge for themselves whether the reviewer should be disqualified. Reviewers should not use knowledge of the work, before its publication, to further their own interests.

Editors and Staff. Editors who make final decisions about manuscripts should have no personal financial involvement in any of the issues they might judge. Other members of the editorial staff, if they participate in editorial decisions, should provide editors with a current description of their financial interests (as they might relate to editorial judgments) and disqualify themselves from any decisions where they have a conflict of interest. Published articles and letters should include a description of all financial support and any conflict of interest that, in the editors' judgment, readers should know about. Editorial staff should not use the information gained through working with manuscripts for private gain.

Corrections, Retractions, and Expressions of Concern about Research Findings

Editors must assume initially that authors are reporting work based on honest observations. Nevertheless, two types of difficulty may arise.

First, errors may be noted in published articles that require the publication of a correction or erratum of part of the work. It is conceivable that an error could be so serious as to vitiate the entire body of the work, but this is unlikely and should be handled by editors and authors on an individual basis. Such an error should not be confused with inadequacies exposed by the emergence of new scientific information in the normal course of research. The latter require no corrections or withdrawals.

The second type of difficulty is scientific fraud. If substantial doubts arise about the honesty of work, either submitted or published, it is the editor's responsibility to ensure that the question is appropriately pursued (including possible consultation with the authors). However, it is not the task of editors to conduct a full investigation or to make a determination; that responsibility lies with the institution where the work was done or with the funding agency. The editor should be promptly informed of the final decision, and if a fraudulent paper has been published, the journal must print a retraction. If this method of investigation does not result in a satisfactory conclusion, the editor may choose to publish an expression of concern with an explanation.

The retraction or expression of concern, so labeled, should appear on a numbered page in a prominent section of the journal, be listed in the contents page, and include in its heading the title of the original article. It should not simply be a letter to the editor. Ideally, the first author should be the same in the retraction as in the article, although under certain circumstances the editor may accept retractions by other responsible people. The text of the retraction should explain why the article is being retracted and include a bibliographic reference to it.

The validity of previous work by the author of a fraudulent paper cannot be assumed. Editors may ask the author's institution to assure them of the validity of earlier work published in their journals or to retract it. If this is not done they may choose to publish an announcement to the effect that the validity of previously published work is not assured.

Confidentiality

Manuscripts should be reviewed with due respect for authors' confidentiality. In submitting their manuscripts for review, authors entrust editors with the results of their scientific work and creative effort, on which their reputation and career may depend. Authors' rights may be violated by disclosure of the confidential details of the review of their manuscript. Reviewers also have rights to confidentiality, which must be respected by the editor. Confidentiality may have to be breached if dishonesty or fraud is alleged but otherwise must be honored.

Editors should not disclose information about manuscripts (including their receipt, their content, their status in the reviewing process, their criticism by reviewers, or their ultimate fate) to anyone other than the authors themselves and reviewers.

Editors should make clear to their reviewers that manuscripts sent for review are privileged communications and are the private property of the authors. Therefore, reviewers and members of the editorial staff should respect the authors' rights by not publicly discussing the authors' work or appropriating their ideas before the manuscript is published. Reviewers should not be allowed to make copies of the manuscript for their files and should be prohibited from sharing it with others, except with the permission of the editor. Editors should not keep copies of rejected manuscripts.

Opinions differ on whether reviewers should remain anonymous. Some editors require their reviewers to sign the comments returned to authors, but most either request that reviewers' comments not be signed or leave the choice to the reviewer. When comments are not signed the reviewers' identity must not be revealed to the author or anyone else.

Some journals publish reviewers' comments with the manuscript. No such procedure should be adopted without the consent of the authors and reviewers. However, reviewers' comments may be sent to other reviewers of the same manuscript, and reviewers may be notified of the editor's decision.

Medical Journals and the Popular Media

The public's interest in news of medical research has led the popular media to compete vigorously to get information about research as soon as possible. Researchers and institutions sometimes encourage the reporting of research in the popular media before full publication in a scientific journal by holding a press conference or giving interviews.

The public is entitled to important medical information without unreasonable delay, and editors have a responsibility to play their part in this process. Doctors, however, need to have reports available in full detail before they can advise their patients about the reports' conclusions. In addition, media reports of scientific research before the work has been peer reviewed and fully published may lead to the dissemination of inaccurate or premature conclusions.

Editors may find the following recommendations useful as they seek to establish policies on these issues.

1. Editors can foster the orderly transmission of medical information from researchers, through peer-reviewed journals, to the public. This can be accomplished by an agreement with authors that they will not publicize their work while their manuscript is under consideration or awaiting publication and an agreement with the media that they will not release stories before publication in the journal, in return for which the journal will cooperate with them in preparing accurate stories (*see* below).

2. Very little medical research has such clear and urgently important clinical implications for the public's health that the news must be released before full publication in a journal. In such exceptional circumstances, however, appropriate authorities responsible for public health should make the decision and should be responsible for the advance dissemination of information to physicians and the media. If the author and the appropriate authorities wish to have a manuscript considered by a particular journal, the editor should be consulted before any public release. If editors accept the need for immediate release, they should waive their policies limiting prepublication publicity.

3. Policies designed to limit prepublication publicity should not apply to accounts in the media of presentations at scientific meetings or to the ab-

stracts from these meetings (*see* Redundant or Duplicate Publication). Researchers who present their work at a scientific meeting should feel free to discuss their presentations with reporters, but they should be discouraged from offering more detail about their study than was presented in their talk.

4. When an article is soon to be published, editors may wish to help the media prepare accurate reports by providing news releases, answering questions, supplying advance copies of the journal, or referring reporters to the appropriate experts. This assistance should be contingent on the media's cooperation in timing their release of stories to coincide with the publication of the article.

Advertising

Most medical journals carry advertising, which generates income for their publishers, but advertising must not be allowed to influence editorial decisions. Editors must have full responsibility for advertising policy. Readers should be able to distinguish readily between advertising and editorial material. The juxtaposition of editorial and advertising material on the same products or subjects should be avoided, and advertising should not be sold on the condition that it will appear in the same issue as a particular article.

Journals should not be dominated by advertising, but editors should be careful about publishing advertisements from only one or two advertisers as readers may perceive that the editor has been influenced by these advertisers.

Journals should not carry advertisements for products that have proved to be seriously harmful to health—for example, tobacco. Editors should ensure that existing standards for advertisements are enforced or develop their own standards. Finally, editors should consider all criticisms of advertisements for publication.

Supplements

Supplements are collections of papers that deal with related issues or topics, are published as a separate issue of the journal or as a second part of a regular issue, and are usually funded by sources other than the journal's publisher. Supplements can serve useful purposes: education, exchange of research information, ease of access to focused content, and improved cooperation between academic and corporate entities. Because of the funding sources, the content of supplements can reflect biases in choice of topics and viewpoints. Editors should therefore consider the following principles.

1. The journal editor must take full responsibility for the policies, practices, and content of supplements. The journal editor must approve the appointment of any editor of the supplement and retain the authority to reject papers.

2. The sources of funding for the research, meeting, and publication should be clearly stated and prominently located in the supplement, preferably on each page. Whenever possible, funding should come from more than one sponsor.

3. Advertising in supplements should follow the same policies as those of the rest of the journal.

4. Editors should enable readers to distinguish readily between ordinary editorial pages and supplement pages.

5. Editing by the funding organization should not be permitted.

6. Journal editors and supplement editors should not accept personal favors or excessive compensation from sponsors of supplements.

7. Secondary publication in supplements should be clearly identified by the citation of the original paper. Redundant publication should be avoided.

The Role of the Correspondence Column

All biomedical journals should have a section carrying comments, questions, or criticisms about articles they have published and where the original authors can respond. Usually, but not necessarily, this may take the form of a correspondence column. The lack of such a section denies readers the possibility of responding to articles in the same journal that published the original work.

Competing Manuscripts Based on the Same Study

Editors may receive manuscripts from different authors offering competing interpretations of the same study. They have to decide whether to review competing manuscripts submitted to them more or less simultaneously by different groups or authors, or they may be asked to consider one such manuscript while a competing manuscript has been or will be submitted to another journal. Setting aside the unresolved question of ownership of data, we discuss here what editors ought to do when confronted with the submission of competing manuscripts based on the same study.

Two kinds of multiple submissions are considered: submissions by coworkers who disagree on the analysis and interpretation of their study, and submissions by coworkers who disagree on what the facts are and which data should be reported.

The following general observations may help editors and others dealing with this problem.

Differences in Analysis or Interpretation. Journals would not normally wish to publish separate articles by contending members of a research team who have differing analyses and interpretations of the data, and submission of such manuscripts should be discouraged. If coworkers cannot resolve their differences in interpretation before submitting a manuscript, they should consider submitting one manuscript containing multiple interpretations and calling their dispute to the attention of the editor so that reviewers can focus on the problem. One of the important functions of peer review is to evaluate the authors' analysis and interpretation and to suggest appropriate changes to the conclusions before publication. Alternatively, after the disputed version is published, editors may wish to consider a letter to the editor or a second manuscript from the dissenting authors. Multiple submissions present editors with a dilemma. Publication of contending manuscripts to air authors' disputes may waste journal space and confuse readers. On the other hand, if editors knowingly publish a manuscript written by only some of the collaborating team, they could be denying the rest of the team their legitimate coauthorship rights.

Differences in Reported Methods or Results.   Workers sometimes differ in their opinions about what was actually done or observed and which data ought to be reported. Peer review cannot be expected to resolve this problem. Editors should decline further consideration of such multiple submissions until the problem is settled. Furthermore, if there are allegations of dishonesty or fraud, editors should inform the appropriate authorities.

The cases described above should be distinguished from instances in which independent, noncollaborating authors submit separate manuscripts based on different analyses of data that are publicly available. In this circumstance, editorial consideration of multiple submissions may be justified, and there may even be a good reason for publishing more than one manuscript because different analytical approaches may be complementary and equally valid.

Members of the International Committee of Medical Journal Editors: Linda Hawes Clever, *Western Journal of Medicine;* Lois Ann Colaianni, U.S. National Library of Medicine; Frank Davidoff, *Annals of Internal Medicine;* Richard Glass, *JAMA;* Richard Horton, *The Lancet;* George Lundberg, *JAMA;* Magne Nylenna, *Tidsskrift for Den Norske legeforening;* Richard G. Robinson, *New Zealand Medical Journal;* Richard Smith, *BMJ;* Bruce P. Squires, *Canadian Medical Association Journal;* Robert Utiger, *The New England Journal of Medicine;* Martin VanDer Weyden, *The Medical Journal of Australia;* and Patricia Woolf, Princeton University.

APPENDIX C

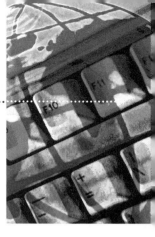

Specialized Databases of The National Library of Medicine

Most literature searches carried out by medical authors are probably carried out adequately using MEDLINE of The National Library of Medicine (NLM) in one of its various forms (PubMed, Internet Grateful Med, and other systems; see Chapter 3). The Library has been planning to incorporate in PubMed the other NLM databases that have been serving more specialized needs. These are described here to indicate the wealth of resources that will eventually be available directly in PubMed rather than in separate accesses to these databases. Details on these are available in the fact sheet "NLM Online Databases and Databanks" available directly at the Internet Web site of the Library (http://www.nlm.nih.gov/pubs/factsheets/online_databases.html). The site can also be consulted for information on the status of the planned conversion. The brief descriptions below are drawn from the fact sheet.

AIDSDRUGS

A dictionary of chemical and biological agents currently being evaluated in the AIDS clinical trials covered in the companion AIDSTRIALS database. Each record represents a single substance and provides information such as standard chemical names, synonyms and trade names, CAS Registry Numbers, protocol ID numbers, pharmacological action, adverse reactions and contraindications, physical and chemical properties, and manufacturers' names. Agents that were tested in closed or completed trials are included. A bibliography of relevant articles is also included.

317

AIDSLINE (AIDS INFORMATION ON LINE)

Bibliographic citations to literature covering research, clinical aspects, and health policy issues relevant to the acquired immunodeficiency syndrome (AIDS) and related topics. The citations are derived from the MEDLINE, CANCERLIT, HealthSTAR, CATLINE, AVLINE, and BIOETHICSLINE files, and the meeting abstracts from the International Conferences on AIDS, and other AIDS-related meetings, conferences, and symposia. Citations and abstracts from newsletters and special AIDS journals are also included. To provide access to additional reference sources, NLM plans to expand the file with records from the POPLINE database as well as with additional meeting abstracts and journal article citations.

AIDSTRIALS

Records of open and closed clinical trials of substances being tested for use against AIDS, HIV infection, and AIDS-related opportunistic diseases. Each record covers a single trial, and provides information such as title and purpose of the trial, diseases studied, patient eligibility criteria, contact persons, agents being tested, and trial locations. Information about trials sponsored by the National Institutes of Health is supplied by the National Institute of Allergy and Infectious Diseases (NIAID), while information about privately sponsored trials is provided by the Food and Drug Administration (FDA). AIDSTRIALS is a part of the AIDS Clinical Trials Information Service (ACTIS), which is a project sponsored by the FDA, the NIAID, the NLM, and the Centers for Disease Control.

AVLINE (AUDIO VISUALS ON LINE)

Bibliographic citations of biomedical audiovisual materials and computer software. Coverage is primarily of English-language items from the United States and represents all audiovisuals and computer software catalogued by the NLM since 1975. Coverage includes motion pictures, videocassettes, slide-cassette programs, filmstrip-cassette programs, computer software, clinical educational materials, and audiovisual-computer software serials. AVLINE also includes bibliographic information for some of the archival motion pictures that form the basis of NLM's National Historical Film Program. Selected citations in the database include abstracts. Procurement information available at the time of cataloging is included.

BIOETHICSLINE (BIOETHICS ON LINE)

Bibliographic citations of English-language journal articles, monographs, analytics (chapters in monographs), newspaper articles, court decisions, bills, laws, audiovisual materials, and unpublished documents relevant to ethics and related public policy issues in health care and biomedical research. Topics include euthanasia and other end-of-life issues, organ donation and transplantation, denial of health care resources, patients' rights, professional ethics, new reproductive technologies, genetic intervention, abortion, behavior control and other mental health issues, AIDS, human experimentation, and animal experimentation. Citations are derived from the literature of law, religion, the social sciences, philosophy, and the popular media as well as that of the health sciences. The file is produced by the Bioethics Information Retrieval Project of the Kennedy Institute at Georgetown University.

CANCERLIT (CANCER LITERATURE)

Bibliographic citations of journal articles, government reports, technical reports, meeting abstracts and papers, monographs, letters, and theses relevant to major cancer topics. Covers primarily English-language items. Comprehensive and international in scope since 1976; some citations published as early as 1963. Since June 1983, most journal literature has been derived from MEDLINE; the file also includes a limited number of foreign-language journals not covered in MEDLINE. Records added since January 1980 have been indexed using the NLM controlled vocabulary (MeSH). CANCERLIT is produced by the National Cancer Institute (NCI) in cooperation with the NLM.

CATLINE (CATALOG ON LINE)

Bibliographic citations of primarily monographs, but also of serials, monographic series, and manuscripts covering the biomedical sciences. All languages; virtually all of the cataloged titles in the NLM collection, from the fifteenth century to the present time. Provides access to NLM's authoritative bibliographic data and is a useful source of information for ordering printed material, verifying interlibrary loan requests, and providing reference services. Much of this information is available in LOCATOR, the NLM online catalog available via the Library's Web site.

CHEMID (CHEMICAL IDENTIFICATION)

A chemical dictionary file for a very large number of compounds of biomedical and regulatory interest. Records include CAS Registry Numbers and other identifying numbers, molecular formulae, generic names, trivial names, other synonyms, MeSH headings, and file locators that lead users to other files on the ELHILL TOXNET systems. In addition, SUPERLIST provides names and other data used to describe chemicals on over 30 federal and state regulatory lists.

CHEMLINE (CHEMICAL DICTIONARY ON LINE)

An online dictionary of chemical substances represented in NLM databases, the Toxic Substances Control Act Inventory of the Environmental Protection Agency, the European Inventory of Existing Commercial Chemical Substances (EINECS), and the Domestic Substances List of Canada. Each record covers a chemical substance, and provides detailed information on the substance's nomenclature, synonyms, and CAS Registry Numbers. NLM file locators direct the user to MEDLARS files that contain more information about the designated substances.

DIRLINE (DIRECTORY OF INFORMATION RESOURCES ON LINE)

A directory of resources providing information services primarily in the United States, with some coverage of international organizations. Focuses primarily on health and biomedical information resources including organizations, government agencies, information centers, professional societies, voluntary associations, support groups, academic research institutions, and research facilities and resources. Records contain resource names, addresses, phone numbers and descriptions of services, publications, and holdings. Much of this information is available in LOCATOR, the NLM online catalog available via the Library's Web site.

HEALTHSTAR (HEALTH SERVICES, TECHNOLOGY, ADMINISTRATION, AND RESEARCH)

Bibliographic citations covering clinical (emphasis on the evaluation of patient outcomes and the effectiveness of procedures, programs, products, services, and processes) and nonclinical (emphasis on health care administration and planning) aspects of health care delivery; combines former HEALTH (Health Planning and Administration) and HSTAR (Health Service–Technology Assessment Research) databases. Citations represent journal articles, technical and government reports, meeting papers and abstracts, books and individual chapters. Contains relevant bibliographic records from MEDLINE (1975 to present) and CATLINE (1985 to present), and unique records from three sources: records emphasizing health care administration selected and indexed by the American Hospital Association (AHA); records emphasizing health planning from the National Health Planning Information Center (only in the backfile); and records emphasizing health services research clinical practice guidelines, and health care technology assessment selected and indexed through NLM's National Information Center on Health Services Research and Health Care Technology (NICHSR). Alternate source information is provided for technical reports and related material selected by NICH that may not be widely held by libraries.

HISTLINE (HISTORY OF MEDICINE ON LINE)

Bibliographic citations of monographs, journal articles, book chapters, and individual chapters in the published proceedings of symposia and congresses. Covers literature in all languages about the history of health-related professions, sciences, specialties, individuals, institutions, drugs, and diseases in all part of the world and all historic periods. It includes virtually all records of secondary historical literature from MEDLINE, CATLINE, and AVLINE. It also contains additional records that have been indexed by the History of Medicine Division that are not available from any other MEDLARS database.

HSRPROJ (HEALTH SERVICES RESEARCH PROJECTS IN PROGRESS)

Descriptions of research projects in health services research including health technology assessment and the development and use of clinical practice guidelines. Provides project records for research in progress funded by federal and private grant contracts. Records include project summaries, names of performing and sponsoring agencies, names and addresses of principal investigator, beginning and ending years of the project; and when available, information about study design. Document types include monographs, journal articles, publications from symposia and congresses.

MESH VOCABULARY FILE

An online dictionary or thesaurus of current biomedical subject headings, subheadings, and supplementary chemical terms used in indexing and searching several MEDLARS databases including MEDLINE, AIDSLINE, AIDSTRIALS, AVLINE, BIOETHICSLINE, CANCERLIT, CATLINE, DIRLINE, HealthSTAR, POPLINE. MeSH heading records typically include synonyms, scope notes, MeSH hierarchical positions, entry dates, and previous indexing information. Records for subheadings include descriptions for their use. The file includes supplementary chemical records that occur in MEDLINE but are not MeSH headings.

OLDMEDLINE

This database contains over 307,000 citations originally published in the 1964 and 1965 editions of *Cumulated Index Medicus*. These citations reflect the MeSH vocabulary and data format used in 1964–65. NLM intends to add more older citations to OLDMEDLINE.

PDQ (PHYSICIAN DATA QUERY)

Detailed information on the prognosis, staging, and treatment of all major tumor types, screening for common cancers, supportive care for common problems encountered in cancer patients; summaries of open and closed clinical trials; directories of physicians and organizations providing cancer care; and information on investigational cancer drugs.

POPLINE (POPULATION INFORMATION ON LINE)

Bibliographic citations, primarily of English-language items, on family planning, population law and policy, and primary health care, including maternal–child health in developing countries, family planning technology and programs, fertility focuses on particular developing-country issues including demography, AIDS and other sexually transmitted diseases, maternal and child health, primary health care communication, and population and environment. Covers publications from 1970 to the present with selected citations dating back to 1886. International in scope.

PREMEDLINE

This database provides basic citation information and abstracts before they are put into MEDLINE. Citations are added daily, remaining in the database only until they have had MeSH terms, publication-type terms, and other indexing data added. Once the indexing is finished, the complete records are added weekly to MEDLINE and the PREMEDLINE records are deleted.

SDILINE (SELECTIVE DISSEMINATION OF INFORMATION ON LINE)

Bibliographic citations from the most recent complete month in MEDLINE, including all citations in the forthcoming printed edition of the monthly *Index Medicus*. Updated monthly. Citations to journal articles from approximately 3900 biomedical journals published in the United States and abroad.

SERLINE (SERIALS ON LINE)

Bibliographic records for all serials in all languages published from 1665 to the present that have been cataloged for the NLM collection, titles ordered or being processed for the NLM, and all serial titles indexed for MEDLINE, HealthSTAR, including titles that do not meet NLM scope and coverage requirements. Also includes titles held by libraries participating in the NLM National Biomedical Serials Holdings Database (SERHOLD). Many records contain locator information which includes major biomedical libraries within the National Network of Libraries of Medicine holding the publication.

SPACELINE

Bibliographic citations of materials relevant to space life-sciences in all languages: journal articles; technical reports; books and book chapters; conference proceedings, conference papers, and meeting abstracts; bibliographies; and audiovisuals. There are many citations in the database to material on basic research related to the space life sciences. Examples of these include basic bone and muscle physiology, psychological effects of isolation, and gravitational effects on plants.

TOXLINE (TOXICOLOGY INFORMATION ON LINE)

Bibliographic citations (primarily of English-language items but with international coverage) of journal articles, monographs, technical reports, theses, letters, and meeting abstracts, papers, reports on toxicological, pharmacological, biochemical, and physiological effects of drugs and other chemicals. Citations may be retrieved by entering free text terms as they may appear in titles, keywords, and abstracts of articles. The portions of the database derived from MEDLINE, DART, and that portion of BIOSIS added since 1985 may be searched using MeSH vocabulary. Chemical substances can be searched by entering their corresponding CAS Registry Numbers and/or synonyms.

TOXLIT (TOXICOLOGY LITERATURE FROM SPECIAL SOURCES)

Bibliographic citations (primarily of English-language items) of journal articles, meeting papers, monographs, and patents relevant to toxicological, pharmacological, biochemical, and physiological effects of drugs and other chemicals. Citations may be retrieved by entering free text terms as they may appear in titles, keywords, and abstracts of articles. Chemical substances can be searched for by entering their corresponding CAS Registry Numbers, synonyms, or both. At present, the citations are derived exclusively from Chemical Abstracts. Royalty charges.

TOXNET (TOXICOLOGY DATA NETWORK)

As part of the MEDLARS system, TOXNET is a computerized collection of files on toxicology, hazardous chemical–related areas. TOXNET contains the following files:

• CCRIS (**C**hemical **C**arcinogenesis **R**esearch **I**nformation **S**ystem): Data and information on carcinogenicity, tumor promotion, tumor inhibition, and mutagenicity test results derived from the scanning of primary journals, current awareness tools, National Cancer Institute (NCI) technical reports, review articles, and International Agency for Research on Cancer monographs published since 1976.

- DART (**D**evelopmental **a**nd **R**eproductive **T**oxicology): Bibliographic citations on teratology and developmental and reproductive toxicology.
- EMIC and EMICBACK (**E**nvironmental **M**utagen **I**nformation **C**enter **BACK**file): Bibliographic citations on chemical, biological, and physical agents that have been tested for genotoxic activity.

APPENDIX D

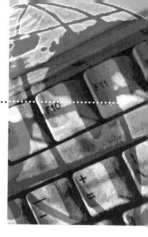

*Searching Index Medicus:
The Print Alternative
to MEDLINE*

In some parts of the world, access to MEDLINE, whether through an online route or a locally maintained version in a local network or a CD-ROM format, is unavailable for reasons of cost or technical limitations. Authors in these settings may, however, have access in medical libraries to *Index Medicus*, the printed index published by the National Library of Medicine. *Index Medicus* has disadvantages when it is compared with access to MEDLINE through, for example, Internet Grateful Med. It covers a smaller number of journals, each indexed paper appears under fewer index terms than are applied in MEDLINE, and it does not carry abstracts. Further, its publication will probably be discontinued by the Library.

INDEX MEDICUS

Index Medicus is a printed subject and author index to over 3200 journals; their titles are listed in the annual publication *List of Journals Indexed in Index Medicus* (1). It began publication in its present form in 1960 and thus covers a big fraction of the medical science literature that most authors are likely to wish to search. *Index Medicus* is issued monthly; the monthly issues are cumulated for each calendar year in *Cumulated Index Medicus*. Each issue includes two main sections, the subject index and the author index. Other sections should also be known by authors, especially the introductory pages on how to use *Index Medicus* and the index to review articles.

Entries in the subject index of *Index Medicus* are arranged under the standard terms known collectively as MeSH (**Me**dical **S**ubject **H**eadings). Searches for papers by subject must, therefore, be carried out using the MeSH terms. To start your search, take the topic terms you have assembled (as discussed above) and go to the MeSH compilation that should be on the library shelf with the *Index Medicus* volumes. *Medical Subject Headings* is published annually as part 2 of the January issue of *Index Medicus* and as a separate publication (2). You should be able to find most of the terms you have jotted down, either in the form you used or in inverted form. If the term appears in large type with a classification number beneath it, this is the term as it is used in the subject index. If the term appears in small type followed by "see" and a synonym, the synonym is the term that is used in the subject index. Under each MeSH term appear synonymous and related terms preceded by X; these are the terms from which cross-reference has been made to the MeSH term. If, for example, you plan to use *AIDS* for your search, you will find from the MeSH compilation that *AIDS* refers you to *acquired immunodeficiency syndrome* as the MeSH term under which to search.

All MeSH terms are arranged in subject groups and hierarchical levels within groups known as "tree structures", included as part of each annual *Medical Subject Headings*. After you have found the MeSH terms that correspond to the topics for your search (identical terms, inverted versions of the terms, or synonyms reached through "see" or "see under" cross-references), inspect the terms in the tree structure around each term you have selected to find other closely related terms which you might also wish to use in searching. Sometimes these closely related terms may yield search results more specific for your needs.

Keep in mind that the indexers always use the most specific term available in MeSH; sometimes this is an inverted form. For example, a paper on cardiogenic shock will be indexed under *shock, cardiogenic,* not under *myocardial infarction;* a paper on involutional depression will be indexed under *depression, involutional,* not under *involutional depression.*

Each annual MeSH compilation includes, in addition to the terms and the tree structures, valuable explanatory introductions that list headings (terms) introduced in that year and terms deleted, with indications of the equivalents (if any) used for the new terms in preceding years. You need to know these changes in indexing and should not assume that current MeSH terms were used for the concepts of your search since the concept first appeared in indexed articles. This introductory section should be read closely by searchers who are not familiar with *Index Medicus.*

INDEX MEDICUS: SEARCHING WITH THE SUBJECT INDEX

You will probably start your search with the most recent monthly issues of *Index Medicus.* Some knowledge of how entries for journal articles are presented under each MeSH term can be useful.

Articles that are of broad interest in relation to the MeSH term or that cannot be subclassified are listed first under the term, followed by article entries classified under subheadings such as COMPLICATIONS, PATHOL-

OGY, THERAPY. Under each heading and subheading, articles in English-language journals are listed before those in foreign-language journals, and within these two groupings entries are listed alphabetically by journal title. The foreign-language grouping is sorted by language.

Articles in foreign-language journals are indicated by square brackets around their titles (presented in English translation), and parenthetic statements indicate the language in which the article is published and whether the article includes an English abstract.

Journal titles are given in the _Index Medicus_ abbreviated form; the full titles are given in the introductory pages of each _Cumulated Index Medicus_. The separately issued list, _List of Journals Indexed in Index Medicus_ (1), also includes titles of the journals covered by _Index Medicus_ arranged by subject and country in which published.

After you have worked your way through the monthly issues of _Index Medicus_ for the current year, you will switch to the annual _Cumulated Index Medicus_ for the previous year; its subject index is organized as in the monthly index.

Understanding how articles are indexed for _Index Medicus_ is a great help to the searcher. The preceding paragraphs have pointed out principles to be kept in mind. The hints below summarize these and additional useful points; these are drawn from a short guide issued some years ago by the National Library of Medicine (3). The most current information relevant to searching _Index Medicus_ can be found in its introductory explanatory section.

- Look for a subject using only the MeSH terms specified in the MeSH list published with each January issue of _Index Medicus_. Articles on "dizziness" cannot be found under this term because it is not a MeSH term; "vertigo" is the MeSH synonym.
- Look for indexed articles under the MeSH term given as a cross-reference by an inappropriate but closely related term, for example, under _SEPTICEMIA_ which is given as a cross-reference at _BACTEREMIA_ in the MeSH list.
- Consider also using MeSH terms related to those you have already selected by examining the categorized list of terms (tree structures) also published with each January issue of _Index Medicus_.
- Look in an alternate location for a subject expressed as a compound concept if you do not find it initially. Some terms are direct; some are arbitrarily inverted. An article on cutaneous tuberculosis is not found under _CUTANEOUS TUBERCULOSIS_, but under _TUBERCULOSIS, CUTANEOUS_. Vinyl ether is under _VINYL ETHER_, not under _ETHER, VINYL_.
- Subjects are divided into more specific breakdowns by subheadings. Look for specific aspects of subjects under the subject as divided by its subheadings. Do not look under a heading that is an exact duplicate of a subheading. An article on the radiography of the pancreas is found under _PANCREAS-radiography_, not under _RADIOGRAPHY_. An article on the me-

tabolism of glucose is found under *GLUCOSE-metabolism,* not under *ME-TABOLISM.* An article on amino acids in the blood is found under *AMINO ACIDS-blood,* not under *BLOOD.* An article on urinalysis in gout is found under *GOUT-urine,* not under *URINE.*

- Look for the most specific term. An article on leishmaniasis is found under *LEISHMANIASIS,* not under *TROPICAL MEDICINE.* An article on neomycin is found under *NEOMYCIN,* not under *ANTIBIOTICS.*
- Look for organs, diseases, and physiologic processes in persons of various ages under the organ, the disease, or the physiologic process, not under the age group. An article on gout in infants is found under *GOUT,* not under *INFANT.* An article on hand injuries in the aged is found under *HAND INJURIES,* not under *AGED.*
- Look for research with laboratory animals under the subject of the research, not under the term for the animal. An article on arthritis induced in rats is found under *ARTHRITIS,* not under *RATS.*
- Look for specific research methods under the specific disease, substance, and so on, not under a term for the method. An article on the chromatography of amino acids is found under *AMINO ACIDS-analysis,* not under *CHROMATOGRAPHY.* An article on the electrophoresis of gamma globulin in syphilis is found under *GAMMA GLOBULINS-analysis* or *SYPHILIS-immunology,* not under *ELECTROPHORESIS* or *BLOOD PROTEIN ELECTROPHORESIS.*
- Look for diseases of various organs under the organ-disease term. If an organ-disease term is not in MeSH, look under the term for the organ. An article on diseases of the cecum is found under *CECAL DISEASES,* not under *CECUM.* An article on diseases of the appendix is sought under *APPENDIX DISEASES,* but because this term is not in MeSH, it is found at *APPENDIX* (specific) and not under *CECAL DISEASES* (general).
- Look for diseases caused by various organisms under the organism-infection term. If an organism-infection term is not in MeSH, locate the organism in the tree structure for MeSH, observe the next level of the hierarchy above it, and then look in *Index Medicus* under the corresponding organism-infection heading. Sometimes an organism-infection term is disguised as a classic disease term. An article on infection with *Escherichia coli* is found under *ESCHERICHIA COLI INFECTIONS,* not under *ESCHERICHIA COLI.* Articles on infection with bacteria not represented directly in MeSH by a genus or species name may be found under a higher taxonomic name, such as a family name. An article on infection with *Clostridium botulinum* is not found under *CLOSTRIDIUM INFECTIONS,* but under *BOTULISM.*
- Look under -ology or -iatrics terms only for articles on the field or specialty of the -ologist or -iatrist. Articles on diseases, organs, or patients will not be found here. An article on dermatologic therapy is found under *SKIN DISEASES-therapy,* not under *DERMATOLOGY,* which covers only articles on dermatology, the field of dermatology, or the dermatologist.

- Look for general pathologic processes of various organs under the organ with the subheading *-pathology*, not under the general pathologic process (*NECROSIS, GANGRENE, INFLAMMATION, HYPERTROPHY, ATROPHY*). An article on necrosis of the pancreas is found under *PANCREAS-pathology*, not under *NECROSIS*.

REFERENCES

1. National Library of Medicine. List of journals indexed in Index Medicus. Bethesda (MD): National Library of Medicine; [annual publication]. Available from Government Printing Office (GPO): Superintendent of Documents, PO Box 371954, Pittsburgh, PA 15250-7954; phone (202) 512-1800; fax (202) 512-2250.
2. National Library of Medicine. Medical subject headings—annotated alphabetic list. Bethesda (MD): National Library of Medicine; [annual publication]. Available from Government Printing Office (GPO): Superintendent of Documents, PO Box 371954, Pittsburgh, PA 15250-7954; phone (202) 512-1800; fax (202) 512-2250. This valuable comprehensive version of the MeSH vocabulary can be usefully supplemented with two other publications: *Medical Subject Headings—Tree Structures* (also published annually) and *Permuted Medical Subject Headings* (also published annually). These three publications can be found in medical libraries.1. National Library of Medicine. Medical subject headings—annotated alphabetic list. Bethesda (MD): National Library of Medicine. Published annually.
3. National Library of Medicine. Hints for Index Medicus users. Bethesda (MD): National Library of Medicine; [undated]. Out-of-print.

APPENDIX E

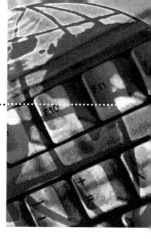

References and Reading: An Annotated Bibliography

Authors in any field often need guides to usage in the many details that make up good prose style. Authors in medicine have to be able to verify the spelling, definition, or correct use of scientific terms. Skills in writing are built largely through self-training, with the help of books that give insights into the characteristics of prose style and into ways of writing more easily and effectively. The books described below will help authors in medicine satisfy these various needs. The titles of the books are given first, rather than the authors' names, to emphasize the subjects of the books.

DICTIONARIES

The American Heritage Dictionary of the English Language. 3rd revised ed. Boston (MA): Houghton Mifflin; 1992.

Merriam-Webster Collegiate Dictionary. 10th ed. Springfield (MA): Merriam-Webster; 1997.

The New Shorter Oxford English Dictionary on Historical Principles. 2 volumes. Oxford: Clarendon Press; 1993.

The Oxford Encyclopedic English Dictionary. Oxford: Clarendon Press; 1991.

For most needs of most authors—other than scientific terms—the smaller dictionaries of the major dictionary publishers (such as the "Collegiate" of Merriam-Webster in the United States) and the more abridged Oxford dictionaries (like the "Encyclopedic" listed above) are entirely adequate. The other two dictionaries listed (the "Heritage" and the "Shorter Oxford") are, for me, at their prices and scopes, the best of the English-language dictionaries. The usage notes of the *American Heritage Dictionary,* a generous part of many of its entries, make more clear than other dictionaries the proper level of usage for a word and the nuances among synonyms. The "Guide to the Dictionary" in the opening pages should be digested by all who are not regular users of any dictionary.

Cambridge International Dictionary of English. Cambridge: Cambridge University Press; 1995.

Collins Cobuild English Dictionary. London: HarperCollins; 1995.

These dictionaries were prepared especially for persons for whom English is a foreign language. They explain in their entries many of the details and nuances of English idiom and usage that are not so explicitly described in standard English dictionaries. The section "Grammar: Parts of Speech" in the introductory pages of the Cambridge dictionary offers an unusually clear and succinct description of grammatical elements. Its "Phrase Index" enables users to quickly find explanations of multiword phrases that are not readily defined as single entries. These dictionaries and the Collins COBUILD guides cited in Chapter 18 can be ordered in the United States from Delta Systems, Inc., 1400 Miller Parkway, McHenry, Illinois, USA; telephone (815) 363-3582, fax (815) 363-2948. Web site http://www.delta-systems.com.

Stedman's Medical Dictionary. 26th ed. Baltimore (MD): Williams & Wilkins; 1995.

International Dictionary of Medicine and Biology. New York (NY): John S. Wiley; 1986.

The major English-language dictionaries of medicine differ little, but among all of them I find *Stedman's* the most attractive, even though I might be accused of a "conflict of interest" because its publisher is also the publisher of this book. But even *Stedman's* has its faults. In its entries for *case* and for *patient* it does not caution against the medical-slang use of *case* to mean *patient.* Indeed, it defines *borderline case* as "a patient, whose clinical findings are suggestive, but not fully convincing, of a specific diagnosis"! *Stedman's* also pays attention in some places to the English preference for digraph spellings like "oestrogen" but does not direct the reader to *hematology* at the point where *haematology* would appear. Thus it may not be the proper dictionary for authors preferring English spellings. The *International Dictionary* is a big 3-volume work particularly useful for its following the proper conventions for italicization of taxonomic terms when they are entry terms (which *Stedman's* does too) and for its wide coverage of biology outside of medicine.

Academic Press Dictionary of Science and Technology. San Diego (CA): Academic Press; 1992.

McGraw-Hill Dictionary of Scientific and Technical Terms. 5th ed. New York (NY): McGraw-Hill; 1996.

Medical dictionaries often cannot answer questions about terms in scientific fields other than clinical and basic-science medicine. These two dictionaries are valuable supplements to the medical dictionaries, but they may seem too expensive to most medical authors because of their probably infrequent use.

GUIDES TO ENGLISH GRAMMAR AND USAGE

A Dictionary of Modern English Usage. HW Fowler. Revised and edited by E Gowers. 2nd ed. New York (NY): Oxford University Press; 1983.

A classic guide, widely known as "Fowler", to myriad details of prose style. Some of Fowler's positions may seem too fastidious, even precious, but his keen judgments rarely fail to make one think more about judgments in writing.

The New Fowler's Modern English Usage. RW Burchfield, editor. Oxford: Clarendon Press; 1996.

"Fowler's" in an updated version. Some of the devotees of the original will wince at some points, but this new "Fowler" does offer helpful guidance.

ESL Resourcebook for Engineers and Scientists. E Campbell. New York (NY): John Wiley and Sons; 1995.

A detailed, thorough discussion of the difficulties likely to be faced by nonanglophone authors. The "ESL" in the title means "English as a second language". It covers potential problems in English-language style, grammar, and vocabulary and in the process of writing. It summarizes differences in American and British spelling. Several chapters suggest how to conduct oneself in North American scientific and technical environments, including meetings.

Modern American Usage: A Guide. W Follett. Edited and completed by J Barzun. New York (NY): Hill & Wang; 1966.

The American equivalent to Fowler's *A Dictionary of Modern English Usage;* not as witty as "Fowler" but the introductory and closing essays offer a well-reasoned argument on the value of careful distinctions in all details of style.

Talking about People. R Maggio. Phoenix (AZ): Oryx Press; 1997.

A guide to, as the author puts it, "fair and accurate language". She considers terms commonly used to describe persons with regard to age, sex, occupation, economic level, religion, "race", ethnicity, physical appearances and difficulties, with analysis of their accuracy, potential offensiveness, and other considerations that should govern choices of terms. Her earlier guides, also published by Oryx Press, include *The Dictionary of Bias-Free Usage: A Guide to Nondiscriminatory Language* (1991) and *The Nonsexist Word Finder: A Dictionary of Gender-Free Usage* (1987).

Merriam-Webster's Dictionary of English Usage. Springfield (MA): Merriam-Webster; 1995.

> An exhaustive survey of historical and contemporary American and English usage in vocabulary, grammar, and syntax. Tends to avoid firm positions but offers thorough discussions and a wealth of examples. Its analyses of possible variations in usage might be regarded as pedantic and indecisive but they have the value of giving its users adequate rationalizations for preferences that can be based on personal values. Probably now the best single source for style decisions in all kinds of American-English prose.

The Words Between: A Handbook for Scientists Needing English, with Examples Mainly from Biology and Medicine. 3rd ed. JM Perttunen. Helsinki: Kustannus oy Duodecim; 1990.

> An exhaustive survey of a great number of details in English prose style often not known to nonanglophone writers in biology and medicine (and even to anglophone writers). Although one chapter focuses specifically on difficulties in Finnish-to-English translation, most of the text will be useful any place in the world of medical and biologic writing.

STYLE MANUALS

The ACS Style Guide: A Manual for Authors and Editors. 2nd ed. JS Dodd, editor. Washington (DC): American Chemical Society; 1997.

> A basic, clear, and authoritative manual of style for all fields of chemistry, with notably detailed sections on chemical names, locants, units, and other conventions. It includes, however, much additional content likely to be useful in other fields of scientific publication, such as guidance on posters and oral presentations, press releases, computer usage, copyrights and copyrights permissions, ethical guidelines, and peer reviewing.

American Medical Association Manual of Style. 9th ed. C Iverson and others, editors. Baltimore (MD): Williams & Wilkins; 1998.

> The comprehensive style manual for the journals of the American Medical Association, much larger in this edition than it was in the preceding eighth edition. It has been notably expanded in its presentation of nomenclature. Some of its conventions differ from standard usage in other medical journals, but in general it adheres to style conventions also set forth in *Scientific Style and Format* of the Council of Biology Editors. The title does not adequately suggest the full range of this manual's content; the coverage is wider than "style", including as it does, for example, a comprehensive chapter on ethical and legal considerations.

ASM Style Manual for Journals and Books. Washington (DC): American Society for Microbiology; 1991.

> Details of style for bacteriology, mycology, virology, and genetic aspects of these fields.

The Chicago Manual of Style. 14th ed. Chicago (IL): University of Chicago Press, 1993.

The standard manual for many fields of scholarly publishing, especially the humanities and social science. Useful to authors of scientific papers for details of style not set forth in some of the more specialized manuals described above. Has discussions of copyright, preparation of tables, mathematics in type, and documentation that supplement related sections in the scientific style manuals.

Medical Style and Format: An International Manual for Authors, Editors, and Publishers. EJ Huth. Philadelphia (PA): ISI Press; 1987. Distribution by Williams & Wilkins. Out of print.

A detailed guide to punctuation, quotation and ellipsis, capitalization, type conventions, word structure, American and British differences in English-language usage, nomenclature, addresses, symbols and abbreviations, degrees and honorific terms, numbers and units of measurement, mathematics, statistics, and style in specific medical fields. Thorough presentation of bibliographic references for a wide range of document types, with principles of reference construction. An appendix on SI units in clinical chemistry and hematology.

Publication Manual of the American Psychological Association. 4th ed. Washington (DC): American Psychological Association, 1994.

A detailed guide for authors preparing papers for publication in journals of the American Psychological Association: organization of manuscripts; prose style; details of manuscript style; procedure for typing and submitting manuscripts; proofreading. Describes the APA journals and their publication process. Lists non-APA journals that use its style specifications. Helpful discussions of ethics in scholarly publishing. Its section on bibliographic references presents formats that, in general, are not used by medical journals, but this section does comprehensively illustrate the data that are likely to be needed in references to documents other than journal articles, for example, legal references. Its section on tables offers a thorough presentation of needed elements and their desirable arrangement.

Scientific Style and Format: The CBE Manual for Authors, Editors, and Publishers. Style Manual Committee, Council of Biology Editors. 6th ed. New York (NY): Cambridge University Press; 1994.

The authoritative guide to manuscript and publication styles in all sciences, including the medical sciences. Particularly valuable in medicine for help with the style conventions for plant sciences, microbiology, animal sciences, chemistry, and biochemistry. The chapter on references gives examples of both the citation-sequence style and formats (often called "Vancouver style" and essentially the references style recommended in Chapter 19 and used throughout this book) and the name–year system and formats (widely known as "Harvard style").

Merriam-Webster Standard American Style Manual. Springfield (MA): Merriam-Webster; 1994.

> A comprehensive general manual. Some of its recommended conventions are not standard in the medical sciences.

SCIENTIFIC DATA AND NOMENCLATURE

How to Report Statistics in Medicine: Annotated Guidelines for Authors, Editors, and Reviewers. T Lang and M Secic. Philadelphia (PA): American College of Physicians; 1997.

> A thorough and detailed manual on what statistical information should be reported for specific kinds of statistical analyses and types of research reports and on how the information should be presented. There are short explanations of types of statistical analyses but this is not a manual on how to carry them out. The 47-page Part 2 defines statistical terms and tests.

The Merck Index: An Encyclopedia of Chemicals, Drugs, and Biologicals. S Budavari, editor. 12th ed. Whitehouse Station (NJ): Merck and Company; 1996.

> An authoritative reference for chemical names. Entry articles include synonymous common names, formal chemical names, molecular formulas and weights, brief descriptions of uses and properties, and other details.

Pharmacological and Chemical Synonyms: A Collection of Names, Drugs, Pesticides & Other Compounds Drawn from the Medical Literature of the World. 10th ed. EEJ Marler. Amsterdam: Excerpta Medica; 1994.

> A dictionary of generic, chemical, and trade names for drugs, pesticides, and other compounds of importance in pharmacology and biochemistry. Draws on International Nonproprietary Names (INN; World Health Organization) and on other nationally approved systems of nomenclature such as United States Adopted Names (USAN; see below).

SI Units for Clinical Measurement. DS Young, EJ Huth. Philadelphia (PA): American College of Physicians; 1998.

> A detailed guide to use of SI units in clinical fields, including cardiology, clinical chemistry, pulmonary medicine, radiology. Comprehensive tables give present metric units and the preferred SI units, conversion factors, and appropriate significant digits and minimal increments for many variables and analytes.

USP Dictionary of USAN and International Drug Names. Rockville (MD): United States Pharmacopeial Convention. Published annually.

> Entries for US Adopted Names, current USP and NF (National Formulary) names, international and other nonproprietary names, brand names, code des-

ignations, Chemical Abstracts Service (CAS) registry numbers, cross-references, and categories of pharmacologic activity. The articles on US Adopted Names typically include year of publication of the USAN, pronunciation, designation of official compendium such as USP, molecular formula, chemical names, CAS registry number, pharmacologic (including therapeutic) activity, brand names, manufacturer or distributor name, code designation, and graphic formula.

GUIDES TO WRITING AND PUBLISHING

Better Medical Writing in India. P Sahni, GK Pande, J Smith, S Nundy, compilers. New Delhi, India: The National Medical Journal of India; 1987. Can be purchased from The National Medical Journal of India, All India Institute of Medical Sciences, New Delhi 11029, India.

Articles by Indian and British authors on many aspects of medical writing but some pay special attention to concerns and potential problems for Indian authors.

Handbook for Academic Authors. 3rd ed. B Luey. New York (NY): Cambridge University Press; 1995.

Especially useful as a guide to developing a proposal for a book, seeking a publisher, negotiating a contract, and writing the book. Individual chapters cover writing journal articles and preparing electronic manuscripts.

How to Write a Paper. George M Hall, editor. London: BMJ Publishing Group; 1994. Also available in the United States from the American College of Physicians, Philadelphia, PA 19106-1572 USA.

Short chapters on the structure of scientific papers, the proper content of introductions, methods, results, and discussions sections, references, writing reviews, case reports, letters, peer reviewing, prose style, and other matters.

How to Write & Publish a Scientific Paper. 4th ed. RA Day. Phoenix (AZ): Oryx Press; 1994.

In addition to covering the writing of scientific papers, it also covers theses, oral presentations, conference reports, and ethical issues. Most of the examples of text, illustrations, and tables are drawn from microbiology. Enlivened with samples of Mr Day's particular brand of wit.

Medical Books in India. P Sahni, S Nundy, editors. New Delhi, India: National Book Trust and The National Medical Journal of India; 1994. Can be purchased from the National Book Trust, A-5, Green Park, New Delhi 110016, India, or The National Medical Journal of India, All India Institute of Medical Sciences, New Delhi 11029, India.

Special attention to the particular opportunities and difficulties of writing and publishing a medical book in India.

Scientific Papers and Presentations. M Davis. San Diego (CA): Academic Press; 1997.

> An extensive guide to bibliographic searches, writing papers and books, writing theses, preparing grant proposals, preparing tables and graphs, revising style and content, ethical issues, scientific presentations, posters, and other topics important in academic settings. The book's breadth necessarily limits its attention to the particular problems in particular disciplines.

Successful Scientific Writing: A Step-by-Step Guide for the Biological and Medical Sciences. JR Matthews, JW Bowen, RW Matthews. New York (NY): Cambridge University Press; 1996.

> A systematic guide to writing papers, revising them, preparing manuscripts, and submitting a paper to a journal. Includes exercises that could be applied in writing courses.

Systematic Reviews: Synthesis of Best Evidence for Health Care Decisions. C Mulrow, D Cook, editors. Philadelphia (PA): American College of Physicians; 1998.

> Book discusses differences between systematic reviews and narrative reviews. Chapter 2, "Locating and Appraising Systematic Reviews", is a valuable supplement to Chapters 3 and 9 of this book.

PROSE STYLE AND STRUCTURE

Clear and Simple as the Truth: Writing Classic Prose. F-N Thomas, M Turner. Princeton (NJ): Princeton University Press; 1994.

> One might guess from the subtitle "Writing Classic Prose" that this book speaks to writers of prose striving to ape the great writers of past masterpieces in the English, French, German, Italian, Spanish, and classical literatures. Not at all; it speaks to writers in any discipline, including science, who simply wish to write prose that speaks directly and efficiently to readers. It is not a book of recipes for writing; it is an analysis of what characteristics define "classic" prose. It draws examples from prose of our time as well as from the "classic" writers of the past.

The Elements of Style. W Strunk Jr, EB White. 3rd ed. New York (NY): Allyn, 1995.

> The short classic on principles of clear writing, widely known as "Strunk and White". Its chief virtue is probably its brevity; it does not come even close to the Williams book described below (*Style: Ten Lessons in Clarity and Grace*) in dealing with the complex weaknesses of prose style that are all too frequent in scientific papers.

English Prose Style. H Read. New York (NY): Pantheon Books; 1983.

> Elegant essays on composition (words, epithets, metaphor, the sentence, the paragraph, arrangement) and rhetoric. Of the eight essays on aspects of rhetoric, that most pertinent to scientific writing is the essay on exposition.

Notes on the Composition of Scientific Papers. TC Allbutt. London: The Keynes Press, British Medical Association; 1984.

This classic short text on clear and direct scientific writing, long out of print, was first published in 1904 and in its third edition in 1923. It is itself a model of clear and direct writing. The flaws it attacks—"woolly style", abstract nouns, meagerness of vocabulary, misused words—still plague us. It should be more widely known and read.

The Reader over Your Shoulder: A Handbook for Writers of English Prose. R Graves, A Hodge. 2nd ed. New York (NY): Random House; 1979.

Twenty-five principles for clear statement and 16 for graceful prose, sharply applied to samples of prose from eminent English writers. This second, abridged edition is not as good as the long out-of-print excellent first edition, which included chapters on the history of English prose style as well as more examinations of prose samples. The most recent edition is *The Use and Abuse of the English Language,* published in 1995 by Marlowe and Company.

Simple & Direct: A Rhetoric for Writers. Revised edition. J Barzun. Chicago (IL): University of Chicago Press; 1994.

In clear essays Barzun works from the smallest elements of style, words, through the elements of linking, tone, and meaning, to paragraphs and the entire composition. The last chapter is on revision. As he goes along, he sets forth 20 principles of clear writing.

Style: Ten Lessons in Clarity and Grace. 5th ed. JM Williams. Chicago (IL): University of Chicago Press; 1995.

A classic didactic text on how to give your prose the qualities of clarity, coherence, emphasis, and concision (economy). Particular attention to rhythm and to punctuation. This may be the best single text now available on how to write clear and effective prose.

ILLUSTRATIONS

Graphics Simplified: How to Plan and Prepare Effective Charts, Graphs, Illustrations, and Other Visual Aids. AJ MacGregor. Toronto (ON): University of Toronto Press; 1979.

Principles of illustration, with examples of various formats.

Illustrating Science: Standards for Publication. Scientific Illustration Committee. Bethesda (MD): Council of Biology Editors; 1988.

A thorough presentation of illustration principles, aesthetic considerations, and technical methods for drawings, photographs, and graphs. Chapter IV, "Graphs and Maps", will be the most useful section for most medical authors.

Preparing Scientific Illustrations: A Guide to Better Posters, Presentations, and Publications. 2nd ed. MH Briscoe. New York (NY): Springer; 1996.

An excellent and thorough guide to preparing photographs, diagrams, tables, graphs, and molecular graphics for publication. Separate chapters cover slides, posters, and computer applications for graphics.

Visualizing Data. WS Cleveland. Summit (NJ): Hobart Press; 1993.

A sophisticated treatise on graphic presentation methods for univariate, bivariate, trivariate, and hypervariate data. An adequate understanding of this text will call for a working knowledge of statistics.

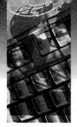

INDEX